1996

ARTERIAL CHEMORECEPTORS
Cell to System

ADVANCES IN EXPERIMENTAL MEDICINE AND BIOLOGY

Recent Volumes in this Series

A Continuation Order Plan is available for this series. A continuation order will bring delivery of each new volume immediately upon publication. Volumes are billed only upon actual shipment. For further information please contact the publisher.

ARTERIAL CHEMORECEPTORS
Cell to System

Edited by

Ronan G. O'Regan
and Philip Nolan

University College Dublin
Dublin, Ireland

Daniel S. McQueen

University of Edinburgh Medical School
Edinburgh, Scotland

and

David J. Paterson

University of Oxford
Oxford, United Kingdom

PLENUM PRESS • NEW YORK AND LONDON

Library of Congress Cataloging-in-Publication Data

Arterial chemoreceptors : cell to system / edited by Ronan G. O'Regan
... [et al.].
        p.   cm. -- (Advances in experimental medicine and biology ; v.
  360)
   Includes bibliographical references and index.
   ISBN 0-306-44824-6
   1. Carotid body--Congresses.   2. Chemoreceptors--Congresses.
 3. Respiration--Regulation--Congresses.   I. O'Regan, R. G. (Ronan
 G.)   II. International Symposium on Arterial Chemoreception (12th :
 1993 : Dublin, Ireland)   III. Series.
   [DNLM: 1. Chemoreceptors--physiology--congresses.   2. Carotid
 Body--physiology--congresses.   3. Oxygen--metabolism--congresses.
 4. Carbon Dioxide--metabolism--congresses.   W1 AD559 v. 360 1994 /
 WL 102.9 A7864 1994]
 QP368.8.A78   1994
 599'.0188--dc20
 DNLM/DLC
 for Library of Congress   94-31472
                                                                  CIP

Proceedings of a meeting of the International Society of Arterial Chemoreception (ISAC) on
Chemoreceptors and Chemoreflexes in Health and Disease, held August 9–13, 1993, in Dublin, Ireland

ISBN 0-306-44824-6

©1994 Plenum Press, New York
A Division of Plenum Publishing Corporation
233 Spring Street, New York, N.Y. 10013

Printed in the United States of America

This volume is dedicated to

Eric Neil

(1918-1990)

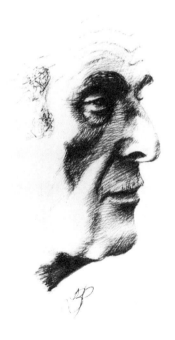

PREFACE

The International Society for Arterial Chemoreception (ISAC) was founded in August 1988 during the 9th International Symposium on Arterial Chemoreception which was held at Park City, Utah, USA. ISAC was established with the aim of providing a framework to support the increasing number of investigators from a wide variety of disciplines (anatomists, pathologists, respiratory physiologists and clinicians, high altitude physiologists, biochemists, biophysicists, physiologists and pharmacologists) who share a common interest in arterial chemoreception.

ISAC took over the co-ordination of the international chemoreceptor meetings, with the membership deciding the venue for forthcoming meetings. During the Park City symposium Dublin was selected to host the 1993 meeting, under the Presidency of Professor Ronan O'Regan. The 12th International Meeting on Arterial Chemoreception, which was held in Dublin in August 1993, was acclaimed as a great success by all those present. The delegates not only shared in a wide-ranging feast of chemoreceptor based science, they had plenty of opportunity during the meeting for renewing acquaintances and establishing new friendships. The location for the meeting at University College Dublin's modern Belfield campus helped to promote such interaction, and the social programme was outstanding.

ISAC greatly appreciates the work of the local organizing committee in making the Dublin meeting such a successful event. This committee worked extremely hard to ensure that the scientific and social programme was varied and interesting. Thanks are also due to the sponsors of the meeting for their financial help, particularly for the substantial contributions given by The Wellcome Trust, Astra Hassle and SmithKline Beecham.

During the Dublin meeting Professor Helmut Acker (Dortmund, Germany) stood down as Hon. Secretary of ISAC. The society is indebted to Helmut for all his hard work in nurturing the society during its early years, and the membership expressed their gratitude to him. Professor Sal Fidone (Salt Lake City, USA) was elected as the new Hon. Secretary, and the meeting wished him well in his duties. Dr. Dan McQueen (Edinburgh, UK) was re-elected as Hon. Treasurer, acknowledging his outstanding contribution to maintaining and enhancing the financial status of the society. It was decided by the members of ISAC that their next meeting would be held in Santiago, Chile, under the Presidency of Professor Patricio Zapata of the Catholic University in Santiago. The precise date has yet to be arranged but it is likely to be around Easter 1996.

In order to provide a wider biomedical audience with an account of the papers that were presented during the Dublin meeting, each contributor was asked to prepare a concise short report for publication in this volume. The Editors took the opportunity of inviting review chapters, and have combined these with the individual papers to give a comprehensive integrated and up-to-date account of arterial chemoreception from cell to system. The quality of this book is a testament to the dedication and hard work of the Editors. David Paterson (Oxford, UK) did much of the initial negotiating with our publishers and the co-ordination of the review chapters, with the assistance of Dan McQueen (Edinburgh, UK). As for the final compilation and editing, using modern word processing techniques, Philip Nolan (Dublin, Ireland) has been outstanding, as can be seen from the content and layout of this book. We would like to thank all the contributors for their prompt submission of manuscripts. We are delighted to be continuing our links with Plenum Publishing Corporation, and are grateful for their assistance in preparing this volume so soon after the Meeting.

CONTENTS

HISTORICAL PERSPECTIVES

MOLECULAR AND IONIC MECHANISMS OF CHEMOTRANSDUCTION

NEUROTRANSMITTERS AND PUTATIVE NEUROTRANSMITTERS
IN THE CAROTID BODY

DEVELOPMENTAL ASPECTS OF ARTERIAL CHEMORECEPTION

MORPHOLOGICAL STUDIES OF THE CAROTID BODY

COMPARATIVE PHYSIOLOGY OF CHEMORECEPTION

AIRWAY RECEPTORS

ERIC NEIL (1918-1990): AN APPRECIATION

In recognition of his outstanding contribution to chemoreceptor research and the stimulus he had given to young researchers in this field of study the International Society for Arterial Chemoreception appropriately associated Eric Neil with Corneille Heymans and Fernando de Castro in naming an award for young investigators. This award, instituted in 1989, is given for the best presentation by a young researcher at each meeting of the Society.

Eric Neil was one of the great pioneers of arterial chemoreceptor research whose experiments were noted for their skill and innovation. His work was truly remarkable for the number of original findings with which he was associated, and to this day workers in certain areas of chemoreceptor science must of necessity refer to his research in their own published work. Among his original observations were the effects of stagnant hypoxia on arterial chemoreceptor activity and the associated reflex effects on the cardiovascular and respiratory systems, the effects of both sympathetic and sinus nerve efferent innervation to the carotid body on the function of this chemoreceptor, the role of adenosine phosphates and mitochondrial metabolism in chemotransduction, and the influences exerted by carbon monoxide on carotid chemoreceptor discharges. He also made a substantial contribution to the study of cholinergic and catecholaminergic neurotransmission in the carotid body.

An outstanding physiologist in the classical mould with a wide range of expertise, extensive knowledge of the biomedical sciences and catholic interests Eric Neil did not limit his research to arterial chemoreceptors. He made major contributions to the study of hypothermia, which greatly influenced the management of acid-base balance in cardiac surgery carried out under hypothermic conditions. He was also responsible for the important findings on the role of pulsatile pressures in modulating the activity of carotid sinus baroreceptors, and the influence of pulse pressure on the effectiveness of baroreflex control of the circulatory system. In addition, he published significant findings on respiratory-cardiovascular interactions in the control of heart rate.

Eric Neil was an author of numerous review articles which included chapters in both the cardiovascular and endocrinology volumes of the Handbook of Physiology. As editor and author he was responsible for the publication of many books on diverse topics within respiratory and cardiovascular science. The classic book "Reflexogenic Areas of the Cardiovascular System", written with Corneille Heymans, was published in 1958. This work, with its wealth of historical and experimental data on cardiovascular mechanoreceptors and arterial chemoreceptors is essential reading for all those involved in cardiovascular and respiratory physiology, especially young scientists embarking on a research career in these fields. With Björn Folkow as co-author he published in 1971 the outstanding volume "Circulation". Eric's prodigious output included one of the best known textbooks of physiology used by generations of medical students this century. Samson Wright's "Applied Physiology" has been

1

translated into many languages and Eric Neil became its main author following the death of Samson Wright in 1956. In collaboration with Cyril Keele, John Jepson and latterly Norman Joels this popular book remained until recently the major textbook in applied physiology used not only by medical students but also by doctors pursuing postgraduate qualifications. It is most unfortunate that the last edition of this book was published more than a decade ago and should a new edition not be forthcoming this textbook seems destined to go out of vogue.

Although born in Cumbria in north-west England in 1918, Eric insisted that his roots were in the island of Barra off the west coast of Scotland. His firm belief that his ancestors were Scandinavian, may account for his strong association with Swedish physiology, which included many productive visits to the Veterinarian Institute in Stockholm where he collaborated in research with, among others, Yngve Zotterman, Bengt Anderson and Sven Landgren. He qualified in medicine in Leeds University in 1942 and following internship joined the Department of Physiology at that University where he came under the influence of Albert Hemingway and Alfred Schweitzer. Subsequently, in 1950, he moved to Samson Wright's department in the Middlesex Hospital Medical School in London, initially as senior lecturer and then as reader. After Samson Wright's death Eric Neil became the John Astor Professor of Physiology, a post he held until his retirement in 1984.

Eric Neil's stamina was truly remarkable. He seemed to need little sleep and was involved not only in teaching, research and publication, but also in activities outside the medical school. Elected as an Ordinary Member of the Physiological Society in 1945 and as an Honorary Member in 1984 he served on the committee of the Society from 1956 with little interruption until 1967. As Honorary Treasurer of the Society (1961-1967) he showed his many-faceted talent in that he quickly grasped the intricacies of financial management, and he left the Society at the end of his stewardship in a much better position than that in which he had found it. On the international scene he was highly respected and admired. It is not surprising therefore that he was elected as Secretary (1968-1974) and subsequently President for an unprecedented two terms (1974-1980) of the International Union of Physiological Sciences. In this capacity he was involved in the successful organization of the Union's Congresses at Paris and Budapest.

On a personal level it was my enormous pleasure and privilege to work in Eric Neil's department from 1965 to 1971. During this time he supervised my work for a Ph.D. degree by thesis and permitted me to use his excellent laboratory facilities including the assistance of skilled technical personnel. Apart from one's immediate family there are few people who can intimately influence the direction of one's career. I was indeed fortunate to work under the guidance of Eric Neil during my formative years as a mammalian physiologist, having come to the Middlesex Hospital Medical School on the recommendation of Joe Donegan, Professor of Physiology at University College Galway, who was a close friend of Eric's. Working in Eric Neil's laboratory was a marvellous experience in being able to participate in experiments of complexity and above all manual dexterity. Eric was a microsurgeon of exceptional skill. His refinement of the technique of measuring the venous outflow of the carotid body, initially undertaken by Daly, Lambertsen & Schweitzer in 1954, demanded microsurgery of a most delicate nature. The technique remains to this day the most effective means of measuring carotid body blood flow. Despite reservations expressed about the use of saline wick electrodes for recording afferent nerve activity, I can vouch that Eric was capable of teasing out single fibre recordings with regularity and these preparations remained active without loss of spike height for many hours. Experiments were conducted with flamboyance, often to the background music of the Beatles; when research was progressing exceptionally well, red wine was supplied to smooth away the long hours of experimentation.

As a mentor Eric Neil was exceptional. His sharp analytical ability coupled with a vast knowledge of all the biomedical sciences singled him out from others. He had an extraordinary memory for all aspects of physiological science and his powers of retention were remarkable. Outside physiology, Eric had wide cultural interests, particularly in history and literature, and he was an accomplished pianist. While he did not suffer fools gladly he was invariably kind and helpful to the many overseas visitors attending his department. A generation of medical, B.Sc. and postgraduate students were greatly influenced by his remarkable ability to impart his knowledge. Moreover, he continued to show a deep and genuine interest in postgraduate students and staff who moved away from his department to take up other posts. Thus, he remained an advisor not only during one's stay in his department but also for many years afterwards. A man of exceptional ability, he is sorely missed by all those with an interest in mammalian physiology.

Eric Neil's attainments were greatly aided by the unstinting support of his family. His wife Anne, whom he met while she was a medical student at Leeds University, proved to be the most compatible of partners. Those who had the pleasure of visiting the Neils' Highgate home were treated to hospitality of the highest order, along with the charming company of Anne, "Ma" (Anne's mother) and Eric and Anne's two daughters Jane and Gina. The relationship between "Ma" and Eric was characterised by wit and tolerance, the opposite of that portrayed by music hall jokes. The warmth of Anne Neil's welcome in Highgate is fondly remembered by all the many visitors to her home.

Not all the editors of this volume had met Eric Neil in person; however his reputation is such that there was unanimous support for the idea of dedicating this book to Eric. It is appropriate that the book contains the proceedings of a meeting held in Dublin, a city frequently visited by Eric. His assistance to Irish physiologists over many years not only as an examiner in our medical schools but also as a friend and advisor will always be appreciated. All of us who have been associated with Eric will remember him with great affection as a most talented, charming, kind and witty man.

Ronan G. O'Regan

INTERNATIONAL MEETINGS ON ARTERIAL CHEMORECEPTORS: HISTORICAL PERSPECTIVES

R. G. O'Regan and P. Nolan

Department of Human Anatomy and Physiology, University College, Earlsfort Terrace, Dublin 2, Ireland

"Historia vero testis temporum, lux veritatis"

Cicero "De oratore" II,9,36

INTRODUCTION

The progression of knowledge in a field of scientific research can be aptly chronicled by a study of the records of scientific meetings on that topic. This review describes the highlights of the first 8 international meetings on arterial chemoreception, and as such provides an interesting historical view of the developments in carotid body research since the 1950's. The success of these meetings culminated in the formation of the International Society for Arterial Chemoreception (ISAC) in 1988. This marked the beginning of a new era with more frequent meetings held within a formal international organizational structure. Four meetings have been held under the auspices of the Society, including the 12th International meeting held in Dublin in September 1993, the proceedings of which form this volume. These meetings are such recent events, and included such a large volume of scientific work, that it would be impossible to accurately describe their place in the history of chemoreceptor research. For this reason, this chapter concentrates largely on the earlier meetings. There is a danger that a review such as this could become a mere catalogue of brief abstracts. Therefore, the focus of this chapter has been further narrowed so that particular attention is paid to work which was the source of controversy or papers which opened new horizons in chemoreceptor research. As a consequence, many excellent experiments and experimenters are not mentioned. We hope, however, that this description of the importance of scientific meetings in the development of carotid body research, while mentioning relatively few individuals, will be taken as a tribute to all those who have participated in such meetings over the years.

STOCKHOLM, 1950

The first International Symposium on Chemoreceptors and Chemoceptive Reactions was held in Stockholm, Sweden, in August 1950, and was organized by Goran Liljestrand, to whom the proceedings of the meeting are dedicated, in collaboration with Ulf von Euler and Yngve Zotterman. These workers had performed some of the earliest studies of chemoreceptor afferents by single unit electroneurographic recording, clearly demonstrating the marked response of these afferents to hypoxia (von Euler et al., 1939), and showing that while the relationship between P_aO_2 and chemoreceptor discharge was hyperbolic, that between S_aO_2 and discharge was linear. The list of those who attended this meeting catalogues the outstanding pioneers of chemoreceptor physiology, and includes Fernando de Castro, Corneille Heymans and Eric Neil.

de Castro discussed at length the microscopic structure of the carotid body, with particular reference to its innervation and the features of the glomic microcirculation. He described direct vision microscopic studies of the carotid body circulation *in vivo,* during which he proposed the concept of autoregulation of carotid body blood flow (de Castro, 1951). This was the only International Chemoreceptor Symposium which de Castro was to attend; he was without doubt the founder of chemoreceptor science. He demonstrated by the classical technique of supra- and infra-petrosal section of the glossopharyngeal nerve the sensory nature of terminals associated with the carotid body type I cells; he also described efferent pathways within this nerve which formed synapses in microganglia in the sinus nerve and within the tissue of the carotid body itself. He is well known to have suggested, in advance of the Heymans' physiological experiments, that the carotid body might 'taste the composition of the blood' and relay this information in afferent fibres in the sinus nerve.

Heymans, in reviewing the importance of chemoreceptors in the control of respiration, discussed the relative roles of peripheral arterial chemoreceptors and direct effects on the medulla in the control of breathing in hypoxia and hypercapnia. Even in these early days, years before the localization of central chemoreceptors, Heymans could forcibly state that "hyperpnoea provoked by acute oxygen deficiency, which had been considered as centrogenic, is brought about exclusively by the chemoreceptors reflex mechanism" (Heymans, 1951). However, hypercapnic hyperpnoea was less well understood: "the importance of the aortic and carotid chemoreflex component as compared with that of the direct central component in the regulation of breathing by CO_2 ... is however still open for investigation" (Heymans, 1951).

Neil discussed the involvement of arterial chemoreceptors in the control of the circulation, particularly in the circumstance of acute haemorrhage (Neil, 1951). He also highlighted a question which received much attention in subsequent years, that is, the physiological importance of changes in carotid body blood flow. His comments were underpinned by the descriptions of the innervation and autoregulation of the carotid body microcirculation presented the previous day by de Castro.

OXFORD, 1966

A lengthy period elapsed before a most distinguished group of scientists assembled at Oxford in July 1966, to discuss again the physiology of arterial chemoreception. Bob Torrance, in his *Prolegomena,* succinctly reviewed the state of knowledge at that time, and posed a series of questions which set the tone for chemoreceptor research for at least the next decade (Torrance, 1968). This review is still widely read and cited, and forms an essential introduction to chemoreceptor physiology for the neophyte student.

The Oxford meeting was marked by many fine contributions on controversial subjects. The role of putative transmitter substances in the initiation of carotid body sensory discharge was examined in the very elegant series of Loewi-type experiments presented by Eyzaguirre & Zapata (1968). They clearly demonstrated that the superfused carotid body, when exposed to asphyxia or electrically stimulated, released a substance capable of exciting a second carotid body placed downstream in the superfusion system. These authors favoured acetylcholine as a transmitter, based, *inter alia,* on their observations that chemoreceptor responses were markedly attenuated (but not abolished) by hemicholinium and mecamylamine. They drew attention to the fact that their inability to completely block

6

carotid body responses using anticholinergic agents was the single most important piece of evidence against acetylcholine as the principal neurotransmitter in chemoreception. They further pointed out the lack of experimental data on the role of catecholamines, and the possibility that multiple neurotransmitters with differing actions could together determine the overall level of chemosensory discharge. Joels and Neil explored some of the problems with the acetylcholine hypothesis (Joels & Neil, 1968). Douglas (1952) had shown that while hexamethonium blocked the vigorous chemoreflex response to acetylcholine, the responses to cyanide and asphyxia remained intact. Joels and Neil could not confirm this observation in the vascularly isolated carotid body perfused with Krebs-Henseleit solution: in these circumstances hexamethonium reduced the chemosensory discharge evoked by 'natural' stimuli as well as that in response to acetylcholine (Joels & Neil 1962, 1963). Pursuing a serendipitous observation, they showed that when even a small amount of blood was added to the solution perfusing the carotid body, hexamethonium then failed to block the chemosensory response to asphyxic stimuli (Joels & Neil, 1968). The relative lack of effect of hexamethonium on hypoxic responsiveness in the blood-perfused (Douglas, 1952) or 'blood-assisted' carotid body preparation suggested that studies involving perfusion with Krebs-Henseleit alone or superfusion were producing misleading results. They concluded that "acetylcholine has little to do with the normal mechanism of transmission of the glomus-sensory complex" (Joels & Neil, 1968). Almost thirty years later, the role in chemotransduction of the acetylcholine known to be synthesised within the carotid body is still the subject of controversy and study (see Prabhakar, this volume; Fitzgerald et al., this volume).

The major thrust of the work presented by Joels and Neil, and a further paper by Krylov and Anichkov, was an examination of the role of high energy phosphates in hypoxic chemotransduction (Joels & Neil, 1968; Krylov & Anichkov, 1968). Neil pointed out that for the early part of his investigations he had been unaware of the important work performed by the Russian group (Anichkov & Belen'kii, 1963), and both groups benefited greatly from the opportunity to compare their results provided by the Oxford meeting. There were some differences in the results obtained in the two laboratories, but they provided convincing evidence for a role for high energy phosphates in the genesis of chemosensory discharge. The fact that uncouplers of oxidative phosphorylation disrupted hypoxic responsiveness but did not affect the chemosensory response to acid brought Krylov and Anichkov to the conclusion that "in the carotid body there may exist at least two independent chemoreceptor mechanisms. One of them is responsible for excitation by CO_2 excess ... the other bears the responsibility of being stimulated by lack of oxygen" (Krylov & Anichkov, 1968). Some years later, with the advent of superior techniques, Lahiri's group fully confirmed this work and greatly advanced the metabolic theory of chemoreception (Mulligan et al., 1981).

The speed of response of the chemoreceptor, and the possibility of dynamic responsiveness, formed the basis of a number of papers (Leitner & Dejours, 1968; Dutton & Permutt, 1968; McCloskey, 1968). These investigations formed part of the lead-up to a great deal of work on the nature and role of oscillatory stimuli in chemoreceptor physiology.

BRISTOL, 1973

Seven years later, in July 1973, Michael Purves convened a meeting in Bristol, which became the forum for yet more controversy. The physiology of 'sinus nerve efferents' was one of the most hotly debated subjects. The was no dispute that such an efferent pathway existed, or that its activation inhibited chemosensory discharge (Neil & O'Regan 1969a,b; Fidone & Sato, 1970; Sampson & Biscoe, 1968,1970), but there was considerable criticism of the appropriateness of using electrical stimulation in the study of this phenomenon (Goodman, 1975). An important question was whether sinus nerve efferent inhibition could be explained solely in terms of changes in carotid body blood flow, or if some non-vascular mechanism also existed. O'Regan (1975) presented evidence for the existence of a physiological efferent inhibition in the absence of blood flow in an ischaemic carotid body preparation. However there was some discussion on whether it could be assumed that there would be absolutely no flow through the carotid body under the conditions of the experiment. Sampson (1975) presented pharmacological evidence that efferent inhibition depended upon dopaminergic mechanisms. Willshaw (1975), demonstrating an efferent inhibition of the arterial chemoreceptors in response to perfusion of the medullary surface with alkaline cerebrospinal fluid, showed that this response occurred with minimal changes in carotid body blood flow, and that the inhibition had similar pharmacological properties to that reported by Sampson (1975). It is fair to say that despite this and much subsequent investigation (O'Regan & Majcherczyk, 1983; Lahiri et al., 1983,1984), the exact mechanism and physiological role of efferent inhibition remain obscure.

It had been asserted, based on a replication of de Castro's original nerve section work (Biscoe et al., 1970), that the majority of sinus nerve terminals on glomus cells were efferent, not afferent in nature. McDonald and Mitchell presented to the meeting the results of what is probably the best analysis of carotid body ultrastructure in the literature (McDonald & Mitchell, 1975). They claimed that the glomus cells were innervated in the main by glossopharyngeal afferent fibres with a small efferent contribution from preganglionic sympathetic fibres. A large volume of subsequent work using a variety of techniques has fully supported their view that the vast majority of endings on type I cells are sensory. These workers also very elegantly demonstrated the existence of reciprocal synapses between sinus nerve afferents and type I cells (Mitchell & McDonald, 1975). They hypothesised "that afferent nerves are chemoreceptors sensitive to hypoxia and glomus cells are dopaminergic interneurons which adjust the sensitivity of the chemoreceptive nerves". They further proposed that unphysiological activation of this inhibitory system accounted for the observations of 'sinus nerve efferent inhibition'. However, it is now generally accepted that type I cells are the primary chemosensor in the carotid body. The role of the reciprocal synapse in the functioning of the chemoreceptor organ remains, therefore, an open question. The complexity of synaptic connections within the carotid body was further emphasised by the description of axo-dendritic connections (Verna, 1975).

Woods (1975) studied the diffusion of horseradish peroxidase into the carotid body and showed that there was no barrier to diffusion; this observation had implications for the speed of response of the chemoreceptors. A physiological investigation of chemoreceptor dynamic responsiveness, with a view to greater understanding of responses to oscillatory stimuli, was presented by Ponte and Purves. These authors found that the resonant frequency of the fastest chemoreceptor response, that to CO_2, was at least an order of magnitude lower than normal respiratory frequency, and hence argued that the chemoreceptors should be relatively unresponsive to oscillations in CO_2/H^+coupled to the respiratory cycle (Ponte & Purves, 1975), at least at normal respiratory rates.

KASHMIR, 1974

Kashmir, in the foothills of the Himalayas, was the idyllic setting for the next gathering, in October 1974, which was organized by Antal Paintal. The meeting was associated with the Krogh Centenary Symposium, and was a satellite to the 26th International Physiological Congress held in New Delhi. These attractions drew a large number of distinguished scientists to India, and made for a very fruitful meeting

The role of respiratory-related oscillations of arterial PO_2, PCO_2 and pH in the control of respiration had been receiving increasing attention from chemoreceptor scientists. The possible importance of such oscillations was first alluded to by Yamamoto (Yamamoto, 1960; Yamamoto & Edwards; 1960). Oscillations in arterial gas tensions (Purves, 1965; Band & Semple, 1967) and chemoreceptor discharge (Biscoe & Purves, 1967; Leitner & Dejours, 1968) secondary to tidal respiration were subsequently unequivocally demonstrated. This topic made appearances at earlier chemoreceptor meetings (Leitner &

Dejours, 1968; Ponte & Purves, 1975), but came to the fore and dominated discussion at Kashmir. A paper presented by Willshaw (Band et al., 1976) challenged the notion that the speed of response of the chemoreceptors was too slow to adequately follow oscillations in arterial gas tensions and pH (Leitner & Dejours, 1968; Ponte & Purves, 1975). They also presented evidence that the chemoreceptor afferents were responsive to the rate of change of arterial pH/PCO_2 (differential or rate sensitivity) as well as the absolute magnitude of pH_a/P_aCO_2 (proportional sensitivity). They asserted that the degree to which rate sensitivity was expressed differed from afferent to afferent and under different experimental conditions. The question whether or not arterial chemoreceptors exhibit rate sensitivity still provokes controversy (see Kumar et al., this volume; Torrance et al., this volume), and the contribution of oscillations in arterial blood gas tensions and chemoreceptor discharge to the control of breathing remains unknown. Theoretical analysis of oscillations in P_aO_2 (Kreuser, 1976) and of the possible role of oscillations in pH_a/P_aCO_2 in the control of respiration in humans (Cunningham & Drysdale, 1976) were presented. Experimental confirmation of such models was elusive: Grant and Semple could not demonstrate a change in ventilation in response to a reduction in the amplitude of the oscillations in pH_a/P_aCO_2 in the anaesthetized cat (Grant & Semple, 1976).

Opposing views on the absolute value of glomus tissue PO_2 (P_tO_2) were presented. When measured in Dortmund, the P_tO_2 varied between 5 and 15 Torr (Acker et al., 1976), whilst in Cleveland, measurements of P_tO_2 averaged 42 Torr deep in the carotid body and 69 Torr nearer the surface, and were greatly affected by changes in carotid body blood flow (Whalen & Nair, 1976). The value of P_tO_2 is of great significance in developing quantitative theories of hypoxic chemotransduction; the more recent results generated using optical techniques (Rumsey et al., 1991) provide an estimate of P_tO_2 somewhere between the two values reported in these earlier studies.

Single fibre electroneurographic studies of carotid chemoreceptor afferents to hypoxia and hypercapnia showed the interaction between these stimuli to be multiplicative (Lahiri & DeLaney, 1976a; Fitzgerald, 1976). It was an unusual event at a chemoreceptor meeting for the results from two laboratories to be in such close agreement.

Bilateral carotid body resection (BCBR) enjoyed a relatively brief vogue as a treatment for asthma and chronic obstructive airways disease in Japan and the United States. The rationale for this operation, which abolishes any meaningful ventilatory or arousal response to hypoxaemia, is obscure, and its benefit to the individual patient has never been adequately documented. Despite these reservations, BCBR patients have provided physiologists with a useful way of determining the contribution of peripheral chemoreceptors to the control of breathing under different circumstances in human subjects. Wasserman and Whipp conducted a comprehensive series of studies on 14 BCBR subjects with near-normal pulmonary function, and provided evidence for an exclusive role for the carotid bodies in the acute respiratory responses to hypoxia and metabolic acidosis (Wasserman & Whipp, 1976). They reported some very interesting results on the control of ventilation in exercise. They clearly showed that the sudden increase in ventilation at the onset of exercise did not depend on the peripheral chemoreceptors. The matching of ventilation to carbon dioxide production in steady-state exercise was also normal in BCBR subjects. However, BCBR subjects achieved steady-state ventilation more slowly than controls, and did not exhibit the normal increase in ventilation in excess of carbon dioxide production in heavy exercise, implying a role for the carotid bodies in these phenomena.

A series of papers concerned with responses to carbon monoxide (CO) clearly demonstrated that the effects of this gas were not mediated by the peripheral chemoreceptors (Fitzgerald et al., 1976; Lahiri & DeLaney, 1976b) but were due to a central excitation of ventilation, perhaps due to a fall in cerebral O_2 delivery causing CNS acidosis (Edelman et al., 1976). The attribution of CO effects to cerebral acidosis encountered opposition, however, based on the observation (Lahiri & DeLaney, 1976b) that ventilation fell rapidly on stopping CO administration in spite of persistent carboxyhaemoglobinaemia. Further investigation of these responses would seen appropriate.

DORTMUND, 1976

The workshop held at the Max-Planck-Institut für Systemphysiologie, Dortmund, in 1976, naturally reflected the host laboratory's interest in carotid body tissue PO_2 and local blood flow. A quantitative study of intercapillary distances in the carotid body (Lubbers et al., 1977) showed that the diffusion distance was not sufficiently long to explain the low P_tO_2 values obtained by Acker and his colleagues (Weigelt & Acker, 1977; Acker & Lubbers, 1977); the authors proposed that plasma skimming and/or differences in blood flow distribution could cause P_tO_2 to be lower than predicted by intercapillary distance. Whalen pointed out that his higher values for P_tO_2 (Whalen & Nair, 1977) agreed very closely with the observed capillary geometry without the need to invoke plasma skimming.

Two major questions initially treated in Dortmund were to reappear at the subsequent meetings in Valladolid and Leicester. The detailed ultrastructural and physiological studies of the early 1970's failed to clarify which of the carotid body structures was the primary chemosensor: there were many who believed the primary afferent was the chemosensitive structure, with type I cells playing a modulatory role. A large series of investigations, presented at these three meetings, attempted to resolve this issue. The study of sinus nerve afferents during regeneration after sinus nerve sectioning and resuturing (Knoche & Kienecker 1977a,b; Bingmann et al., 1977) appeared to show that chemosensitivity required the carotid body vasculature but not specific connections between the afferent and type I cells. Later studies from these workers (Bingmann et al., 1981a,b) detected hypoxic and hypercapnic responses from sinus nerve fibres re-implanted into the wall of the external carotid artery. These experiments implied that the afferent fibre was the chemosensitive structure. Zapata, however, presented data to show that the time taken for recovery of chemoresponsiveness after crushing the sinus nerve depended on the distance of the crush site from the glomus, and that recovery of chemoreceptor function coincided with the re-establishment of connections with type I cells (Zapata et al., 1977). Furthermore, a broader group of experiments involving cryodestruction of the glomus tissue (Leitner et al., 1981), glomectomy (Mills & Smith, 1981), cross-anastomosis of the carotid sinus and lingual nerves (Dinger et al., 1984) and carotid body transplantation (Monti-Bloch et al., 1984) all pointed to an essential role for the type I cell in the genesis of chemoreceptor activity in response to changes in blood gas tensions.

Dortmund saw an explosion of interest in the biochemistry and physiology of catecholamines in the carotid body (Belmonte et al., 1977; Hanbauer, 1977; Hellstrom, 1977; Gronblad & Korkala, 1977; Starlinger, 1977) which was continued at the Valladolid and Leicester meetings (Stensaas et al., 1981; Gonzalez et al, 1981a,b; Fidone et al.,1981; Hellstrom & Hanbauer, 1981; Starlinger & Acker, 1981; Monti-Bloch & Eyzaguirre, 1981; Hess et al.,1981; Lahiri, 1981; Mir et al., 1984; McQueen, 1984; Zapata et al., 1984; Horn et al., 1984; Gonzalez et al., 1984; Dawes et al., 1984; Eyzaguirre et al., 1984). These studies clearly demonstrated that the type I cells contained the necessary enzymatic apparatus to synthesise catecholamines, that catecholamines were stored in the carotid body (dopamine being the most plentiful, followed by noradrenaline, with very small amounts of adrenaline detected), and that catecholamine synthesis is induced by hypoxia. The effects of catecholamines on carotid body chemosensory discharge varied between species and preparation, but the balance of evidence at the time pointed to an inhibitory role for dopamine, whereas noradrenaline could evoke both excitatory and inhibitory effects. However, despite the large volume of detailed and rigorous work which has been done to elucidate the role of classical and novel neurotransmitters in carotid body function, we still have little idea of the mechanisms by which glomus cells communicate with chemoreceptor afferents.

The history of this meeting must include mention of one far-sighted paper. Demonstrating a vigorous chemosensory discharge in response to perfusion of the carotid body with solutions containing ruthenium red or lanthanum, Roumy and Leitner proposed that a rise in cytosolic calcium, as a result of decreased mitochondrial uptake, was the stimulus to transmitter release in hypoxia, and therefore central to hypoxic chemotransduction (Roumy & Leitner, 1977). In view of the prominent part played by intracellular calcium in current models of chemotransduction (see Buckler & Vaughan-Jones, this volume; Peers, this volume) this was, in retrospect, a landmark observation which may not have received the credit it deserves.

VALLADOLID, 1979

At the end of the Dortmund workshop, Bob Torrance and Carlos Eyzaguirre suggested that a symposium be held in Spain to celebrate the 50th anniversary of Fernando de Castro's 1928 publication on the microscopic structure and possible physiological function of the carotid body. This symposium was organized by Carlos Belmonte and held, albeit one year late, in Valladolid, in September 1979. The meeting was opened by Antonio Gallego, who gave an appraisal of the work of his long-time friend, Fernando de Castro (Gallego, 1981), describing his formidable contribution to the study of carotid body structure and function. Carlos Eyzaguirre, in the second invited lecture, described his investigations of the electrophysiological properties of the glomus cells and primary nerve endings, including his attempts to record from these endings, and endeavoured to integrate his findings into an overall model of carotid body function (Eyzaguirre, 1981). The Valladolid meeting contained many fine papers on the necessity of glomus cells for normal chemoreceptor function and on the role of catecholamines in chemotransduction; these have been mentioned above. In addition, the demonstration that the relatively impermeant carbonic anhydrase inhibitor benzolamide is much less effective than the permeant acetazolamide in inhibiting CO_2/H^+ chemoreception (Hanson et al., 1981) generated the hypothesis that the chemoreceptor response to CO_2/H^+ depends on changes in intracellular pH. This observation is the basis of the most recent hypotheses on this aspect of carotid body chemotransduction (see Buckler & Vaughan-Jones, this volume). A final noteworthy paper described a more thorough approach to the possible metabolic mechanisms underlying hypoxic chemosensitivity, with the use of oligomycin (Mulligan & Lahiri, 1981), work which at the time was described by Mills as "a lovely dissection of the transport chain function in the carotid body."

LEICESTER, 1982

The scientific content of the meeting held in Leicester in September, 1982, organized by David Pallot developed many of the themes that had been prominent at the preceding meetings, with many reports on the contribution of glomus cells and the catecholamines they contained to the detection of O_2, CO_2 and acid. In particular, as described above, the observations on re-innervation of the carotid body by foreign nerves (Dinger et al., 1984) and carotid body transplantation (Monti-Bloch et al., 1984) were the death knell for the hypothesis that the primary afferent endings are the site of chemotransduction.

Studies of changes in extracellular ion concentration and their role in the functioning of the carotid body had been presented at earlier meetings, and were discussed in Leicester also (O'Regan & Acker, 1984; Delpiano & Acker, 1984) In studies of the ionic mechanisms of chemoreceptor responses, these technically very difficult experiments have been superseded by isolated cell and patch clamp approaches.

OEIRAS, 1985

The Gulbenkian Institute of Science in Oeiras, Portugal was the setting for the 8th International symposium on Arterial Chemoreception, organized by Jose Ribeiro. The meeting was dominated by presentations on neurotransmitters and putative neurotransmitters. Particularly notable was the growing interest in novel agents outside the traditional acetylcholine and catecholamines (McQueen & Kirby, 1987; Ribiero & McQueen, 1987; Monteiro & Ribeiro, 1987).

The great bulk of work on reflexes involving the peripheral arterial chemoreceptors has involved detailed examination of afferent or efferent elements outside the central nervous system. David Jordan, Michael Spyer and their associates are amongst the few investigators who have (Jordan et al., 1987) and still are (see Jordan, this volume) attempting to uncover the brain stem and hypothalamic pathways through which chemoreflex responses are elaborated. A second area of expanding knowledge is the developmental biology of chemoreception. Pioneering work on the function of chemoreceptors in late fetal and early neonatal life (Blanco et al., 1987a,b; Eden & Hanson, 1987) showed the importance developmental aspects of chemoreceptor physiology to the understanding of respiratory adaptations in infants.

The study of carotid body morphology in human disease was the subject of a number of interesting papers (Heath et al., 1987; Smith et al., 1987; Hurst et al., 1987). Finally, a series of studies where the selective peripheral chemoreceptor stimulant, almitrine, was employed to study carotid body physiology, were presented. (Pequignot et al., 1987; O'Regan et al., 1987; Gordon et al., 1987).

CONCLUSION

There have been four further meetings held under the auspices of the International Society for Arterial Chemoreception: in Salt Lake City (1988), Warsaw (1989), Cheiti (1991) and Dublin (1993). We do not feel it appropriate to try to assess these meetings from a historical perspective. However, some trends are obvious and deserve comment. These meetings have been dominated by molecular physiological and biochemical approaches to the study of chemoreceptor function. In particular, the application of patch clamp and microflourimetric techniques to the carotid body has provided a great volume of data on the functioning of type I cells. We feel confident that these approaches are slowly but surely piecing together a comprehensive model of the molecular biology of chemoreception. The elucidation of the roles of the different neurotransmitters known to be present in the carotid body is an elusive goal, made even more difficult by the recent description of neurotransmitter roles for substances like nitric oxide and carbon monoxide (see Prabhakar, this volume). New techniques, such as the electrochemical detection of catecholamines within the carotid body using microelectrodes, promise insights into the role of neurotransmission in chemoreceptor function, which we now realise must involve a dynamic interaction between a number of chemical transmitters.

However, the remarkable success of these approaches may have drawn attention away from the study of how chemoreceptor responses are integrated into the normal functioning of the intact organism. This is an area where there is a great dearth of knowledge. Little is known about how the brain stem organizes the broad range of cardiorespiratory responses to chemoreceptor stimuli. Developmental physiologists continue to struggle with the mechanisms underlying and the significance of the changes in chemoreceptor and chemoreflex function in fetal and neonatal life. Finally, the contribution of the peripheral chemoreceptors to respiratory and cardiovascular control in the unanaestheised animal or human, whether awake or asleep, infant or adult, is in many ways incompletely understood.

The detailed description of the mechanisms by which the carotid body "tastes the composition of the blood" is one of the greatest challenges faced by respiratory physiologists this century. It is an equally daunting task to explain how the afferent input from the carotid body is manipulated, interpreted, and translated into an appropriate output by the central nervous system, and how such integrated responses are employed to subserve the ultimate goal of respiratory and metabolic homeostasis. Future meetings on arterial chemoreception are promise to be exciting events as the answers to these questions are slowly uncovered.

REFERENCES

Acker, H., Weigelt, H., Lubbers, D.W., Bingmann, D. & Caspers, H. (1976) Effect of changes in Ca^{++} and K^+ activity upon tissue PO_2 and chemoreceptor activity of the cat carotid body. In "Morphology and Mechanisms of Chemoreceptors." A.S. Paintal, ed., Vallabhbhai Patel Chest Institute, University of Delhi, Delhi, India. pp. 103-112

Acker, H. & Lubbers, D.W. (1977) Relationship between local flow, tissue PO_2 and total flow of the cat carotid body. In "Chemoreception in the Carotid Body", H. Acker, S. Fidone, D. Pallot, C. Eyzaguirre, D.W. Lubbers & R. W Torrance, eds., Springer-Verlag, Berlin, Germany. pp 271-276

Anichkov, S.V. & Belen'kii, M.L. (1963) "Pharmacology of the Carotid Body Chemoreceptors" Permagon, Oxford, UK.

Band, D.M. & Semple, S.J.G. (1967) Continuous measurement of blood pH with an indwelling glass electrode. J. Appl. Physiol. 22:854-857

Band, D.M., Willshaw, P. & Wolff, C.B. (1976) The speed of response of the carotid body chemoreceptor. In "Morphology and Mechanisms of Chemoreceptors." A.S. Paintal, ed., Vallabhbhai Patel Chest Institute, University of Delhi, Delhi, India. pp. 197-208

Belmonte, C., Gonzalez, C. & Garcia, A.G. (1977) Dopamine beta-hydroxylase activity in the cat carotid body. In "Chemoreception in the Carotid Body", H. Acker, S. Fidone, D. Pallot, C. Eyzaguirre, D.W. Lubbers & R. W Torrance, eds., Springer-Verlag, Berlin, Germany. pp 99-105

Bingmann, D., Kienecker, E.-W. & Knoche, H. (1977) Chemoreceptor activity in the rabbit carotid sinus nerve during regeneration. In "Chemoreception in the Carotid Body", H. Acker, S. Fidone, D. Pallot, C. Eyzaguirre, D.W. Lubbers & R. W Torrance, eds., Springer-Verlag, Berlin, Germany. pp 36-43

Bingmann, D., Kienecker, E.W., Caspers, H., & Knoche, H. (1981a) Chemoreceptor activity of sinus nerve fibres after their implantation into the wall of the external carotid artery. In "Arterial Chemoreceptors", C. Belmonte, D.J. Pallot, H. Acker & S. Fidone, eds., Leicester University Press, Leicester, UK. pp 92-104

Bingmann, D., Kienecker, E.W., Caspers, H., & Knoche, H. (1981) Receptive properties of regenerating sinus nerve endings in the wall of the external carotid artery. In "Arterial Chemoreceptors", C. Belmonte, D.J. Pallot, H. Acker & S. Fidone, eds., Leicester University Press, Leicester, UK. pp 105-114

Biscoe, T.J., Lall, A. & Sampson, S.R. (1970) Electron microscopic and electrophysiological studies on the carotid body following intracranial section of the glossopharyngeal nerve. J. Physiol. 208:133-152

Biscoe, T.J. & Purves, M.J. (1967) Observations on the rhythmic variation in the cat carotid body chemoreceptor activity which has the same period as respiration. J. Physiol. 190:389-412

Blanco, C.E., Hanson, M.A., McCooke, H.B. & B.A. Williams (1987a) The effect of premature delivery on chemoreceptor sensitivity in the lamb. In "Chemoreceptors in Respiratory Control", J.A. Ribeiro & D.J. Pallot, eds., Croom Helm, Kent, UK. pp 216-220

Blanco, C.E., Hanson, M.A., McCooke, H.B. & B.A. Williams (1987b) Studies of chemoreceptor resetting after hyperoxic ventilation of the fetus in utero. In "Chemoreceptors in Respiratory Control", J.A. Ribeiro & D.J. Pallot, eds., Croom Helm, Kent, UK. pp 221-227

Cunningham, D.J.C. & Drysdale, D.B. (1976) The role of human arterial chemoreceptors in normal respiratory regulation, and some factors which may influence the responses to dynamic stimulation. In "Morphology and Mechanisms of Chemoreceptors." A.S. Paintal, ed., Vallabhbhai Patel Chest Institute, University of Delhi, Delhi, India. pp. 209-221

Dawes, G.S., Hanson, M.A., Holman, R.B. & McCooke, H.B. (1984) Preliminary observations on the concentrations of catecholamines and their metabolites in the carotid bodies of newborn lambs. In "The Peripheral Arterial Chemoreceptors", D.J.Pallot, ed., Croom Helm, London, UK. pp 365-372

de Castro, F. (1951) Sur la structure de la synapse dans les chemocepteurs: leur mechanisme d'excitation et role dans la circulation sanguine locale. Acta. Physiol. Scand. 22:14-43

Delpiano, M.A. & Acker, H. (1984) The extracellular Ca^{++} and K^+ activities in the cat carotid body and their relationship to chemoreception. In "The Peripheral Arterial Chemoreceptors", D.J.Pallot, ed., Croom Helm, London, UK. pp 101-110

Dinger, B.G., Stenaas, L.J. & Fidone S.J. (1984) Chemosensory end organs re-innervated by normal and foreign nerves. In "The Peripheral Arterial Chemoreceptors", D.J.Pallot, ed., Croom Helm, London, UK. pp 225-234

Douglas, W.W. (1952) The effect of a ganglion-blocking drug, hexamethonium, on the response of the cat's carotid body to various stimuli. J. Physiol. 118:373-383

Dutton, R.E. & Permutt, S. (1968) Ventilatory responses to transient changes in carbon dioxide. In "Arterial Chemoreceptors.", R.W. Torrance, ed., Blackwell, Oxford, UK, pp 373-385

Edelman, N.H., T.V. Santiago & Doblar, D. (1976) Mechanism of the ventilatory response to carbon monoxide of unanaesthetized goats. In "Morphology and Mechanisms of Chemoreceptors." A.S. Paintal, ed., Vallabhbhai Patel Chest Institute, University of Delhi, Delhi, India. pp. 317-326

Eden, G.J. & Hanson, M.A. (1987) Effects of chronic hypoxia on chemoreceptor function in the newborn. In "Chemoreceptors in Respiratory Control", J.A. Ribeiro & D.J. Pallot, eds., Croom Helm, Kent, UK. pp 369-377

Eyzaguirre, C. (1981) An overview of mechanisms associated with the onset of sensory discharges in the carotid nerve. In "Arterial Chemoreceptors", C. Belmonte, D.J. Pallot, H. Acker & S. Fidone, eds., Leicester University Press, Leicester, UK. pp 20-44

Eyzaguirre, C. & Zapata, P. (1968) A discussion of possible transmitter or generator substances in carotid body chemoreceptors. In "Arterial Chemoreceptors.", R.W. Torrance, ed., Blackwell, Oxford, UK, pp 213-251

Eyzaguirre, C., Monti-Bloch, L. & Hayashida, Y. (1984) The effects of putative neurotransmitters on the glomus cell membrane and carotid nerve discharges. In "The Peripheral Arterial Chemoreceptors", D.J.Pallot, ed., Croom Helm, London, UK. pp 373-382

Fidone, S.J. & Sato, A. (1970) Efferent inhibition and antidromic depression of chemoreceptor A-fibres from the cat carotid body. Brain Res. 22:181-193

Fidone, S., Gonzalez, C. & Yoshikazi, K. (1981) A study of the relationship between dopamine release and chemosensory discharge from rabbit carotid body in vitro: preliminary findings. In "Arterial Chemoreceptors", C. Belmonte, D.J. Pallot, H. Acker & S. Fidone, eds., Leicester University Press, Leicester, UK. pp 209-219

Fitzgerald, R.S. (1976) Single fiber chemoreceptor responses of carotid and aortic bodies. In "Morphology and Mechanisms of Chemoreceptors." A.S. Paintal, ed., Vallabhbhai Patel Chest Institute, University of Delhi, Delhi, India. pp. 27-35

Fitzgerald, R.S., Traystman, R.J., Sylvester, J.T. & Permutt, S. Comparison of the effects of hypoxic hypoxia and carbon monoxide: a review. In "Morphology and Mechanisms of Chemoreceptors." A.S. Paintal, ed., Vallabhbhai Patel Chest Institute, University of Delhi, Delhi, India. pp. 327-334

Gallego, A. (1981) Fernando de Castro: contributions to the discovery and study of the vascular baroreceptors and the blood chemoreceptors. In "Arterial Chemoreceptors", C. Belmonte, D.J. Pallot, H. Acker & S. Fidone, eds., Leicester University Press, Leicester, UK. pp 1-19

Gonzalez, C., Kwok, Y., Gibb, J. & Fidone, S. (1981a) Regulation of tyrosine hydroxylase activities in carotid body, superior cervical ganglion and adrenal gland of rat rabbit and cat. In "Arterial Chemoreceptors", C. Belmonte, D.J. Pallot, H. Acker & S. Fidone, eds., Leicester University Press, Leicester, UK. pp 187-197

Gonzalez, C., Yoskikazi, Y. & Fidone, S. (1981b) Catecholamine synthesis from tyrosine and dopa in rabbit carotid body: effects of natural stimulation. In "Arterial Chemoreceptors", C. Belmonte, D.J. Pallot, H. Acker & S. Fidone, eds., Leicester University Press, Leicester, UK. pp 198-208

Gonzalez, E., Rigual, R., Gonzalez, C. & Fidone, S. (1984) Uptake and metabolism of dopamine by the carotid body. In "The Peripheral Arterial Chemoreceptors", D.J.Pallot, ed., Croom Helm, London, UK. pp 353-364

Goodman, N.W. (1975) Efferent inhibition of arterial chemoreceptors and stimulation of the sinus nerve. In "The Peripheral Arterial Chemoreceptors" M.J. Purves, ed., Cambridge University Press, London, UK, pp. 241-251

Gordon, B.H., Pallot, D.J., Mir, A., Ings, R.M.J., Evrard, Y. & Campbell, D.B. (1987) Kinetics of almitrine bismesylate and its metabolites in the carotid body and other tissues of the rat. In "Chemoreceptors in Respiratory Control", J.A. Ribeiro & D.J. Pallot, eds., Croom Helm, Kent, UK. pp 394-407

Grant, B. & Semple, S.J.G. (1976) Mechanisms whereby oscillations in arterial carbon dioxide tension might affect pulmonary ventilation. In "Morphology and Mechanisms of Chemoreceptors." A.S. Paintal, ed., Vallabhbhai Patel Chest Institute, University of Delhi, Delhi, India. pp. 191-208

Gronblad, M. & Korkola, O. (1977) Loss of histochemically demonstrable catecholamines in the glomus cells of the carotid body after α-methylparatyrosine treatment. In "Chemoreception in the Carotid Body", H. Acker, S. Fidone, D. Pallot, C. Eyzaguirre, D.W. Lubbers & R. W Torrance, eds., Springer-Verlag, Berlin, Germany. pp 130-135

Hanbauer, I. (1977) Molecular biology of chemoreceptor function: induction of tyrosine hydroxylase in the rat carotid body elicited by hypoxia. In "Chemoreception in the Carotid Body", H. Acker, S. Fidone, D. Pallot, C. Eyzaguirre, D.W. Lubbers & R. W Torrance, eds., Springer-Verlag, Berlin, Germany. pp 114-121

Hanson, M.A., Nye, P.C.G., & Torrance, R.W. (1981) The exodus of an extracellular bicarbonate theory and the genesis of an intracellular one. In "Arterial Chemoreceptors", C. Belmonte, D.J. Pallot, H. Acker & S. Fidone, eds., Leicester University Press, Leicester, UK. pp 417-429

Horn, N.M., Hasan, F.F. & Waters, R. (1984) Dopamine receptors in the peripheral chemoreceptors of the rat. In "The Peripheral Arterial Chemoreceptors", D.J.Pallot, ed., Croom Helm, London, UK. pp 345-352

Heath, D., Smith, P. & Hurst, G. (1987) The carotid bodies in coarctation of the aorta. In "Chemoreceptors in Respiratory Control", J.A. Ribeiro & D.J. Pallot, eds., Croom Helm, Kent, UK. pp 247.253

Hellstrom, S. (1977) Effects of hypoxia on carotid body type I cells and their catecholamines. A biochemical and morphologic study. In "Chemoreception in the Carotid Body", H. Acker, S. Fidone, D. Pallot, C. Eyzaguirre, D.W. Lubbers & R. W Torrance, eds., Springer-Verlag, Berlin, Germany. pp 122-129

Hurst, G., Heath, D. & Smith, P. (1987) Histological changes associated with ageing of the human carotid body. In "Chemoreceptors in Respiratory Control", J.A. Ribeiro & D.J. Pallot, eds., Croom Helm, Kent, UK. pp 262-270

Hellstrom, S. & Hanbauer, I. (1981) Modification of the dopamine content in the rat carotid body by metacholine and hypoxia. In "Arterial Chemoreceptors", C. Belmonte, D.J. Pallot, H. Acker & S. Fidone, eds., Leicester University Press, Leicester, UK. pp 220-230

Heymans, C. (1951) Chemoreceptors and regulation of respiration. Acta. Physiol. Scand. 22:4-13

Hess, A., Mishra, J. & Sapru, H.N. (1981) Dopamine stimulation and preliminary studies on the presence and localisation of dopaminergic receptors in the rat carotid body. In "Arterial Chemoreceptors", C. Belmonte, D.J. Pallot, H. Acker & S. Fidone, eds., Leicester University Press, Leicester, UK. pp 266-276

Joels, N. & Neil, E. (1962) The action of high tensions of carbon monoxide on the carotid chemoreceptors. Arch Int. Pharmacodyn. Ther. 139:528-534

Joels, N. & Neil, E. (1963) The excitation mechanism of the carotid body. Br. Med. Bull. 19:21-24

Joels, N. & Neil, E. (1968) The idea of a sensory transmitter. In "Arterial Chemoreceptors.", R.W. Torrance, ed., Blackwell, Oxford, UK, pp 153-177

Jordan, D., Donoghue, S., Felder, R.B. & Spyer, K.M. (1987) Central terminations of carotid body chemoreceptor afferents. In "Chemoreceptors in Respiratory Control", J.A. Ribeiro & D.J. Pallot, eds., Croom Helm, Kent, UK. pp 29-38

Knoche, H. & Kienecker, E.-W. (1977a) Degenerative changes in rabbit carotid body following systematic denervation and preliminary results about the morphology of sinus nerve neuromas. In "Chemoreception in the Carotid Body", H. Acker, S. Fidone, D. Pallot, C. Eyzaguirre, D.W. Lubbers & R. W Torrance, eds., Springer-Verlag, Berlin, Germany. pp 25-29

Knoche, H. & Kienecker, E.-W. (1977b) Regeneration of nerves and nerve terminals in rabbit carotid body following carotid nerve sectioning and suturing. In "Chemoreception in the Carotid Body", H. Acker, S. Fidone, D. Pallot, C. Eyzaguirre, D.W. Lubbers & R. W Torrance, eds., Springer-Verlag, Berlin, Germany. pp 30-35

Kreuser, F. (1976) Transmission of alveolar oxygen pressure oscillations. In "Morphology and Mechanisms of Chemoreceptors." A.S. Paintal, ed., Vallabhbhai Patel Chest Institute, University of Delhi, Delhi, India. pp. 176-190

Krylov, S.S. & Anichkov, S.V. (1968) The effect of metabolic inhibitors on carotid chemoreceptors. In "Arterial Chemoreceptors.", R.W. Torrance, ed., Blackwell, Oxford, UK, pp 103-113

Lahiri, S. (1981) Dopamine and chemoreception in carotid and aortic bodies. In "Arterial Chemoreceptors", C. Belmonte, D.J. Pallot, H. Acker & S. Fidone, eds., Leicester University Press, Leicester, UK. pp 277-288

Lahiri, S. & DeLaney, R.G. (1976a) The nature of response of single chemoreceptor fibres of carotid body to changes in arterial PO_2 and PCO_2-H^+. In "Morphology and Mechanisms of Chemoreceptors." A.S. Paintal, ed., Vallabhbhai Patel Chest Institute, University of Delhi, Delhi, India. pp. 18-26

Lahiri, S. & DeLaney, R.G. (1976b) Effect of carbon monoxide on carotid chemoreceptor activity and ventilation. In "Morphology and Mechanisms of Chemoreceptors." A.S. Paintal, ed., Vallabhbhai Patel Chest Institute, University of Delhi, Delhi, India. pp. 340-344

Lahiri, S. Smatresk, N., Pokorski, M., Barnard, P., Mokashi, A. & McGregor, K.H. (1983) Efferent inhibition of carotid body chemoreceptors in chronically hypoxic cats. Am. J. Physiol. 247:R24-R28

Lahiri, S., Smatresk, N., Pokorski, M., Barnard, P., Mokashi, A. & McGregor, K.H. (1984) Dopaminergic efferent inhibition of carotid body chemoreception in chronically hypoxic cats. Am. J. Physiol. 245:R678-R683

Leitner, L.-M. & Dejours, P. (1968) The speed of response of chemoreceptors. In "Arterial Chemoreceptors.", R.W. Torrance, ed., Blackwell, Oxford, UK, pp 79-90

Leitner, L.-M., Roumy, M. & Verna, A. (1981) Further studies on the cryodestruction of the rabbit carotid body. In "Arterial Chemoreceptors", C. Belmonte, D.J. Pallot, H. Acker & S. Fidone, eds., Leicester University Press, Leicester, UK. pp 85-91

Lubbers, D.W., Teckhaus, L. & Seidl, E. (1977) Capillary distances and oxygen supply to the specific tissue of the carotid body. In "Chemoreception in the Carotid Body", H. Acker, S. Fidone, D. Pallot, C. Eyzaguirre, D.W. Lubbers & R. W Torrance, eds., Springer-Verlag, Berlin, Germany. pp 62-68

McCloskey, D.I. (1968) Carbon dioxide and the carotid body. In "Arterial Chemoreceptors.", R.W. Torrance, ed., Blackwell, Oxford, UK, pp 279-295

McDonald, D.M. & Mitchell, R.A. (1975) A quantitative analysis of synaptic connections in the rat carotid body In "The Peripheral Arterial Chemoreceptors" M.J. Purves, ed., Cambridge University Press, London, UK, pp. 101-131

McQueen, D.S. (1984) Effects of selective dopamine receptor agonists and antagonists on carotid body chemoreceptors. In "The Peripheral Arterial Chemoreceptors", D.J.Pallot, ed., Croom Helm, London, UK. pp 325-335

McQueen, D.S. & Kirby, G.C. (1987) Pharmacological studies on opioid receptors in the cat carotid body. In "Chemoreceptors in Respiratory Control", J.A. Ribeiro & D.J. Pallot, eds., Croom Helm, Kent, UK. pp 296-304

Mills, E. & Smith, P.G. (1981) Carotid sinus nerve function and reflexes after glomectomy. In "Arterial Chemoreceptors", C. Belmonte, D.J. Pallot, H. Acker & S. Fidone, eds., Leicester University Press, Leicester, UK. pp 166-175

Mir, A.K., Pallot, D.J. & Nahorski, S.R. (1984). Catecholamines: their receptors and cyclic AMP generating mechanisms in the carotid body. In "The Peripheral Arterial Chemoreceptors", D.J.Pallot, ed., Croom Helm, London, UK. pp 311-324

Mitchell, R.A. & McDonald, D.M. (1975) Adjustment of chemoreceptor sensitivity in the cat carotid body by reciprocal synapses. In "The Peripheral Arterial Chemoreceptors" M.J. Purves, ed., Cambridge University Press, London, UK, pp. 269-291

Monteiro, E.C. & Ribeiro, J.S. (1987) Adenosine modulation of respiration mediated by carotid body chemoreceptors. In "Chemoreceptors in Respiratory Control", J.A. Ribeiro & D.J. Pallot, eds., Croom Helm, Kent, UK. pp 314-321

Monti-Bloch, L. & Eyzaguirre, C. (1981) Different effects of putative neurotransmitters on cat and rabbit chemoreceptors. In "Arterial Chemoreceptors", C. Belmonte, D.J. Pallot, H. Acker & S. Fidone, eds., Leicester University Press, Leicester, UK. pp 254-265

Monti-Bloch, L., Stenaas, L.J. & Eyzaguirre, C. (1984) Induction of chemosensitivity in muscle nerve fibres by carotid body transplantation. In "The Peripheral Arterial Chemoreceptors", D.J.Pallot, ed., Croom Helm, London, UK. pp 235-242

Mulligan, E. & Lahiri, S. (1981) Mitochondrial oxidative metabolism and chemoreception in the carotid body. In "Arterial Chemoreceptors", C. Belmonte, D.J. Pallot, H. Acker & S. Fidone, eds., Leicester University Press, Leicester, UK. pp 316-326

Mulligan, E., Lahiri, S. & Storey, B.T. (1981) Carotid body O_2 chemoreception and mitochondrial oxidative phosphorylation. J. Appl. Physiol. 51:438-446

Neil, E. (1951) Chemoreceptor areas and chemoreceptor reflexes. Acta. Physiol. Scand. 22:54-65

Neil, E. & O'Regan, R.G. (1969a) Effects of sinus and aortic nerve efferents on arterial chemoreceptor function. J. Physiol. 200: 69P-71P

Neil, E. & O'Regan, R.G. (1969b) Efferent and afferent impulse in the 'intact' sinus nerve. J. Physiol. 205:20P-21P

O'Regan, R.G., (1975) The influences exerted by the centrifugal innervation of the carotid sinus nerve. In "The Peripheral Arterial Chemoreceptors" M.J. Purves, ed., Cambridge University Press, London, UK, pp. 221-240

O'Regan, R.G. & Majcherczyk, S. (1983) Control of peripheral chemoreceptors by efferent nerves. In "Physiology of the Peripheral Arterial Chemoreceptors.", H. Acker & R.G. O'Regan, eds., Elsevier, Amsterdam, pp. 257-298

O'Regan, R.G. & Acker, H. (1984) Effects of sympathetic stimulation and catecholamines on extracellular calcium and potassium activities in the cat carotid body. In "The Peripheral Arterial Chemoreceptors", D.J.Pallot, ed., Croom Helm, London, UK. pp 75-86

O'Regan, R.G., Kennedy, M. & Przybyszewski, A.W. (1987) In "Chemoreceptors in Respiratory Control", J.A. Ribeiro & D.J. Pallot, eds., Croom Helm, Kent, UK. pp 386-393

Pequignot, J.M., Tavitian, E., Boudet, C. & Peyrin, L. (1987) Reduction in dopaminergic activity in the rat carotid body after acute or chronic almitrine. In "Chemoreceptors in Respiratory Control", J.A. Ribeiro & D.J. Pallot, eds., Croom Helm, Kent, UK. pp 378-385

Ponte, J.C.M.R. & Purves, M.J. (1975) On the speed of response of the chemoreceptors. In "The Peripheral Arterial Chemoreceptors" M.J. Purves, ed., Cambridge University Press, London, UK, pp. 357-371

Purves, M.J. (1965) Oscillations of oxygen tension in arterial blood. J. Physiol. 176:7P

Ribeiro, J.A. & McQueen, D.S. (1987) Chemoexcitation evoked by adenosine. Pharmacological characterisation of the receptor. In "Chemoreceptors in Respiratory Control", J.A. Ribeiro & D.J. Pallot, eds., Croom Helm, Kent, UK. pp 305-313

Roumy, M. & Leitner, L.-M. (1977) Role of calcium ions in the mechanism of arterial chemoreceptor excitation. In "Chemoreception in the Carotid Body", H. Acker, S. Fidone, D. Pallot, C. Eyzaguirre, D.W. Lubbers & R. W Torrance, eds., Springer-Verlag, Berlin, Germany. pp 257-263

Rumsey, W.L., R. Iturriaga, D. Spergel, S. Lahiri & D.F. Wilson. (1991) Optical measurements of the dependence of chemoreception on oxygen pressure in the cat carotid body. Am. J. Physiol. 261(30):C614-C622

Sampson, S.R. (1975) Pharmacology of feedback inhibition of carotid body chemoreceptors in the cat. In "The Peripheral Arterial Chemoreceptors" M.J. Purves, ed., Cambridge University Press, London, UK, pp. 207-217

Sampson, S.R. & Biscoe, T.J. (1968) Rhythmical and non-rhythmical activity recorded from the central cut end of the sinus nerve. J. Physiol. 196:327-338

Sampson, S.R. & Biscoe, T.J. (1970) Efferent control of the carotid body chemoreceptor. Experientia. 26:261-262

Smith, P., Hurst, G., Heath, D. & Drewe, R. (1987) The carotid bodies in a case of ventricular septal defect. In "Chemoreceptors in Respiratory Control", J.A. Ribeiro & D.J. Pallot, eds., Croom Helm, Kent, UK. pp 254-261

Starlinger, H. (1977) Enzymes and inhibitors of the catecholamine metabolism in the cat carotid body. In "Chemoreception in the Carotid Body", H. Acker, S. Fidone, D. Pallot, C. Eyzaguirre, D.W. Lubbers & R. W Torrance, eds., Springer-Verlag, Berlin, Germany. pp 136-141

Starlinger, H & Acker, H. (1981) In vivo formation of octopamine in the cat carotid body and superior cervical ganglion under the influence of different respiratory gases. In "Arterial Chemoreceptors", C. Belmonte, D.J. Pallot, H. Acker & S. Fidone, eds., Leicester University Press, Leicester, UK. pp 245-253

Stenaas, L.J. Stenaas, S.S., Gonzalez, C. & Fidone, S.J. (1981) Analytical electron microscopy of granular vesicles in the carotid body of the normal and reserpinized cat. In "Arterial Chemoreceptors", C. Belmonte, D.J. Pallot, H. Acker & S. Fidone, eds., Leicester University Press, Leicester, UK. pp 176-186

Torrance, R.W. (1986) Prolegomena. In "Arterial Chemoreceptors.", R.W. Torrance, ed., Blackwell, Oxford, UK, pp 1-40

von Euler, U.S., Liljestrand, G. & Zotterman, Y. (1939) Skand. Arch. Physiol. 83:132

Wasserman, K. & Whipp, B.J. (1976) The carotid bodies and respiratory control in man. In "Morphology and Mechanisms of Chemoreceptors." A.S. Paintal, ed., Vallabhbhai Patel Chest Institute, University of Delhi, Delhi, India. pp. 156-175

Weigelt, H. & Acker, H. (1977) Comparative measurements of tissue PO_2 in the carotid body. In "Chemoreception in the Carotid Body", H. Acker, S. Fidone, D. Pallot, C. Eyzaguirre, D.W. Lubbers & R. W Torrance, eds., Springer-Verlag, Berlin, Germany. pp 244-249

Whalen, W.J. & Nair, P. (1976) Factors affecting the tissue PO_2 in the carotid body of the cat. In "Morphology and Mechanisms of Chemoreceptors." A.S. Paintal, ed., Vallabhbhai Patel Chest Institute, University of Delhi, Delhi, India. pp. 91-102

Whalen, W.J. & Nair, P. (1977) Factors affecting O_2 consumption of the cat carotid body. In "Chemoreception in the Carotid Body", H. Acker, S. Fidone, D. Pallot, C. Eyzaguirre, D.W. Lubbers & R. W Torrance, eds., Springer-Verlag, Berlin, Germany. pp 233-239

Willshaw, P. (1975) Sinus nerve efferents as a link between central and peripheral chemoreceptors. In "The Peripheral Arterial Chemoreceptors" M.J. Purves, ed., Cambridge University Press, London, UK, pp. 253-267

Woods, R.I. (1975) Penetration of horseradish peroxidase between all elements of the carotid body. In "The Peripheral Arterial Chemoreceptors" M.J. Purves, ed., Cambridge University Press, London, UK, pp. 195-205

Yamamoto, W.S. (1960) Mathematical analysis of the time course of alveolar CO_2 J. Appl. Physiol. 15:215-219

Yamamoto, W.S. & Edwards, McIver W. Jr. (1960) Homeostasis of carbon dioxide during intravenous infusion of carbon dioxide. J. Appl. Physiol. 15:807-818

Zapata, P., Stenaas, L.J. & Eyzaguirre, C. (1977) Recovery of chemosensory function of regenerating carotid nerve fibres. In "Chemoreception in the Carotid Body", H. Acker, S. Fidone, D. Pallot, C. Eyzaguirre, D.W. Lubbers & R. W Torrance, eds., Springer-Verlag, Berlin, Germany. pp 44-50

Zapata, P. Serani, A., Cardenas, H. & Lavados, M. (1984) Characterisation of dopaminoceptors in carotid body chemoreceptors. In "The Peripheral Arterial Chemoreceptors", D.J.Pallot, ed., Croom Helm, London, UK. pp 335-344

OXYGEN SENSING IN THE CAROTID BODY : IDEAS AND MODELS

H. Acker

Max Planck Institut für molekulare Physiologie, Rheinlanddamm 201,
D-44139, Dortmund

The carotid body is able to respond to changes of the arterial PO_2 in a range between 100 Torr and 30 Torr with the chemoreceptor nervous discharge peaking at the low arterial PO_2 values (Lahiri & DeLaney, 1975). It is not the scope of this article to review and speculate on the main neurotransmitter which is released in hypoxia from type I cells to excite adjacent nerve endings, nor on the different biophysical properties of the type I cells to facilitate this transmitter release. However, it is the aim of this article to review and to speculate on the different possibilities as to how oxygen changes might be sensed in the carotid body tissue leading to a nervous response. There are three different views concerning the oxygen sensing mechanism in the carotid body that should be mentioned:

1.) The mitochondria are the site of the oxygen sensing, i.e. when the tissue PO_2 in the carotid body tissue approaches values close to the critical mitochondrial PO_2 ($PO_2 < 1$ Torr) the hypoxia-induced decrease of cellular ATP serves as a triggering signal.

2.) Cytochrome aa_3 of carotid body mitochondria has an unusually low affinity for oxygen ($PO_2 > 90$ Torr) and redox changes of this cytochrome dependent on PO_2 serve as a signal.

3.) Hemeproteins not involved in the energy producing process by the cytochromes of the mitochondrial respiratory chain undergo redox changes dependent on PO_2, inducing the nervous chemoreceptor response.

1.) Recent studies as published by Rumsey et al. (1991) favour the involvement of the first mechanism. Using a newly developed optical method they measured, under normoxic conditions of the inflowing medium (PO_2: 111 ± 15 Torr), intercapillary PO_2 values of about 23 ± 3 Torr in the carotid body tissue, confirming finally after about 20 years PO_2 measurements with microelectrodes in the carotid body tissue as published by Acker et al. (1971). In the experiments published by Rumsey et al. (1991) chemosensory discharge rose slowly as intercapillary PO_2 steadily declined to values of 10 Torr. Between 10 and 3 Torr, chemosensory discharge increased strikingly, concomitant with an enhanced rate of oxygen disappearance. As PO_2 fell below 3 Torr, oxygen disappearance slowed and neural activity decayed. This low range of PO_2 would be expected to affect oxygen metabolism and thus the metabolic state in the cells of the carotid body (Wilson et al., 1988). It is conceivable that the decrease in the tissue PO_2 of the carotid body produces a decline in the cytosolic phosphorylation potential and consequent adjustments in the redox state of the intramitochondrial pyridine nucleotides (Rumsey et al., 1991). A fall in the cytosolic phosphorylation potential will stimulate, in the presence of oxygen, oxidative phosphorylation to meet the energy demands of the different ATP-driven reactions inside the cells necessary to initiate and maintain nervous chemoreceptor activity. Blocking the energy production of the respiratory chain by different drugs, Mulligan et al. (1981) could impede the hypoxic responsiveness of the carotid body. Measuring an enhanced glucose uptake by the neurotransmitter-containing type I cells of the carotid body under low PO_2, Obeso et al. (1993) confirmed that the utilization of metabolic energy is an integral component of the chemoreceptor response to hypoxia. Furthermore, Donnelly (1993) underlined the importance of unimpaired oxidative metabolism for chemoreception in the carotid body by showing that chemoreceptor discharge and catecholamine release of the rat carotid body increase concomitantly with falling PO_2 but that chemoreceptor discharge declines while catecholamine release further increases when PO_2 reaches very low levels. One should conclude from these experiments that energy production by the respiratory chain is necessary for a regular nervous response curve of carotid body cells to hypoxia; however this does not necessarily imply that the mitochondrial respiratory chain also functions as an oxygen sensor. It seems reasonable to assume that the chemoreceptor process needs a stable energetic base which is guaranteed by mitochondrial ATP production.

2.) The membrane depolarisation necessary for transmitter release in hypoxia could be accomplished by the recently described outward-rectifying potassium currents of type-I cells, which are reduced under hypoxic conditions (Hescheler et al., 1989; Lopez-Lopez et al., 1989; Stea & Nurse, 1991). Observations that the open-probability of K^+-channels in type-I cells decreased under hypoxia (Delpiano & Hescheler, 1989; Ganfornina & Lopez-Barneo, 1991) substantiated the importance of these findings for understanding PO_2 chemoreception in the carotid body. Membrane depolarisation would open voltage-dependent Ca^{2+} channels, increasing cytosolic calcium and facilitating transmitter release (Biscoe et al., 1989; Pietruschka, 1985; Sato et al., 1991). However, the role of intracellular calcium stores in regulating the cytosolic calcium concentration, especially that of the mitochondria, has also been discussed (Duchen & Biscoe 1992a). In their classical paper, Mills and Jöbsis (1972) detected photometrically a cytochrome aa_3 with a low as well as with a high O_2 affinity component in the carotid body which could generate a decrease of the mitochondrial membrane potential with a concomitant calcium release, which is necessary for transmitter release to start at relatively high PO_2. This idea is in accordance with tissue PO_2 measurements in the carotid body as published by Nair et al. (1986) with values between 60 and 90 Torr. Duchen and Biscoe (1992b) supported the idea of a specialized cytochrome aa_3 by a model which located the O_2 sensor in the carotid body mitochondria, responding to oxygen changes due to a low O_2 affinity far above the critical mitochondrial PO_2, causing mitochondrial membrane depolarization and subsequent calcium release. Under most conditions the control of electron flux by oxygen concentration in both mitochondria and cells appears to be minimal. The apparent K_m of respiration for oxygen in cells and in isolated mitochondria is less than 0.7 Torr., although respiratory chain intermediates do show redox responses to changes in PO_2 of 70 Torr or even higher (Brand & Murphy,

1987). Chance (1988) pointed out that alternative explanations of apparent cytochrome responses to high PO_2 (20-70 Torr) observed by spectroscopy are provided by the following factors: interference from hemoglobin deoxygenation, high O_2 gradients particularly in rapidly metabolizing tissues and aggregated cells, non-steady states of control chemicals and mitochondrial substrates as well as another pigment, not cytochrome aa_3, that is present. I would like to question, therefore, the evidence supporting the existence of a specialized cytochrome aa_3 with low PO_2 affinity as an oxygen sensing mechanism.

3.) The molecular mechanism of the inhibitory effect of low PO_2 on K^+-channel conductivity and thus on the chemoreceptor properties of type-I cells is unknown, but the involvement of a heme-type PO_2 sensor protein has been suggested (Acker et al., 1989). The idea of heme proteins acting as PO_2 sensors in the carotid body has been published by several groups (Lloyd et al., 1968; Lahiri & DeLaney, 1975). Cross et al. (1990) carried out a detailed photometric analysis of the rat carotid body to gain more information about hemeprotein characteristics in this tissue. They detected a measurable heme signal with absorbance maxima at 559 nm, 518 nm and 425 nm suggesting the presence of a b-type cytochrome. This was confirmed by pyridine hemochrome and CO spectra. This heme protein is capable of H_2O_2 formation and seems to possess, therefore, similarities with cytochrome b_{558} of the NAD(P)H oxidase in neutrophils (Jones et al., 1991). Cytochrome b_{558} consisting of 91 kDa ($gp91_{phox}$) and 22 kDa ($p22_{phox}$) subunits resides in the plasma membrane and the membrane of neutrophil-specific granules, where it serves as the terminal electron carrier of the oxidase. Two additional cofactors, $p47_{phox}$ and $p67_{phox}$ are cytosolic and may exist as preformed complexes which translocate to the plasma membrane upon phagocyte activation, becoming integral parts of the active oxidase (Bokoch, 1993). The four proteins $p22_{phox}$, $gp91_{phox}$, $p47_{phox}$ and $p67_{phox}$, could be identified immunohistochemically in type I cells of the human carotid body (Kummer et al., 1993) recently highlighting the probable involvement of an NAD(P)H oxidase or a related isoform in the cellular oxygen sensing of the carotid body. Of special interest in this context are findings as published by Lopez-Lopez and González (1992) showing that the hypoxia-induced decrease in type I cell potassium channel activity can be inhibited by CO. This might be interpreted as being due to CO inducing an oxidation of a hemeprotein which interacts with potassium channels in the cell membrane of type I cells. The following discussion tries to give a model for the involvement of a H_2O_2 generating NAD(P)H oxidase in the cellular oxygen sensing process influencing potassium channels. Hydrogen peroxide produced by this oxidase is supposed to act as a second messenger on different targets inside the cell. The scavenging of hydrogen peroxide by catalase can lead to the formation of the heme-containing catalase-compound I complex which activates the heme containing guanylate cyclase (GC) by interaction of the two heme groups as described for smooth muscle cells of the lung vasculature (Cherry et al., 1990). The enhanced cGMP level might lead to an activation of the different cytosolic activator proteins of the NAD(P)H oxidase (Bockoch, 1993). The availability of oxygen provided by the oxygen supply determines the amount of hydrogen peroxide formed by the oxidase with a declining formation under hypoxia. This mechanism would also lead to a PO_2 dependent cGMP level, which is known to vanish in carotid body type I cells under hypoxic conditions (Wang et al., 1991), decreasing perhaps the open probability of potassium channels. Type I cells as well as smooth muscle cells of the lung vasculature might depolarise under hypoxia by this mechanism leading to transmitter secretion or vasoconstriction. Hydrogen peroxide can also be scavenged by glutathione peroxidase (Sies et al., 1972), changing the ratio 2GSH/GSSG. The higher level of GSH under hypoxia could lead to a closing of GSH-sensitive potassium channels (Ruppersberg et al., 1991). A change in the 2GSH/GSSG ratio, and a concomitant variation of the chemoreceptor discharge, can be induced by H_2O_2 or organic hydroperoxides, as demonstrated by Acker et al. (1992) in the superfused rat carotid body in vitro.

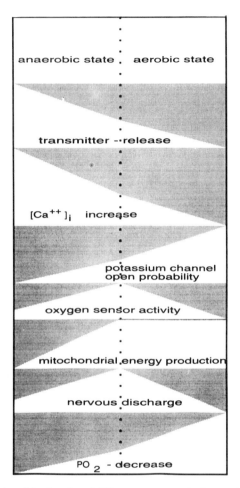

Figure 1: Schematic drawing of the function of different parameters in the carotid body tissue during anaerobic and aerobic conditions. As explained in the text more in detail this figure demonstrates that regular function of the carotid body is possible only under aerobic conditions whereas during the anaerobic state which is often reached with in vitro experiments the strong interplay between the four different parameters is lost rendering more difficult the interpretation of the main mechanism.

Figure 1 tries to reconcile the different views of the oxygen sensing process in the carotid body. From the discussion above it seems to be important to distinguish between an anaerobic and an aerobic state in which the carotid body oxygen sensor operates. The PO_2 decrease in the carotid body tissue determines the transition between these two states. From the above cited literature it seems to be obvious that the chemoreceptor nervous discharge increases with falling PO_2 and then declines when the PO_2 approaches very low levels. It is also very well documented that mitochondrial energy production remains stable over a wide PO_2 range but is then impaired when PO_2 reaches low levels. I would like to hypothesize that the oxygen sensor function exhibits also a PO_2 dependence peaking at an PO_2 optimum. Both nervous activity, as well as the oxygen sensor function, demand for a steadily increasing response a certain energy supply which seems to be available under aerobic conditions only. The PO_2 dependence of the open probability of the potassium channels as published by Ganfornina and Lopez-Barneo (1992) indicates a steeper decrease of the open probability at higher PO_2 values and significantly less decrease at low PO_2 values. Intracellular calcium as well as transmitter release which depend strongly on the membrane depolarisation induced by closing of potassium channels reach their optimum at very low PO_2 values indicating an anaerobic state; however, at these very low PO_2 values, nerve endings cannot respond to the higher concentration of transmitters anymore due to lack of energy necessary for fuelling different ion pumps in the cells. In the aerobic state, however, each of the parameters act in concert on the stable base of an undisturbed mitochondrial energy production to give rise to a chemoreceptor response curve which is able to stimulate respiration and the circulation to counteract tissue hypoxia.

REFERENCES

Acker, H., D.W. Lübbers, & M.J.Purves. (1971) Local oxygen tension field in the glomus caroticum of the cat and its change at changing arterial PO_2. Pflüg. Arch. 329:136-155

Acker, H., E. Dufau, J. Huber, & D. Sylvester. (1989) Indications to an NAD(P)H oxidase as a possible PO_2 sensor in the rat carotid body. FEBS Lett. 256:75-78

Acker, H., B. Bölling, M.A. Delpiano, E. Dufau, A. Görlach & G. Holtermann. (1992) The meaning of H_2O_2 generation in carotid body cells for PO_2 chemoreception. J. Auton. Nerv. Syst. 41:41-52

Biscoe, T.J., M.R. Duchen, D.A. Eisner, S.C O'Neill & M.Valdeolmillos. (1989) Measurements of intracellular Ca^{2+} in dissociated type I cells of the rabbit carotid body. J. Physiol 416:421-434

Bokoch, G.M. (1993) Biology of the Rap proteins, members of the ras superfamily of GTP-binding proteins. Biochem. J. 289:17-24

Brand, M.D., & M.P. Murphy. (1987) Control of electron flux through the respiratory chain in mitochondria and cells. Biol. Rev. 62:141-193

Chance, B. (1988) Early reduction of cytochrome c in hypoxia. FEBS Lett. 226:343-346

Cherry, P.D., H.A. Omar, K.A. Farrell, J.S. Stuart & M.S. Wolin. (1990) Superoxide anion inhibits cGMP associated bovine pulmonary relaxation. Am. J. Physiol. 259(28):H1056-H1062

Cross, A.R., L. Henderson, O.T.G. Jones, M.A. Delpiano, J. Hentschel & H. Acker. (1990) Involvement of an NAD(P)H oxidase as a PO_2 sensor protein in the rat carotid body. Biochem. J. 272:743-747

Donnelly, D.F. (1993) Electrochemical detection of catecholamine release from rat carotid body in vitro. J. Appl. Physiol. 74:2330-2337

Duchen, M.R., & T.J. Biscoe. (1992a) Relative mitochondrial membrane potential and [Ca^{2+}] in type I cells isolated from the rabbit carotid body. J. Physiol. 450:33-61

Duchen, M.R., & T.J. Biscoe. (1992b) Mitochondrial function in type I cells isolated from rabbit arterial chemoreceptors. J. Physiol. 450:13-31

Ganfornina, M.D., & J. López-Barneo. (1992) Potassium channel types in arterial chemoreceptor cells and their selective modulation by oxygen. J. Gen. Physiol. 100:401-426

Hescheler, J., M.A. Delpiano, H. Acker & F. Pietruschka. (1989) Ionic currents on type-I cells of the rabbit carotid body measured by voltage clamp experiments and the effect of hypoxia. Brain Res. 486:79-88

Jones, O.T.G., A.R. Cross, J.T. Hancock, L.M. Henderson & V.B. O'Donnell. (1991) Inhibitors of NAD(P)H oxidase as guides to its mechanism. Biochem. Soc. Trans. 19:70-72

Kummer, W., J.O. Habeck, D. Koesling, M. Quinn, & H. Acker. (1993) Immunohistochemical analysis of components of the oxygen sensing cascade in the human carotid body. Pflüg. Arch. 422:R129

Lahiri, S., & R.G. DeLaney. (1975) Stimulus interaction in the response of carotid body chemoreceptor single afferent fibers. Respir.Physiol. 24:249-266

Lloyd, B.B., D.J.C. Cunningham & R.C. Goode. (1968) Depression of hypoxic hyperventilation in man by sudden inspiration of carbon monoxide. In: "Arterial chemoreceptors" R.W. Torrance, ed., Blackwell, Oxford, pp.145-148.

Lopez-Lopez, J., C. Gonzalez, J. Urena, & J. Lopez-Barneo. (1989) Low PO_2 selectively inhibits K channel avtivity in chemoreceptor cells of the mammalian carotid body. J. Gen. Physiol. 93:1001-1015

López-López, J.R., & C.González. (1992) Time course of K^+ current inhibition by low oxygen in chemoreceptor cells of adult rabbit carotid body. Effects of carbon monoxide. FEBS Lett. 299:251-254

Mills, E., & F.F. Jöbsis. (1972) Mitochondrial respiratory chain of carotid body and chemoreceptor response to changes in oxygen tension. J. Neurophysiol. 35:405-428

Mulligan, E, S. Lahiri, & B.T.Storey. (1981) Carotid body O_2 chemoreception and mitochondrial oxidative phosphorylation. J. Appl. Physiol. 51:438-446

Nair, P.K., D.G. Buerk & W.J. Whalen. (1986) Cat carotid body oxygen metabolism and chemoreception described by a two cytochrome model. Am. J. Physiol. 19:H202-H207

Obeso, A., C. Gonzalez, R. Rigual, B. Dinger & S. Fidone. (1993) Effect of low O_2 on glucose uptake in rabbit carotid body. J. Appl. Physiol. 74:2387-2393

Pietruschka, F. (1985) Calcium influx in cultured carotid body cells is stimulated by acetylcholine and hypoxia. Brain Res. 347:140-143

Rumsey, W.L., R. Iturriaga, D. Spergel, S. Lahiri & D.F. Wilson. (1991) Optical measurements of the dependence of chemoreception on oxygen pressure in the cat carotid body. Am. J. Physiol. 261(30):C614-C622

26

Ruppersberg, J.P., M. Stocker, O. Pongs, St.H. Heinemann, R. Frank, & M. Koenen. (1991) Regulation of fast inactivation of cloned mammalian IK(A) channels by cysteine oxidation. Nature. 352:711

Sato, M., K. Ikeda, K. Yoshizaki & H. Koyano. (1991) Response of cytosolic calcium to anoxia and cyanide in cultured glomus cells of newborn rabbit carotid body. Brain Res. 551:327-330

Sies, H., C.H. Gerstenecker, H. Menzel, & L. Flohé. (1972) Oxidation in the NADP system and release of GSSG from hemoglobin free perfused rat liver during peroxidatic oxidation of glutathione by hydroperoxides. FEBS Lett. 171-175

Stea, A. & C.A. Nurse. (1991) Whole cell and perforated patch recordings from O_2-sensitive rat carotid body cells grown in short and long term culture. Pflügers Arch. 418:93-101

Wang, Z.Z., L.J. Stensaas, J. de Vente, B. Dinger & S.J. Fidone. (1991) Immunocytochemical localization of cAMP and cGMP in cells of the rat carotid body following natural and pharmacological stimulation. Histochem. 96:523-530

Wilson, D.F., W.L. Rumsey, T.J. Green & J.M. Vanderkooi. (1988) The oxygen dependence of mitochondrial oxidative phosphorylation measured by a new optical method for measuring oxygen concentration. J. Biol. Chem. 263:2712-2718

IONIC CHANNELS IN TYPE I CAROTID BODY CELLS

Chris Peers

Department of Pharmacology, Leeds University, Leeds, UK

INTRODUCTION

Over many years, a wealth of neurochemical and histological studies have established that type I (or glomus) cells, which lie in synaptic contact with afferent chemosensory nerve endings within the carotid body, are the primary sites of chemodetection. These cells contain various neurotransmitters (dopamine generally being accepted as the most important) which are released in response to both physiological and pharmacological stimuli. The good correlation between stimulus intensity, transmitter release and afferent chemosensory nerve discharge strongly suggests that release of transmitter(s) from type I cells is a fundamental step in the transduction of chemostimuli in the carotid body (Fidone & Gonzalez, 1986; Fidone et al., 1990; Gonzalez et al., 1992).

In recent years, it has been shown that type I cells can be enzymatically and mechanically dispersed, maintained in tissue culture and still retain chemoreceptor properties (Fishman et al., 1985; Pietruschka, 1985). This breakthrough has allowed the study of type I cell physiology without the complicating influence of other cells, such as afferent nerve endings themselves, type II (sustentacular) cells, vascular endothelial cells and autonomic neurones. Undoubtedly these other cells all exert modulatory influences which are of great physiological importance, but our lack of understanding of chemotransduction at a cellular level necessitates the development of a simple system: if we can establish how the individual components of this complex organ function, we will be better equipped to examine the integration of the different cell types and, ultimately, form a more complete picture of chemotransduction.

Isolation of type I cells has allowed them to be studied with the relatively new and powerful techniques of patch clamping and microfluorimetry which can be applied either alone or in combination. Microfluorimetric techniques use fluorescent, ion-sensitive dyes to measure intracellular ion levels in intact cells, and results of experiments on type I cells using such methodology are described by Buckler & Vaughan-Jones elsewhere in this volume. The aim of this article is to review the results of groups who have used patch clamp techniques to examine ion channels in type I cells. Patch clamping (Hamill et al., 1981) can be used to examine single ion channels in patches of membrane which are either still attached to the cell or have been excised (therefore isolated from the cell cytosol). Whole-cell patch clamp recordings can be used to study all the ion channels in the cell membrane under conditions of good voltage-clamp (type I cells are small and reasonably spherical) and the composition of the cytosol can be controlled by dialysis from the patch pipette. Alternatively, the perforated-patch technique (Horn & Marty, 1988) can be used to record whole-cell currents without dialysis of the cell interior. This technique has the advantage of retaining small diffusible molecules (which might be crucial to the normal functioning of ion channels) inside the cell.

The first report of ionic currents in isolated type I cells came from the laboratory of Gonzalez in Valladolid, Spain. This group used whole-cell recordings to demonstrate three separate ionic currents in cells isolated from adult rabbit carotid bodies (Na^+, Ca^{2+} and K^+ currents), of which the K^+ current was selectively inhibited by hypoxia (Lopez-Barneo et al., 1988). Since the publication of that report other laboratories have published single channel and whole-cell recordings from type I cells of rats and rabbits of differing ages. Below, I give a brief account of the various ionic channels / currents that have been described in type I cells, and discuss the ways in which they may be involved in chemotransduction.

POTASSIUM CHANNELS

K^+ channels or currents in type I cells have received by far the most attention to date, and it is becoming increasingly clear that they constitute an important site of modulation by carotid body stimuli. In neurones and other cell types, different populations of K^+ channels co-exist (e.g. Rudy, 1988), and the type I cell is no exception; all groups who have studied K^+ currents have reported the co-existence of at least two sub-populations of channels. In adult rabbit cells, whole-cell recordings revealed both Ca^{2+}-dependent (IK_{Ca}) and Ca^{2+}-independent (IK_v) K^+ currents (Duchen et al., 1988; Lopez-Lopez et al., 1989). Recently, single channels studies have extended these observations to report three distinct K^+ channels: a high-conductance Ca^{2+}-activated K^+ channel (210pS in symmetrical 140mM K^+) and two Ca^{2+}-independent channels with conductances of 40pS and 16pS (Ganfornina & Lopez-Barneo, 1991, 1992). Duchen et al. (1988) have also reported apamin-sensitive (therefore presumably low conductance Ca^{2+}-activated) K^+ currents. Cultured embryonic rabbit type I cells also possess Ca^{2+}-activated and Ca^{2+}-independent K^+ currents (Hescheler et al., 1989), and cell-attached single channel recordings have revealed a high-conductance K^+ channel with inwardly rectifying properties (Delpiano & Hescheler, 1989). In neonatal rat type I cells, Ca^{2+}-dependent and Ca^{2+}-independent, voltage-gated K^+ currents (the latter being sensitive to 4-aminopyridine) have been identified (Peers, 1990a,b,c). The Ca^{2+}-activated component has been shown to be inhibited by charybdotoxin, indicative of a high conductance K_{Ca} current (Peers, 1990a), and this has recently been confirmed at the single channel level (Wyatt & Peers, 1993; also this volume).

Despite one report to the contrary (Biscoe & Duchen, 1989), there is a superficial consensus of opinion that chemostimuli inhibit K^+ channels in type I cells. However, there is a lack of consensus as to which subtype of K^+ channel is inhibited. For adult rabbit type I cells, hypoxia and acidity both inhibit a 4-aminopyridine sensitive, Ca^{2+}-independent K^+ current (Lopez-Lopez et al., 1989; however, see also Biscoe & Duchen, 1990a,b). Hypoxic suppression is extremely rapid and can be reversed by carbon monoxide, suggesting the involvement of a haem-protein (Lopez-Lopez & Gonzalez, 1992). It appears that this putative haem-protein must be tightly coupled to the K^+ channel, since hypoxic inhibition of this channel is observed in cell-free excised patches of membrane (Ganfornina & Lopez-Barneo, 1991a). Ganfornina and Lopez-Barneo (1992) also report a lack of effect of hypoxia on high conductance Ca^{2+}-activated K^+ channels. This is in marked contrast to results obtained in neonatal rat type I cells, where the Ca^{2+}-activated K^+ channel is selectively inhibited by hypoxia (Peers, 1990b,c) and also a variety of other natural and pharmacological chemostimuli (Peers, 1990a, 1991; Peers & Green, 1991; Wyatt & Peers, 1992), a finding which suggests an important role for this K^+ channel type in the rat. Other groups have not as yet clearly identified the sub-type of K^+ channel which is sensitive to chemostimuli, or indeed whether inhibition is selective at all between K^+ channel types (Hescheler et al., 1989; Stea & Nurse, 1991a).

The hypoxic inhibition of K^+ channels in adult rabbit type I cells has been studied in greatest detail to date, but one aspect of these studies has brought into question the relevance of such an effect in hypoxic chemotransduction. Both whole-cell (Lopez-Lopez et al., 1989) and single channel recordings (Ganfornina & Lopez-Barneo, 1992) have demonstrated that the relationship between hypoxia and current / channel inhibition is steepest over the PO_2 range of approximately 100 to 150mmHg. These authors have suggested several reasons as to why there is such a discrepancy between to the PO_2 range over which the channel is most sensitive, and the PO_2 range which excites the intact organ, as seen in carotid sinus nerve recordings (see e.g. Fidone & Gonzalez, 1986; Gonzalez et al., 1992). Perhaps the most appealing (yet still quite tentative) idea involves the second messenger cyclic AMP (cAMP). The concentration of this intracellular messenger is well known to be elevated during hypoxia, and pharmacological interventions which elevate cAMP levels can enhance transmitter release in response to chemostimuli (Delpiano & Acker, 1991; Perez-Garcia et al., 1991; Wang et al., 1991). Furthermore, cAMP has recently been demonstrated to inhibit the O_2-sensitive K^+ current in adult rabbit type I cells (Lopez-Lopez et al, 1993). If both cAMP and hypoxia act and interact at the level of the K^+ channel, then perhaps we may obtain a more understandable relationship between PO_2 and K^+ channel activity. Interactive studies, varying both PO_2 and intracellular cAMP levels whilst recording K^+ channel activity, remain to be reported and are awaited with interest.

Acidity has also been reported to inhibit K^+ channels (Lopez-Lopez et al., 1989; Peers, 1990a; Peers & Green, 1991; Stea et al., 1991) and this has been studied in greatest detail in type I cells of the neonatal rat. Importantly, extracellular and intracellular acidification selectively inhibit Ca^{2+}-activated K^+ currents in these cells without affecting Ca^{2+} channels (Peers & Green, 1991). Furthermore, elevations in intracellular $[Ca^{2+}]$ seen in response to acidic stimuli (Buckler & Vaughan-Jones, 1993b) can be abolished by voltage-clamping cells at their initial, pre-stimulus value (Buckler & Vaughan-Jones, 1993a), suggesting that acidity, like hypoxia, may depolarize type I cells and so trigger Ca^{2+} influx via voltage-gated Ca^{2+} channels. However, as outlined later in this article, there are alternative mechanisms suggested for both hypoxic and acidic / hypercapnic transduction mechanisms in type I cells of the adult rabbit carotid body.

CALCIUM CHANNELS

Hypoxia stimulates Ca^{2+} influx into type I cells (Pietruschka, 1985), and evoked catecholamine release from type I cells is dependent on the presence of extracellular Ca^{2+} (Fishman et al., 1985). There is good evidence to suggest voltage-gated Ca^{2+} channels may provide the route for Ca^{2+} entry that is required to trigger transmitter release in response to chemostimuli (Obeso et al., 1987; 1992). Voltage-gated Ca^{2+} channels in other tissues can be crudely divided into four classes, termed T-, N-, L-, and P-type, of which L-type are the most widely distributed, and N- and P-type appear to be confined to neuronal tissue (see e.g. Tsien et al., 1988; Llinas et al., 1989). The earlier experiments distinguishing Ca^{2+} channel subtypes used both whole-cell and single channel recordings, and the presence of subtypes was based largely (although not exclusively) on differences in the voltage-dependence of both activation and steady-state inactivation, the kinetics of current inactivation during depolarizing voltage steps and on single channel properties (Nowycky et al., 1985; see also Tsien et al., 1988). This work quickly led to an explosion of publications on coexistent Ca^{2+} channel subtypes in various tissues, but in more recent times classification of different Ca^{2+} channels based on kinetic analysis and even single channel properties has been brought into question (Swandulla et al., 1989). Instead, current opinion seems to favour a pharmacological approach to the dissection and identification of different types of Ca^{2+} channels.

In the carotid body, it is likely that L-type Ca^{2+} channels play an important role in chemotransduction since agents such as organic Ca^{2+} channel antagonists (e.g. dihydropyridines), which block or enhance these channels, can modulate responses of intact carotid bodies to hypoxia both in vitro and in vivo (Shaw et al., 1989; Shirahata & Fitzgerald, 1991; Obeso et al., 1992). Ca^{2+} channels in isolated type I cells have only been studied at the macroscopic level, using conventional whole-cell or perforated patch recordings. Studies in adult rabbit (Duchen et al., 1988; Lopez-Barneo et al., 1988) and neonatal rat (Peers & Green, 1991) type I cells have revealed sustained inward Ca^{2+} currents. These currents can be enhanced by the dihydropyridine agonist Bay K 8644 (Peers & Green, 1991), suggesting that they are attributable (at least in part) to L-type Ca^{2+} channels. In type I cells cultured from embryonic rabbits, Ca^{2+} currents show partial inactivation during depolarizations, but can still be inhibited by approximately 80% with the organic Ca^{2+} channel antagonists D600 or PN 200-110 (Hescheler et al., 1989), again indicative of the presence of L-type Ca^{2+} channels. Thus there is reasonable agreement that L-type Ca^{2+} channels can be recorded in isolated type I cells and this is accordance with observations that organic Ca^{2+} channel blockers inhibit elevated carotid sinus nerve discharge from intact carotid bodies (Shaw et al., 1989; Shirahata & Fitzgerald, 1991; Obeso et al., 1992). However, it is impossible to say at present whether other subtypes of Ca^{2+} channels are present: pharmacological separation of different subtypes has not yet been thoroughly investigated and although organic compounds which inhibit L-type channels do have profound effects in type I cells, they have not been shown to fully inhibit the Ca^{2+} current even at high concentrations ($>1\mu M$) (Hescheler et al., 1989). This might suggest that a small fraction of Ca^{2+} current may be carried by channels other than L-type. Indeed the possibility of co-existent Ca^{2+} channel subtypes has been tentatively suggested in adult rabbit type I cells (Urena et al., 1989), on the basis of the analysis of tail-current kinetics. Clearly there is a need for a more comprehensive characterization of Ca^{2+} channels in order to determine whether or not a single population can account for the macroscopic Ca^{2+} currents of type I cells.

Although the potent carotid body stimulus cyanide has been shown to partially inhibit Ca^{2+} currents in type I cells (Biscoe & Duchen, 1989; Hescheler et al., 1989), other more physiological stimuli do not affect these currents. For example, Hescheler et al. (1989) demonstrated a lack of effect of hypoxia at levels which inhibit K^+ currents, and in type I cells of neonatal rats Ca^{2+} currents are unchanged by reductions in pH_o or pH_i which block K^+ currents (Peers & Green, 1991). Thus it is unlikely that a direct action of physiological stimuli on Ca^{2+} channels is important in chemotransduction. Nevertheless, Ca^{2+} channel activity may be indirectly modulated by chemostimuli, as a result of a primary action of such agents on K^+ channels (see below).

SODIUM CHANNELS

Voltage-gated Na^+ channels have been characterized in type I cells from adult rabbits at the whole-cell level (Duchen et al., 1988, Lopez-Barneo et al., 1989), and microfluorimetric studies have provided evidence that they are also present in newborn rabbit cells (Sato et al., 1991). However, in cells isolated from embryonic rabbits, there is no evidence for Na^+ currents (Hescheler et al., 1989). Although some reports have not identified Na^+ channels in neonatal rat type I cells (Peers, 1990a; Peers & Green, 1991) other workers have indicated that they are present at low density (Stea & Nurse, 1991a) and interestingly that their expression can be induced by prolonged exposure in culture to hypoxia or a membrane-permeable analogue of cyclic AMP (Stea et al., 1992). Wherever seen, Na^+ channels have always been shown to be blocked by tetrodotoxin (TTx).

Given these mixed reports, it is perhaps not surprising that there is no clear evidence for the role of Na^+ channels in type I cell chemotransduction. Lopez-Lopez et al. (1989) have demonstrated that type I cells can generate action potentials spontaneously, and that their frequency increases in hypoxia. Presumably these action potentials are attributable to the activity of Na^+ channels (which are not themselves affected by hypoxia; Lopez-Barneo et al., 1988), but this has not been demonstrated. Nevertheless, hypoxia-induced release of catecholamines has been shown to be reduced by TTx in adult rabbit carotid bodies (Rocher, Obeso, Herreros & Gonzalez, this volume). In contrast, Sato et al. (1991) have shown that although Na^+ channels are present in newborn rabbit type I cells, they are not involved in the rise of intracellular $[Ca^{2+}]$ seen in response to anoxia, which involves Ca^{2+} influx via voltage-gated Ca^{2+} channels (i.e. presumably via cell depolarization). Thus even where Na^+ channels are present, it is not clear whether they are of importance in hypoxic chemotransduction. Indeed, action potential generation is not essential for activation of Ca^{2+} channels; Delpiano and Hescheler (1989) have shown that embryonic rabbit type I cells depolarize in hypoxia sufficiently strongly to activate Ca^{2+} channels directly, without inducing action potentials (see also Buckler & Vaughan-Jones, this volume).

CHLORIDE CHANNELS

Direct evidence for the presence of Cl⁻ channels has been provided by Stea and Nurse (1989, 1991b), using both whole-cell and single channel recordings from rat carotid body type I cells. These channels were of high conductance (approximately 300pS) and had a high open probability regardless of membrane potential (ranging from -50mV to +50mV). These findings support the observation that type I cell membrane potential is influenced by chloride ions (Oyama et al., 1986). Stea and Nurse (1989) also reported that these channels were unaffected by changes in intracellular Ca^{2+}, pH, ATP, cyclic AMP or cyclic GMP which would indicate that they are probably not affected directly by chemostimuli. However, the channels were seen to be highly permeable to HCO_3^-, suggesting that they may play a role in regulating pH_i in type I cells, along with other pH_i-regulatory mechanisms (Buckler et al., 1991a). Regulation of pH_i in type I cells is central to the response of the carotid body to acidic / hypercapnic stimuli (Buckler et al., 1991b), and so it seems likely that HCO_3^- flux through these anion-selective channels is of importance in chemotransduction.

ROLES FOR IONIC CHANNELS IN HYPOXIC CHEMOTRANSDUCTION

Possible mechanisms by which hypoxia might elevate intracellular $[Ca^{2+}]$ levels in (and hence presumably trigger transmitter release from) type I cells are shown schematically in Figure 1. Of fundamental importance is the observation that hypoxia can inhibit K^+ channels, but exactly how this channel is regulated by PO_2 remains to be clarified. K^+ channel inhibition can occur directly (Ganfornina & Lopez-Barneo, 1992), but may also be influenced by the fact that hypoxia also elevates cAMP which can itself inhibit K^+ channels in these cells (Lopez-Lopez et al, 1993; also Wyatt & Peers, unpublished observations). In addition, hypoxic inhibition of K^+ channels in rabbit type I cells may involve a haem-like protein, since inhibition can be reversed by carbon monoxide (Lopez-Lopez & Gonzalez, 1992). In rat type I cells, the presence of a b-type cytochrome has been identified, and this haem can generate H_2O_2 (Cross et al., 1990). Inhibition of H_2O_2 formation also leads to reduced carotid sinus nerve discharge and the reduction of $NAD(P)^+$, leading the authors to suggest that an oxidase such as NAD(P)H oxidase may act as an oxygen sensor in these cells which may in turn regulate K^+ channels via changes in the redox state of mobile thiol groups (Cross et al., 1990).

As indicated earlier, the nature of this K^+ channel is different in adult rabbit cells (a voltage-gated, 4-aminopyridine sensitive channel; Lopez-Lopez et al, 1993) as compared with neonatal rat cells (a high- conductance, Ca^{2+}-activated K^+ channel; Peers, 1990b). If, as has been demonstrated in embryonic rabbit type I cells (Delpiano & Hescheler, 1989), K^+ channel activity is an important determinant of type I cell resting potential (maintaining a hyperpolarizing influence), then closure of this channel leads to cell depolarization. Whether or not depolarization triggers action potential generation or increases the frequency of spontaneous action potentials by increasing the depolarizing rate of a pacemaker potential (Lopez-Lopez et al., 1989), an increase in the open probability of voltage-gated (presumably L-type) Ca^{2+} channels will ensue, providing a pathway for Ca^{2+} influx into the type I cell, and hence will trigger transmitter release.

Figure 1 also illustrates an alternative mechanism by which hypoxia might lead to elevated $[Ca^{2+}]$ in the type I cell. In a series of reports, Biscoe and Duchen have provided evidence that a specialized mitochondrial electron transport accounts for type I cell chemosensitivity (Duchen & Biscoe, 1992a,b). These authors used microfluorimetric measurements to demonstrate that hypoxia can elevate intracellular $[Ca^{2+}]$ not by stimulating influx across the plasma membrane, but by causing its release primarily from mitochondrial stores (Biscoe & Duchen, 1990a,b); anoxia was seen to raise internal $[Ca^{2+}]$ even in the absence of extracellular Ca^{2+} (although to a lesser degree), and exposure of cells to the mitochondrial uncoupler FCCP, which itself raised intracellular $[Ca^{2+}]$, excluded the anoxic effect suggesting that FCCP and anoxia release Ca^{2+} from the same mitochondrial store (Biscoe & Duchen, 1990a,b).

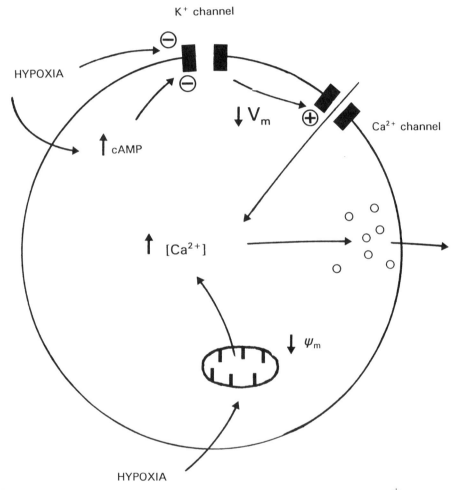

Figure 1. Mechanisms for hypoxic chemotransduction by the type I cell. Hypoxia inhibits K^+ channel activity. This can occur directly (or via a closely associated haem protein), but may also involve increased cyclic AMP levels (see text for further details). Closure of K^+ channels leads to cell membrane depolarization (reduced V_m) which in turn increases the activity of voltage-gated Ca^{2+} channels. This results in increased Ca^{2+} influx, triggering neurosecretion. Alternatively, hypoxia has been shown to release Ca^{2+} from mitochondrial stores, by reducing the mitochondrial membrane potential (ψ_m) which is normally required to sequester Ca^{2+}. Again, this would lead to a rise in cytosolic Ca^{2+} levels which would trigger transmitter release.

ROLES FOR IONIC CHANNELS IN TRANSDUCTION OF ACIDIC STIMULI

In rat type I cells, there is good evidence that acidic / hypercapnic stimuli elevate intracellular $[Ca^{2+}]$ via a mechanism involving K^+ and Ca^{2+} channels which appears at least superficially like the actions of hypoxia (Fig. 2). Reducing external pH, or selectively reducing internal pH using weak acid-containing solutions, inhibits Ca^{2+}-dependent K^+ channels in these cells without affecting Ca^{2+} channels (Peers, 1990a; Peers & Green, 1991). Furthermore, exposure of cells to hypercapnic or acidic solutions raises intracellular $[Ca^{2+}]$ (Buckler & Vaughan-Jones, 1993a,b), and this effect is blocked if cells are voltage-clamped at their resting potential (Buckler & Vaughan-Jones, 1993a), which raises the attractive possibility that the inhibition of K^+ channels depolarizes type I cells and consequently opens voltage-gated Ca^{2+} channels to allow Ca^{2+} influx and so transmitter release. Indeed, intracellularly acting protons have long been known to inhibit this class of K^+ channel (e.g. Cook et al., 1984).

For adult rabbit type I cells, a completely different mechanism has been proposed for transduction of acidic stimuli (Rocher et al., 1991). In brief, cytosolic acidification stimulates proton extrusion via Na^+-dependent exchangers in the plasma membrane, leading to accumulation of Na^+ inside type I cells. This rise in intracellular $[Na^+]$ is sufficient to reverse the action of the sodium-calcium exchanger, which normally operates to remove Ca^{2+} from the cytosol. Hence Ca^{2+} enters type I cells via this transporter (and not via voltage-dependent Ca^{2+} channels; Rocher et al., 1991; Obeso et al., 1992) to trigger transmitter release.

Thus the transduction mechanisms proposed to date for both hypoxic (Fig. 1) and acidic (Fig. 2) stimuli are contested. It remains to be determined whether the differing reports arise because the relative importance of ion channels, membrane transporters and intracellular Ca^{2+} stores vary according to the age or species of animals used for study, or whether there are differences in tissue isolation and culture procedures which may influence the behaviour of type I cells in different laboratories.

FUTURE DIRECTIONS

Despite the advances made in carotid body chemotransduction at the cellular level over the past five years, many perhaps unexpected problems have arisen and there is obviously a great deal of scope for further studies. Indeed, the ideas I have related here for both hypoxic and acidic chemotransduction in type I cells have been based on the central idea that a rise in intracellular $[Ca^{2+}]$ concentration is a prerequisite for elevated transmitter release. Although this does not seem unreasonable, it has been brought into question recently by a report from Donnelly & Kholwadwala (1992) which demonstrates that hypoxia *decreases* intracellular $[Ca^{2+}]$ in rat type I cells. There is a clear need to monitor simultaneously changes in $[Ca^{2+}]$, membrane potential and K^+ channel activity in order to examine the interrelationship of these variables and so determine the importance of ion channels in chemotransduction. Furthermore, we need to study the relationship between changes in $[Ca^{2+}]$ and transmitter release. A recent report by Donnelly (1993) has indicated that it is possible to monitor release of catecholamines from intact carotid bodies using the carbon-fibre electrochemical technique, and this methodology holds great promise for the real-time resolution of catecholamine release from isolated type I cells.

As indicated elsewhere (e.g. Fidone & Gonzalez, 1986; Fidone et al., 1990), numerous neurotransmitters other than catecholamines are present and active within the carotid body. These transmitters are not always located in the type I cell and their roles in chemotransduction await definitive description (again species variations have been apparent). Indeed, the roles of released catecholamines in transduction is still poorly defined. Furthermore, the importance of the other cellular elements of the carotid body await description. Nevertheless, the recent progress made in understanding the activity of ion channels (as well as membrane transporters and intracellular Ca^{2+} stores) in the type I cell

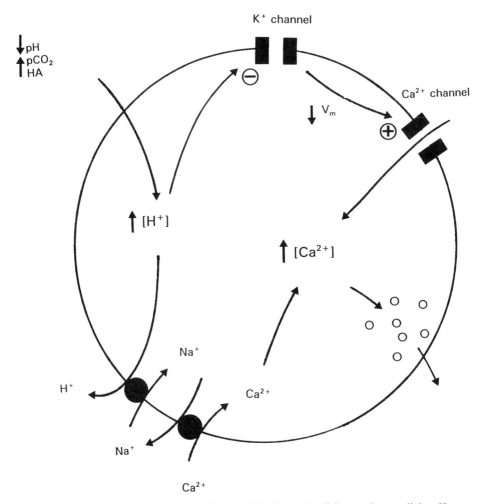

Figure 2. Mechanisms for transduction of acidic stimuli by the type I cell. Lowered extracellular pH, hypercapnia or application of weak acids (HA) leads to cytosolic acidification. The raised levels of intracellular protons can then inhibit the activity of K^+ channels. If these channels are important in determining resting cell membrane potential (V_m), channel inhibition will lead to depolarization. This will increase voltage-gated Ca^{2+} channel activity and lead to Ca^{2+} influx to trigger transmitter release. In adult rabbit type I cells (see text for further details) acidic stimuli have been shown to stimulate Na^+-dependent acid extrusion mechanisms (e.g. Na^+-H^+ exchange), leading to a rise in intracellular Na^+ levels. This rise in cytosolic Na^+ is sufficient to reverse the operation of the Na-Ca exchanger which normally operates to remove Ca^{2+} to the extracellular environment. Reversal of the exchanger leads to a rise of intracellular Ca^{2+} which triggers neurosecretion.

brings closer the possibility that we will be able to piece together the cellular elements of the carotid body and form a more complete, integrative understanding of this complex organ. Many of the findings reported here, including those to which I have contributed, were supported by The Wellcome Trust.

REFERENCES

Biscoe, T. J. & Duchen, M. R. (1989). Electrophysiological responses of dissociated type I cells of the rabbit carotid body to cyanide. J. Physiol. 413: 447-468.

Biscoe, T. J. & Duchen, M. R. (1990a). Responses of type I cells dissociated from the rabbit carotid body to hypoxia. J. Physiol. 428: 39-59.

Biscoe, T. J. & Duchen, M. R. (1990b). Monitoring pO_2 by the carotid chemoreceptor. News in Physiol. Sci. 5:229-233.

Buckler, K.J. & Vaughan-Jones, R.D. (1993a). Increasing pCO_2 raises $[Ca^{2+}]_i$ through voltage-gated Ca^{2+} entry in isolated carotid body glomus cells of the neonatal rat. J. Physiol. 459:272P.

Buckler, K.J. & Vaughan-Jones, R.D. (1993b). Effects of acidic stimuli on intracellular calcium in isolated type-I cells of the neonatal rat carotid body. Pflugers Archiv. (in press).

Buckler, K.J., Vaughan-Jones, R.D., Peers, C. & Nye, P. C. G. (1991a). Intracellular pH and its regulation in isolated type I carotid body cells of the neonatal rat. J. Physiol. 436:107-129.

Buckler, K.J., Vaughan-Jones, R.D., Peers, C. Lagadic-Gossmann, D. & Nye, P. C. G. (1991b). Effects of extracellular pH, pCO_2 and HCO_3^- on intracellular pH in isolated type-I cells of the neonatal rat carotid body. J. Physiol. 444:703-721.

Cook, D. L., Ikeuchi, M. & Fuyimoto, D. W. (1984). Lowering of pH inhibits Ca^{2+}-activated K^+ channels in pancreatic beta cells. Nature 311:269-271.

Cross, A. R., Henderson, L., Jones, O. T. G., Delpiano, M. A., Hentschel, J. & Acker, H. (1990). Involvement of an NAD(P)H oxidase as a pO_2 sensor protein in the rat carotid body. Biochem. J. 272:743-747.

Delpiano, M.A. & Acker, H. (1991). Hypoxia increases the cyclic AMP content of the cat carotid body in vitro. J. Neurochem. 57:291-297.

Delpiano, M.A. & Hescheler, J. (1989). Evidence for a pO_2-sensitive K^+ channel in the type-I cell of the rabbit carotid body. FEBS Lett. 249:195-198.

Donnelly, D. F. (1993). Electrochemical detection of catecholamine release from rat carotid body in vitro. J. Appl. Physiol. 74:2330-2337.

Donnelly, D. F. & Kholwadwala, D. (1992). Hypoxia decreases intracellular calcium in adult rat carotid body glomus cells. J. Neurophysiol. 67:1543-1551.

Duchen, M. R. & Biscoe, T. J. (1992a). Mitochondrial function in type I cells isolated from rabbit arterial chemoreceptors. J. Physiol. 450:13-31.

Duchen, M. R. & Biscoe, T. J. (1992b). Relative mitochondrial membrane potential and $[Ca^{2+}]_i$ in type I cells isolated from the rabbit carotid body. J. Physiol. 450:33-61.

Duchen, M. R., Caddy, K. W. T., Kirby, G. C., Patterson, D. L., Ponte, J. & Biscoe, T. J. (1988). Biophysical studies of the cellular elements of the rabbit carotid body. Neuroscience 26: 291-311.

Fidone, S. & Gonzalez, C. (1986). Initiation and control of chemoreceptor activity in the carotid body. In "The Respiratory System", Handbook of Physiology, N. S. Cherniack & J. G. Widdicombe, eds., Am Physiol. Soc., Bethesda, MD.

Fidone, S., Gonzalez, C., Obeso, A., Gomez-Nino, A. & Dinger, B. (1990). Biogenic amine and neuropeptide transmitters in carotid body chemotransmission: Experimental findings and perspectives. In "Hypoxia: The Adaptations" J. R. Sutton, G. Coattes & J. E. Remmers, eds., Marcel-Decker, London.

Fishman, M. C., Greene, W. L. & Platika, D. (1985). Oxygen chemoreception by carotid body cells in culture. Proc. Natl. Acad. Sci. USA 82:1448-1450.

Ganfornina, M. D. & Lopez-Barneo, J. (1991). Single K^+ channels in membrane patches of arterial chemoreceptor cells are modulated by O_2 tension. Proc. Natl. Acad. Sci. USA 88:2927-2930.

Ganfornina, M. D. & Lopez-Barneo, J. (1992). Potassium channel types in arterial chemoreceptor cells and their selective modulation by oxygen. J. Gen. Physiol. 100:401-426.

Gonzalez, C., Almarez, L., Obeso, A. & Rigual, R. (1992). Oxygen and acid chemoreception in the carotid body chemoreceptors. Trends in Neurosci. 15: 146-153.

Hamill, O. P., Marty, A., Neher, E., Sakmann, B. & Sigworth, F. J. (1981). Improved patch-clamp techniques for high resolution current recording from cells and cell-free membrane patches. Pflugers Archiv. 391:85-100.

Hescheler, J., Delpiano, M. A., Acker, H. & Pietruschka, F. (1989). Ionic currents on type-I cells of the rabbit carotid body measured by voltage-clamp experiments and the effect of hypoxia. Brain Res. 486:79-88.

Horn, R. & Marty, A. (1988). Muscarinic activation of ionic currents measured by a new whole-cell recording method. J. Gen. Physiol. 92:145-159.

Kholwadwala, D. & Donnelly, D.F. (1992). Maturation of carotid chemoreceptor sensitivity to hypoxia: in vitro studies in the newborn rat. J. Physiol. 453:461-474.

Llinas, R., Sugimori, M., Lin, J. W., & Chrksey, B., (1989). Blocking and isolation of a calcium channel from neurons in mammals and cephalopods utilizing a toxin fraction (FTX) from funnel-web spider poison. Proc. Natl. Acad. Sci. USA 86:1689-1693.

Lopez-Barneo, J., Lopez-Lopez, J.R., Urena, J. & Gonzalez, C. (1988). Chemotransduction in the carotid body: K^+ current modulation modulated by pO_2 in type I carotid body cells. Science 241:580-582.

Lopez-Lopez, J. & Gonzalez, C. (1992). Time course of K^+ current inhibition by low oxygen in chemoreceptor cells of adult rabbit carotid body. Effect of carbon monoxide. FEBS Lett. 299:251-254.

Lopez-Lopez, J., Gonzalez, C., Urena, J. & Lopez-Barneo, J. (1989). Low pO_2 selectively inhibits K channel activity in chemoreceptor cells of the mammalian carotid body. J. Gen. Physiol. 93:1001-1015.

Lopez-Lopez, J., De Luis, D. A. & Gonzalez, C. (1993). Properties of a transient K^+ current in chemoreceptor cells of rabbit carotid body. J. Physiol. 460:15-32.

Nowycky, M. C., Fox, A. P. & Tsien, R. W. (1985). Three types of neuronal calcium channel with different calcium agonist sensitivity. Nature 316:440-443.

Obeso, A., Fidone, S. & Gonzalez, C. (1987). Pathways for calcium entry into type I cells: significance for the secretory response. In "Chemoreceptors in Respiratory Control." J. A. Ribeiro & D. J. Pallot eds, Croom Helm, London.

Obeso, A., Rocher, A., Fidone, S. & Gonzalez, C. (1992). The role of dihydropyridine-sensitive Ca^{2+} channels in stimulus-evoked catecholamine release from chemoreceptor cells of the carotid body. Neuroscience 47:463-472.

Oyama, Y., Walker, J. L. & Eyzaguirre, C. (1986). The intracellular chloride activity of glomus cells in the isolated rabbit carotid body. Brain Res. 368:167-169.

38

Peers, C. (1990a). Selective effect of lowered extracellular pH on Ca^{2+}-dependent K^+ currents in type I cells isolated from the neonatal rat carotid body. J. Physiol. 422: 381-395.

Peers, C. (1990b). Hypoxic suppression of K^+ currents in type I carotid body cells: selective effect on the Ca^{2+}-activated K^+ current. Neurosci. Lett. 119:253-256.

Peers, C. (1990c). Effects of D600 on hypoxic suppression of K^+ currents in isolated type I carotid body cells of the neonatal rat. FEBS Lett. 271: 37-40.

Peers, C. (1991). Effects of doxapram on ionic currents in isolated type I cells of the neonatal rat. Brain Res. 568:116-122.

Peers, C. & Green, F.K. (1991). Intracellular acidosis inhibits Ca^{2+}-activated K^+ currents in isolated type I cells of the neonatal rat carotid body. J. Physiol. 437:589-602.

Peers, C. & O'Donnell, J. (1990). Potassium currents recorded in type I carotid body cells isolated from the neontal rat and their modulation by chemoexcitatory agents. Brain Res. 522:259-266.

Perez-Garcia, M. T., Almaraz, L. & Gonzalez, C. (1991). Cyclic AMP modulates differentially the release of dopamine induced by hypoxia and other stimuli and increases dopamine synthesis in the rabbit carotid body. J. Neurochem. 57:1992-2000.

Pietruschka, F. (1985). Calcium influx in cultured carotid body cells is stimulated by acetylcholine and hypoxia. Brain Res. 347:140-143.

Rigual, R., Gonzalez, E., Fidone, S. & Gonzalez, C. (1984). Effects of low pH on synthesis and release of catecholamines in the cat carotid body in vitro. Brain Res. 309:178-181.

Rocher, A., Obeso, A., Gonzalez, C. & Herreros, B. (1991). Ionic mechanisms for the transduction of acidic stimuli in rabbit carotid body glomus cells. J. Physiol. 433:533-548.

Rudy, B. (1988). Diversity and ubiquity of K channels. Neurosci. 25:729-749.

Sato, M., Ikeda, K., Yoshizaki, K. & Koyano, H. (1991). Response of cytosolic calcium to anoxia and cyanide in cultured glomus cells of newborn rabbit carotid body. Brain Res. 551: 327-330.

Shaw, K., Montague, W. & Pallot, D. J. (1989). Biochemical studies on the release of catecholamines from the rat carotid body in vitro. Biochim. Biophys. Acta 1013:42-46.

Shirahata, M. & Fitzgerald, R. S. (1991). Dependency of hypoxic chemotransduction in cat carotid body on voltage-gated calcium channels. J. Appl. Physiol. 71:1062-1069.

Stea, A., Alexander, S. A. & Nurse, C. A. (1991). Effects of pH_i and pH_e on membrane currents recorded with the perforated-patch method from cultured chemoreceptors of the rat carotid body. Brain Res. 567:83-90.

Stea, A., Jackson, A. & Nurse, C. A. (1992). Hypoxia and $N^6,O^{2'}$-dibutyryladenosine 3',5'-cyclic monophosphate, but not nerve growth factor, induce Na^+ channels and hypertrophy in chromaffin-like arterial chemoreceptors. Proc. Natl. Acad. Sci. USA 89:9469-9473.

Stea, A. & Nurse, C. A. (1989). Chloride channels in cultured glomus cells of the rat carotid body. Am. J. Physiol. 257:C174-C181.

Stea, A. & Nurse, C. A. (1991a). Whole-cell and perforated-patch recordings from O_2-sensitive rat carotid body cells grown in short- and long-term culture. Pflugers Arch. 418:93-101.

Stea, A. & Nurse, C. A. (1991b). Contrasting effects of HEPES vs HCO$_3$--buffered media on whole-cell currents in cultured chemoreceptors of the rat carotid body. Neurosci. Lett. 132:239-242.

Swandulla, D., Carbone, E. & Lux, H. D. (1991). Do calcium channel classifications account for neuronal calcium channel diversity? Trends in Neurosci. 14:46-51.

Tsien, R. W., Lipscombe, D., Madison, D. V., Bley, K. R. & Fox, A.P. (1988). Multiple types of neuronal calcium channels and their selective modulation. Trends in Neurosci. 11:431-438.

Urena, J., Lopez-Lopez, J., Gonzalez, C. & Lopez-Barneo, J. (1989). Ionic currents in dispersed chemoreceptor cells of the mammalian carotid body. J. Gen. Physiol. 93:979-999.

Wang, W.-J., Cheng, G.-F., Yoshizaki, K., Dinger, B. & Fidone, S. (1991). The role of cyclic AMP in chemoreception in the rabbit carotid body. Brain Res. 540:96-104.

Wyatt, C.N. & Peers, C. (1992). Modulation of ionic currents in isolated type I cells of the neonatal rat carotid body by p-chloromercuribenzenesulfonic acid. Brain Res. 591:341-344.

Wyatt, C.N. & Peers, C. (1993). Actions of doxapram on Ca^{2+}-activated K^{+} channels from isolated type I carotid body cells of the neonatal rat. Br. J. Pharmacol. (in press).

ROLE OF INTRACELLULAR pH AND $[Ca^{2+}]_i$ IN ACID CHEMORECEPTION IN TYPE-I CELLS OF THE CAROTID BODY

Keith J. Buckler and Richard D. Vaughan-Jones

University Laboratory of Physiology
Parks Road
Oxford, OX1 3PT

INTRODUCTION

Early theories of acid chemotransduction proposed that a fall in blood pH or rise in PCO_2 excited afferent discharge from the carotid body through a direct action of extracellular pH upon the type-I cell or upon the nerve ending. This hypothesis was later amended to propose that the site of chemoreception was an intracellular one (Hanson et al., 1981). The shift in the proposed site of chemotransduction was based upon the key observation that the rate at which afferent discharge increased in response to a respiratory acidosis was dramatically slowed by membrane permeant carbonic anhydrase inhibitors (but not by impermeant ones). This suggested that the hydration of CO_2 intracellularly to yield H^+_i and $HCO_3^-_i$ was an important step in transduction. Torrance and colleagues (Hanson et al., 1981) also noted an interesting correlation between the transient effects of isohydric hypercapnia upon chemoreceptor discharge and the transient effects of this manoeuvre upon pH_i in snail neurones. The similarities in behaviour between these two different systems led to the proposal that it was changes in pH_i which drove the chemoreceptor response. These authors further speculated that a fall of pH_i in the type-I cell might cause a rise in $[Ca^{2+}]_i$ which would promote neurosecretion from the type-I cell, thus stimulating the nerve ending. It is now generally accepted that the type-I cell is the primary transducing element. Indeed acidic stimuli (as well as hypoxia) promote neurosecretion from the cell (Rigual et al., 1986). This chapter reviews the results of recent experiments into the regulation of pH_i and the effects of acidic stimuli upon pH_i, $[Ca^{2+}]_i$ and electrical excitability in type-I cells. There is much new evidence to support Torrance's original hypothesis and we present a model which delineates certain steps in the acid transduction pathway from a fall in pH_i through to a rise in $[Ca^{2+}]_i$.

pH-REGULATION IN TYPE-I CELLS

Despite the obvious potential importance of intracellular pH-regulation to sensory transduction in the type-I cell, such regulation has only recently been studied. This has undoubtedly been due to technical difficulties. The use of pH-sensitive microelectrodes in the small type-I cell although possible (He et al., 1991), is extremely difficult and not

Arterial Chemoreceptors: Cell to System
Edited by R. O'Regan *et al*, Plenum Press, New York, 1994

without considerable risk of cell injury. It is therefore only with the advent of fluorescent pH-sensitive indicators which can be easily introduced into cells, that much of the work on pH-regulation in the type-I cell has been possible. The two indicators most commonly used are BCECF and carboxy-SNARF-1. These indicators can be readily introduced into cells by incubation with the membrane permeant acxtoxy-methyl ester form of the indicator. Once inside the cell the ester bonds are hydrolysed by cellular esterases thereby releasing the native pH-sensitive indicator. Intracellular pH can then be determined from the fluorescence of the intracellularly trapped indicator which is measured in a microspectrofluorimeter. This technique allows the non-destructive investigation, at the single cell level, of pH_i-regulation and its response to chemostimuli (see e.g. Buckler & Vaughan-Jones, 1990).

Resting pH_i in type-I cells

In physiological salines (i.e. those containing HCO_3^- and CO_2) most estimates of resting pH_i for rat type-I cells are in the region of 7.2 to 7.3 (Buckler et al., 1991a; Wilding et al., 1992); these values are typical of a great many mammalian cells. In the absence of CO_2/HCO_3^-, however, the pH_i may be very different with values of 6.9 reported for acutely isolated rabbit type-I cells (Biscoe et al., 1989) and up to 7.8 for short term cultured (24 hr)

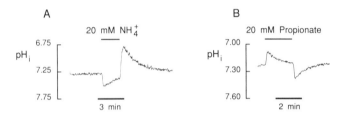

Figure 1. pH_i-regulation in Type-I cells (pH_i was measured using carboxy-SNARF-1). i) Acid-recovery, type-I cells were acidified by **A**) the NH_4^+-prepulse technique (see Roos & Boron, 1981), and **B**) the addition of a weak acid, weak acids rapidly diffuse across biological membranes and once inside the cell dissociate releasing H^+. After this initial acidification there follows a period of net acid extrusion from the cell, returning pH_i to the resting level. ii) Alkaline-recovery, the removal of propionate causes a rapid cellular alkalinization (due to the efflux of propionate as propionic acid). This alkalinization is followed by a net alkali extrusion as pH_i again returns to the control level.

neonatal rat type-I cells (Buckler et al., 1991a). The reasons for these differences are unknown but the observations should serve as a caution against the use of HCO_3^--free media in studies of chemoreceptor function.

The ability of these cells to regulate pH_i can readily be demonstrated. The imposition of an intracellular acid load, either by the ammonium chloride prepulse technique or by the addition of a membrane permeant weak acid, is swiftly met by the activation of mechanisms which effect net extrusion of the excess acid from the cell. Similarly the imposition of an intracellular alkaline load is met by the activation of net alkali extrusion from the cell (see Fig. 1).

What are the mechanisms responsible for this pH_i-regulation? At present there are only a few studies of pH_i-regulation in the type-I cell so that what follows is a combination of what has been established in type-I cells and what can be surmised from studies of pH_i-regulation in other tissues. In general pH_i is regulated through a number of ion transport mechanisms which are designed to remove acid or alkali (or their ionic equivalent e.g. HCO_3^-) from the cell. In the type-I cell there appear to be at least two mechanisms which are capable of pumping acid out of the cell. These mechanisms are the Na^+/H^+-exchanger and a Na^+-HCO_3^--dependent process.

42

Na$^+$/H$^+$-Exchange

The first pH$_i$-regulatory mechanism to be described in the type-I cell was the Na$^+$/H$^+$-exchanger (identified by its amiloride sensitivity and dependence upon Na^+_o; Buckler & Vaughan-Jones, 1990; Buckler et al., 1991a; Wilding et al., 1992). There are now known to be at least 4 different isoforms of the Na$^+$/H$^+$ exchanger expressed in various mammalian cells (Counillon & Pouyssegur, 1993). Although it is not yet known which of these isoforms are expressed in the type-I cell, NHE-1 so far seems to be ubiquitous to all cells studied. Na$^+$/H$^+$-exchangers mediate an electroneutral (1:1) exchange of internal protons for external Na$^+$ (Aronson, 1985), the driving force for the expulsion of protons being provided by the sodium chemical gradient.

In keeping with its role as a pH$_i$-regulatory mechanism, the activity of Na$^+$/H$^+$-exchange is pH$_i$-sensitive. In the type-I cell, a fall of pH$_i$ markedly enhances Na$^+$/H$^+$-exchange-mediated acid extrusion (Buckler et al., 1991a). Regulation of exchanger activity by pH$_i$, in some cells, displays steep sigmoidal kinetics which suggests that exchange activity is not modulated simply by substrate availability (ie H$^+$) but that there are also regulatory binding sites for protons (e.g. Aronson et al., 1982).

In addition to being modulated by changes in internal pH, Na$^+$/H$^+$-exchange activity in many other cell types is also sensitive to changes in external pH. Changes in external pH however have opposite effects to those of internal pH, i.e. extracellular acidity <u>inhibits</u> the exchanger whereas intracellular acidity <u>stimulates</u> the exchanger (see e.g. Aronson, 1985; Vaughan-Jones & Wu 1990). The importance of this modulation of Na$^+$/H$^+$-exchange by both internal and external pH will be dealt with later.

Na$^+$-HCO$_3^-$-dependent acid efflux

The second mechanism involved in acid extrusion from the type-I cell is dependent upon both Na$^+$ and HCO$_3^-$ (Buckler et al., 1991a). The precise nature of this transporter is unknown, but it is thought to mediate a co-influx of Na$^+$ and HCO$_3^-$ into the cell. This HCO$_3^-$-influx is equivalent to a H$^+$-efflux in its effect on pH$_i$. In common with Na$^+$/H$^+$-exchange, HCO$_3^-$-dependent acid extrusion in the type-I cell is also activated by a fall in pH$_i$ (Richmond & Vaughan-Jones, personal communication). The possible involvement of other ions such as Cl$^-$ in this transport process and the question as to whether the carrier is electrogenic have yet to be addressed. The relative importance of the two acid extruders (Na$^+$/H$^+$-exchange and Na$^+$-HCO$_3^-$-influx) in controlling pH$_i$ in the type-I cell also remains to be determined but initial estimates suggest that they contribute about equally to acid extrusion following an acid load (Buckler et al., 1991a; Richmond & Vaughan-Jones, personal communication).

The precise control of pH$_i$ under a variety of acidifying and alkalinising influences requires more than just acid extruders, mechanisms which can bring acid or its equivalent into the cell are also required. The study of alkaline-regulation in general has not been as extensive as acid regulation. There are nevertheless a number of mechanisms which are believed to participate in alkaline regulation. In the type-I cell three potential mechanisms have been identified.

Cl$^-$/HCO$_3^-$-Exchange

The presence of Na$^+$-independent, DIDS-sensitive, Cl$^-$/HCO$_3^-$-exchange has been identified in the neonatal rat type-I cell (Buckler et al., 1991a). The exchange mechanism is probably similar to that found in many other mammalian cells, where at least 3 genes for anion exchangers have been found (for review see Alper, 1991). Anion exchangers mediate a tightly coupled electroneutral 1:1 exchange of Cl$^-$ for HCO$_3^-$. Unless [Cl$^-$]$_i$ is exceptionally high (or pH$_i$ exceptionally low) the normal mode of action is a net exchange of external Cl$^-$ for internal HCO$_3^-$ ie. this mechanism serves as an acid loader. In other tissues, the activity of anion exchange is known to be pH$_i$ dependent, it is activated by alkalosis (see e.g. Alper,

1991). It is important to note that the effects of pH_i upon the alkali extruding (HCO_3^--efflux) Cl^--HCO_3^- exchange are opposite to its effects upon Na^+/H^+-exchange or Na^+-HCO_3^--cotransport. Thus the acid extruders and the anion exchange complement each other, with acid extrusion being switched on by intracellular acidity and alkali extrusion by intracellular alkalinity.

Anion Channels

An anion permeable channel has been identified in inside-out membrane patches from cultured rat type-I cells (Stea & Nurse, 1989). This channel is insensitive to voltage, calcium and pH but has a large unitary conductance (296 pS) and is very permeant to HCO_3^- as well as Cl^- ($PHCO_3/PCl =0.7$). Assuming that the resting membrane potential of the type-I cell is around -50 mV such a channel would permit a net efflux of HCO_3^- and could therefore be a major route for acid-equivalent entry into the cell. Although this channel is pH_i-insensitive it could still play an important role in pH_i regulation and not just as a constant background acid leak since the magnitude of the net HCO_3^--flux may vary with the transmembrane HCO_3^--gradient (= pH gradient). The presence of such an acidifying HCO_3^- leak from the type-I cell and its role in pH_i-regulation remains to be formally demonstrated however.

K^+/H^+-Exchange

The presence of a K^+/H^+ exchanger has been suggested in the adult rat type-I cell (Wilding et al., 1992). The detailed properties of this exchanger have not yet been characterised but it seems to be electroneutral. Given a reasonably high intracellular K^+-concentration this mechanism would be expected to catalyse the net exchange of intracellular K^+ for extracellular H^+ ie. it would function as an acid-influx (alkali-efflux) pathway. Similar mechanisms have recently been reported in a number of other tissues (e.g. Bonanno, 1991). Caution in accepting this as a new pH-regulatory system is, however, advised. In the neonatal rat type-I cell, endogenous K^+/H^+ exchange seems to be absent (Richmond & Vaughan-Jones, 1993). More importantly, it has been observed that in this cell type (and presumably others) that K^+/H^+-exchange activity is easily introduced *in situ* via contamination with the K^+/H^+-ionophore nigericin (Richmond & Vaughan-Jones, 1993). Nigericin is used extensively for the calibration of pH-sensitive fluoroprobes and it is difficult to remove all traces of nigericin from superfusion systems. The K^+/H^+-exchange identified in the type-I cell may therefore be an experimental artefact arising from nigericin contamination.

Cytoplasmic H^+-buffering

In addition to the above transport processes, which both set and correct resting pH_i through the controlled efflux and influx of acid or HCO_3^-, major excursions in pH_i, in response to acidifying or alkalinising influences, are also opposed by the cells buffering capacity. Type-I cells possess an intrinsic buffering capacity (as do all cells) due, for example, to H^+ binding sites on intracellular proteins. This intrinsic buffering is supplemented by CO_2/HCO_3^--dependent buffering. Given an open system for CO_2 (ie. where PCO_2 is maintained constant), intracellular CO_2/HCO_3^--buffering capacity is optimal and is given by the simple relation βCO_2 (mMoles/pH) $= 2.3[HCO_3^-]_i$. At a pH_i of 7.2 and in the presence of 5% CO_2 the CO_2/HCO_3^--buffering capacity amounts to about 31 mMoles/pH, whereas the intrinsic buffering capacity is about 12 mMoles/pH. The contribution of CO_2/HCO_3^--dependent buffering to total cellular buffering capacity is therefore substantial. It is worth noting, however, that the CO_2/HCO_3^--buffering system cannot protect against changes in pH_i which result from changes in PCO_2.

In summary the type-I cell possesses a number of mechanisms which, under normal conditions, serve to maintain the pH of the intracellular environment more or less constant.

EFFECTS OF ACIDIC STIMULI ON TYPE-I CELL pH_i

In view of the apparent ability of the type-I cell to clamp its pH_i to a predetermined level, one might question whether pH_i can have any role in acid-chemotransduction. Fortunately, whilst the type-I cell is able to defend pH_i against internal acid/base challenges, the steady state level for pH_i is sensitive to changes in pH_o (Buckler et al., 1990; Buckler et al., 1991b; He et al., 1991; Wilding et al., 1992). This is true irrespective of whether pH_o is changed by varying PCO_2 or by varying $[HCO_3^-]_o$ (Buckler et al., 1991b) or even when pH_o is varied in a nominally CO_2/HCO_3^--free medium (Wilding et al., 1992). This dependence of steady state pH_i upon extracellular pH is not exclusive to the type-I cell. In most cells studied, lowering pH_o lowers pH_i and raising pH_o raises pH_i. What is unusual about the type-I cell is the *sensitivity* of pH_i to changes in pH_o. In many other cell types, e.g. nerve (Tolkovsky & Richards, 1987), mammalian skeletal muscle (Aickin & Thomas, 1977), heart muscle (Ellis & Thomas, 1976; Vaughan-Jones 1986), and some smooth muscles (Aickin, 1984) steady state pH_i only changes by some 30% of the change in pH_o. In rat type-I cells the figure is between 65 and 82% (Buckler et al., 1991b; Wilding et al., 1992) ie. a fall in pH_o of 0.2 would cause a fall in steady state pH_i of up to 0.16 (NB. the relationship between pH_i and pH_o in the type-I cell is approximately linear over a wide range of pH_o). Although such an extreme sensitivity to changes in pH_o is not unique (some smooth muscles are similarly sensitive see Austin & Wray, 1993) it does suggest a functional specialisation of pH_i-regulation in the type-I cell.

How is this pH_o-sensitivity brought about? The simple answer is we don't yet know, but the known dependency of Na^+/H^+-exchange upon both pH_o and pH_i (see above) may provide a clue. Consider the situation in which the normal resting pH_i results from a balance between a fixed acid leak into the cell and an acid efflux mediated by Na^+/H^+-exchange. If pH_o is suddenly lowered, this will inhibit Na^+/H^+-exchange leading to an initial imbalance between acid influx and efflux, so that the cell will acidify. As pH_i falls it progressively reactivates Na^+/H^+-exchange. Eventually a pH_i is reached at which Na^+/H^+-exchange activity balances acid influx, and pH_i although now lower, is stable. In the cardiac Purkinje fibre this effect of pH_o upon Na^+/H^+-exchange appears to be sufficient to account for the modest dependence of pH_i upon pH_o (Vaughan-Jones & Wu, 1991). To account for the relationship in the type-I cell, however, either the Na^+/H^+ exchanger must be even more sensitive to pH_o or other acid/alkali transport systems must also be modulated by pH_o. The explanation of the steep pH_i/pH_o relationship in the type-I cell may therefore lie in the effects of both pH_i and pH_o upon the kinetics of the acid-equivalent transport systems in the surface membrane. A definitive explanation must await a detailed characterisation of the kinetics of all the pH-regulatory mechanisms in type-I cells.

DOES pH_i PLAY A ROLE IN TRANSDUCTION?

Having established that changes in extracellular pH cause large changes in intracellular pH in the type-I cell, what is the evidence that pH_i plays a role in chemotransduction? There are three lines of evidence.

(**1**) It was established by Torrance that membrane-permeant carbonic anhydrase inhibitors can substantially slow the speed of the chemoreceptor's response to a respiratory acidosis (Hanson et al., 1981). It has also been shown more recently that acetazolamide substantially slows the rate of intracellular acidification in type-I cells following a sudden increase in PCO_2 (Buckler et al., 1991a). This implies that the hydration of CO_2 and subsequent production of H^+ plays an important role in the transduction of a respiratory acidosis.

(**2**) Gray (1968) has shown that the chemoreceptor is responsive to a variety of acidic stimuli ie. a hypercapnic acidosis, an isocapnic acidosis and an isohydric hypercapnia. These stimuli are associated with changes of pH, $[HCO_3^-]$ and CO_2. However, as shown in Table

1, the only *common* feature of these stimuli is a *decrease of pH$_i$* (see also Figure 2), no other single factor changes consistently with all three acidic stimuli.

(3) There are some interesting correlations between the detailed nature of the effects of the above acid-stimuli upon both chemoreceptor discharge and type-I cell pH$_i$ (see Buckler et al., 1991b). The most significant of these is that, whereas both a hypercapnic and an isocapnic acidosis cause a sustained fall in pH$_i$ and a sustained increase in chemoreceptor activity, an isohydric hypercapnia only induces *transient* changes in pH$_i$ (Fig. 2 and Buckler et al., 1991b) and discharge (Gray, 1968). In other words the chemoreceptor response is maintained only if the fall in pH$_i$ is also maintained.

Table 1. Relative changes of pH, [HCO$_3^-$] and PCO$_2$ during acidic-stimulation of the type-I cell.

	Hypercapnic Acidosis	Isocapnic Acidosis	Isohydric Hypercapnia
pH$_O$	Decrease	Decrease	No change
PCO$_2$	Increase	No change	Increase
[HCO$_3^-$]$_O$	No change	Decrease	Increase
[HCO$_3^-$]$_i$	Increase	Decrease	Increase
pH$_i$	**Decrease**	**Decrease**	**Decrease**

The above considerations all make a powerful case for a central role of pH$_i$ in acid chemotransduction and provide considerable support for much of Torrance's original hypothesis (Hanson et al., 1981). There are, however, some differences. Firstly, in his original hypothesis, Torrance suggested that the processes of cellular pH$_i$-regulation might account for the adaptation of the response to a respiratory acidosis. From what evidence is available, it would seem that in simple HCO$_3^-$-buffered solutions the type-I cell responds to all but the most severe of hypercapnic acidoses with a monophasic decline in pH$_i$ (see Fig. 2 & Buckler et al., 1991b) yet neural discharge from the isolated carotid body when exposed to similar stimuli shows a clear adaptation (Iturriaga & Lahiri, 1991). One possibility is that the rapid adaptation of the response seen with a respiratory or a hypercapnic acidosis, results from processes that occur subsequent to the fall in pH$_i$ (we return to this point later). Secondly, Torrance proposed that hypoxic stimuli might also be transduced through changes of pH$_i$ produced via the inhibition of pH$_i$-regulatory mechanisms. Whilst hypoxia can inhibit some cellular pH$_i$-regulatory systems (Fonteriz et al., 1993), all the available data indicates that hypoxia induces only a very small or no change in type-I cell pH$_i$ (Buckler, Richmond & Vaughan-Jones, unpublished; Wilding et al., 1992). Hypoxic chemotransduction must therefore proceed via other pathways and will not be considered further in this chapter.

ROLE OF [Ca^{2+}]$_i$ IN ACID CHEMOTRANSDUCTION

If a fall in pH$_i$ in the type-I cell is the initial event in the acid-chemoreception pathway, how does this lead to the excitation of afferent nerve fibres? The most likely explanation is that intracellular acidosis promotes the release of neurotransmitter substances from the type-I which then excite the sensory nerve endings. In support of this hypothesis, the secretion of catecholamines from type-I cells is stimulated by acidosis (Rigual et al., 1991) and hypoxia (Rigual et al., 1986; Fidone et al., 1982) and this secretion correlates closely with an increase of chemoreceptor discharge. What promotes this neurosecretion? One could hypothesise that the fall of pH$_i$ acts directly upon the exocytotic machinery to increase vesicular transmitter release. However the observation that acid-induced neurosecretion is dependent upon extracellular Ca^{2+} (Rocher et al., 1991) suggests a prominent role for intracellular Ca^{2+} in mediating the secretory response.

The most likely scenario for transduction is therefore that a fall in pH_i induces a rise of $[Ca^{2+}]_i$ which then triggers neurosecretion. Two previous studies however have either found that acidosis decreases type-I cell $[Ca^{2+}]_i$ (Donnelly & Kholwadwala, 1992) or that it only increases $[Ca^{2+}]_i$ under hypoxic conditions (Biscoe & Duchen, 1990).

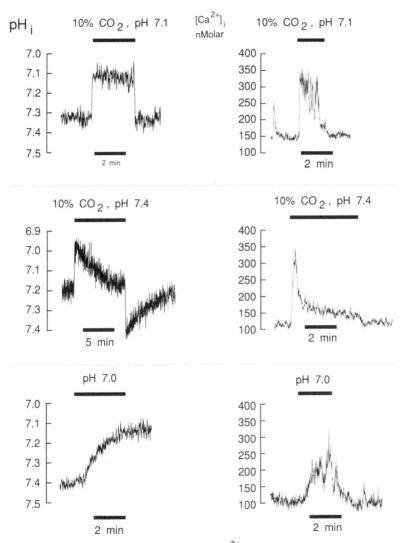

Figure 2. Effects of various acidic stimuli upon pH_i and $[Ca^{2+}]_i$ in type-I cells. **Left:** pH_i measured using carboxy-SNARF-1. **Right:** $[Ca^{2+}]_i$, measured with Indo-I (NB all recordings from different type-I cell clusters). **Top row:** effects of a hypercapnic acidosis (an increase in CO_2 from 5% to 10% at constant $[HCO_3^-]_o$). **Middle row:** effects of an isohydric hypercapnia (an increase in CO_2 from 5% to 10% at constant pH_o, $[HCO_3^-]_o$ increased from 23 to 46 mM). **Bottom row:** effects of an isocapnic acidosis (decrease in $[HCO_3^-]_o$ from 23 to 8.1 mM). Note that i) all manoeuvres lower pH_i and raise $[Ca^{2+}]_i$, ii) the effects of hypercapnia (top & middle) are more rapid in onset than that of an isocapnic acidosis (bottom), iii) the response to a isohydric hypercapnia is mostly transient (both pH_i and $[Ca^{2+}]_i$).

Effects of acidic stimuli on $[Ca^{2+}]_i$

More recently we have re-investigated the effects of a number of acidic stimuli upon $[Ca^{2+}]_i$ in type-I cells from the neonatal rat (Buckler & Vaughan-Jones, 1993). We found that all three of the acidic stimuli described above (i.e. a hypercapnic acidosis, isocapnic acidosis and an isohydric hypercapnia) raise $[Ca^{2+}]_i$ (see Figure 2). In single isolated cells, the rise of $[Ca^{2+}]_i$ consisted of an increase in the mean frequency and size of repetitive $[Ca^{2+}]_i$ fluctuations. In cell clusters, however, although fluctuations of $[Ca^{2+}]_i$ were still evident they were to some degree fused forming a more smooth $[Ca^{2+}]_i$ response (e.g. Fig 2). There are at least two possible reasons for theses differences between recordings form individual cells verses clumps: (i) the recordings obtained from clusters may represent the averaging out of asynchronous $[Ca^{2+}]_i$ fluctuations in individual uncoupled cells within the cluster and (ii) if there is cell-to-cell coupling within a cluster, this may somehow cause a decrease in $[Ca^{2+}]_i$ fluctuations in individual cells in favour of a more tonic, co-ordinated $[Ca^{2+}]_i$ response. It was also observed that not all single type-I cells respond to acidic stimuli, whereas almost all clusters do. The reason for this is unknown but it is possible that different cells have different thresholds of responsiveness.

Taken as a whole, these results (see Buckler & Vaughan-Jones, 1993) provide compelling evidence that acidic stimuli elevate $[Ca^{2+}]_i$ in type-I cells of the carotid body.

Correlations between the $[Ca^{2+}]_i$ signal in the type-I cell and chemoreceptor discharge

It was notable, both in recordings from cell clusters (e.g. Fig. 2) and in the averages of a number of recordings (Buckler & Vaughan-Jones, 1993), that the $[Ca^{2+}]_i$ response to each stimulus had a characteristic pattern. The averaged $[Ca^{2+}]_i$ response to a hypercapnic acidosis was biphasic, displaying a rapid initial rise in $[Ca^{2+}]_i$ followed by a secondary exponential decline towards a plateau level. The averaged $[Ca^{2+}]_i$ response to an isohydric hypercapnia was similarly biphasic with a rapid initial rise, but followed by a more pronounced secondary decline in which $[Ca^{2+}]_i$ approached the previous control level i.e. there was little or no sustained elevation of $[Ca^{2+}]_i$. Finally the averaged $[Ca^{2+}]_i$ response to an isocapnic acidosis displayed a slower initial rise with little secondary decline.

These patterns of response bear a striking resemblance to the effects of these same three acidic stimuli upon chemoreceptor discharge in that (i) the initial response to hypercapnia is more rapid than that to an isocapnic acidosis (Gray, 1968), (ii) the response to both a hypercapnic acidosis (Black et al., 1971) and an isohydric hypercapnia (Gray, 1968) display marked adaptation and (iii) the response to an isohydric hypercapnia is mostly transient with little or no sustained increase in discharge (Gray, 1968). The nature of the rise of type-I cell $[Ca^{2+}]_i$ seen in response to all three types of acidic stimulus (hypercapnic acidosis, isohydric hypercapnia and isocapnic acidosis) is therefore consistent with a central role for type-I cell $[Ca^{2+}]_i$ in acid chemotransduction.

Role of $[Ca^{2+}]_i$ in sensory adaptation

A characteristic feature of the carotid body's afferent discharge in response to a respiratory acidosis is the rapid and marked adaptation that occurs (Black et al., 1971). Although the cause of this adaptation is unknown and likely to be complex, the biphasic $[Ca^{2+}]_i$ response seen with a hypercapnic acidosis may well provide at least part of the explanation. Although there is some disparity between the time course for the decline of the $[Ca^{2+}]_i$ signal ($t_{1/2}$=24s, Buckler & Vaughan-Jones, 1993) and the rate of adaptation of afferent discharge ($t_{1/2}$=5-10 s, Black et al., 1971), this is to be expected since (a) only the average whole cell $[Ca^{2+}]_i$ was measured whereas $[Ca^{2+}]$ at the sites of exocytosis are what govern secretion and (b) the relationship between $[Ca^{2+}]_i$ and secretion is unlikely to be first order. A decline in the intensity of the $[Ca^{2+}]_i$ signal to neurosecretion is therefore a plausible part explanation of sensory adaptation in this tissue. What is the cause of the secondary decline of $[Ca^{2+}]_i$? Since we have previously noted that, in simple HCO_3^--buffered solutions, the changes in type-I cell pH_i are mostly monophasic, it must result from the events coupling changes in pH_i to $[Ca^{2+}]_i$.

THE COUPLING OF CHANGES IN pH_i TO CHANGES IN $[Ca^{2+}]_i$

As described above, it is likely that the increase in $[Ca^{2+}]_i$ during acid-stimulation is triggered by a fall in pH_i. How is this coupling achieved? One could envisage a number of possibilities e.g. (i) displacement from internal binding sites, (ii) release from internal stores or (iii) influx from the external medium.

Evidence for Ca^{2+}-influx

A role for Ca^{2+}-influx in acid chemotransduction is suggested by the observations that the increase in catecholamine secretion, in response to acidic stimuli, is dependent upon the presence of extracellular Ca^{2+} (Rocher et al., 1991). This hypothesis is also supported by the following observations. In neonatal rat type-I cells, the rise in $[Ca^{2+}]_i$ induced by a hypercapnic acidosis is abolished in Ca^{2+}_o-free media, and substantially inhibited by 2mM Ni^{2+} (Fig. 3; Buckler & Vaughan-Jones, 1993; Buckler & Vaughan-Jones, 1994: NB 2mM Ni^{2+} will inhibit both voltage activated Ca^{2+}-channels and Na^+/Ca^{2+}-exchange). A hypercapnic acidosis also dramatically increases the permeability of type-I cells to Mn^{2+} (Buckler & Vaughan-Jones, 1994). As many Ca^{2+}-channels, including voltage operated Ca^{2+}-channels, are permeable to Mn^{2+}, the increase in Mn^{2+} permeability suggests an increase in Ca^{2+}-channel opening. Together, these data argue convincingly that the rise of $[Ca^{2+}]_i$ during acidic stimulation of the type-I cell results from Ca^{2+}-entry from the external medium.

Cause of Ca^{2+}-influx

Two mechanisms linking a fall in pH_i to a rise in $[Ca^{2+}]_i$ have been proposed, one (the Na^+-Ca^{2+}-exchange hypothesis) is based on measurements of catecholamine secretion in the rabbit type-I cell and the other (the membrane potential hypothesis) is based on direct Ca^{2+} and electrophysiological measurements made in the rat type-I cell. The Na^+-Ca^{2+}-exchange hypothesis (Rocher et al., 1991) has been reviewed recently (Gonzalez et al., 1992). In brief, the following steps are proposed to lead to the rise of $[Ca^{2+}]_i$; (i) acid stimuli induce a fall in pH_i which activates Na^+-dependent acid extrusion mechanisms (i.e. Na^+/H^+-exchange and $Na^+-HCO_3^-$-co-influx), (ii) the resultant increase in Na^+-influx raises $[Na^+]_i$, and (iii) the rise in $[Na^+]_i$ promotes reverse mode Na^+/Ca^{2+}-exchange which brings Ca^{2+} into the cell.

The basic concepts of the membrane potential hypothesis is that acidic stimuli inhibit K^+-channels in type-I cells which leads to membrane depolarisation and Ca^{2+}-entry through voltage activated Ca^{2+}-channels (Peers, 1990; Peers & Green, 1991; Stea et al., 1991). Evidence that K^+-channels in type-I cells are inhibited by acidic stimuli has come from a number of laboratories (Lopez-Lopez et al., 1989; Peers, 1990; Stea et al., 1991). In the rat type-I cell, this effect appears to be specific for the large conductance Ca^{2+}-activated K^+-channel (Peers, 1990; Peers & Green, 1991). Until recently, however, there has been no direct demonstration that the rise of $[Ca^{2+}]_i$ is directly related to depolarisation and to voltage-gated Ca^{2+}-entry.

Two lines of evidence point directly to both the role of depolarisation and voltage activated Ca^{2+}-channels in mediating the Ca^{2+}-response to a hypercapnic acidosis. Firstly, pharmacological evidence shows that the Ca^{2+}-response is partially inhibited by the L-type Ca^{2+}-channel antagonists, nicardipine and D600 (Fig. 3 and Buckler & Vaughan-Jones, 1994). Secondly direct, simultaneous recordings of membrane potential (using the perforated patch technique) with $[Ca^{2+}]_i$ measurement have established (i) that acidosis promotes membrane depolarisation and electrical activity in type-I cells (Fig. 4), and (ii) that preventing these electrical responses to acidosis by voltage-clamping eliminates the $[Ca^{2+}]_i$-response (Buckler & Vaughan-Jones, 1994). Thus the rise of $[Ca^{2+}]_i$ is dependent upon membrane depolarisation.

Although depolarisation could theoretically promote Ca^{2+}-entry through a voltage sensitive Na^+-Ca^{2+}-exchanger, there are three pieces of evidence which weigh against such a mechanism in the rat type-I cell (see Buckler & Vaughan-Jones, 1994). (i) A $[Ca^{2+}]_i$-

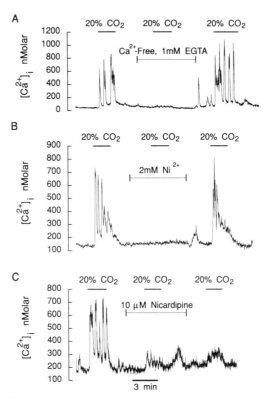

Figure 3. The rise in $[Ca^{2+}]_i$ induced by a hypercapnic acidosis is inhibited (**A**) by removal of extracellular Ca^{2+}, (**B**) by 2 mM Ni^{2+} and (**C**) is substantially attenuated by nicardipine.

response to a hypercapnic acidosis can be elicited in Na^+-free solutions (under appropriate conditions). (ii) The removal of extracellular Na^+ has little effect upon either resting $[Ca^{2+}]_i$ or upon the removal of Ca^{2+} from the cytoplasm following a brief depolarisation. This suggests that Na^+/Ca^{2+}-exchange contributes little to the control of $[Ca^{2+}]_i$ in rat type-I cells. (iii) The rise of $[Ca^{2+}]_i$ in response to direct depolarisation (using the voltage clamp technique) displayed a voltage sensitivity inconsistent with exchange mediated Ca^{2+}-influx but entirely consistent with channel mediated Ca^{2+}-influx (Buckler & Vaughan-Jones, 1994). The conclusion, therefore, is that the main route for Ca^{2+}-entry during depolarisation is through voltage activated Ca^{2+}-channels including, but not necessarily exclusively, L-type Ca^{2+}-channels.

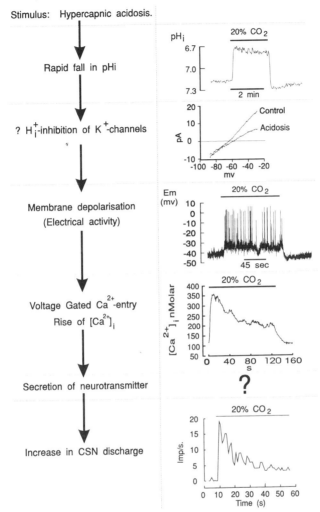

Figure 4. Schematic diagram of proposed acid transduction pathway. Right hand column summarises data supporting each step in the pathway (where available). From the top, the effects of a 20% CO_2 hypercapnic acidosis upon (i) type-I cell pH_i, (ii) membrane conductance in type-I cell, measured using 2s voltage ramps from -90 to -30 mV (perforated patch clamp) (iii) membrane potential, figure shows a membrane depolarisation or receptor potential and the generation of action potentials in the type-I cell in response to the stimulus (iv) type-I cell $[Ca^{2+}]_i$, figure is an average of many recordings which shows characteristic response pattern, (v) secretion of neurotransmitter, no direct evidence as to nature of excitatory transmitter's, (vi) changes in carotid sinus nerve discharge in intact ventilated cat (redrawn from Black et al., 1971). For further details of experiments see Buckler & Vaughan-Jones (1993; 1994).

What is the cause of the depolarisation and electrical excitability. As was stated above, there is direct evidence that acidosis inhibits Ca^{2+}-activated K^+-channels in rat type-I cells. What has been unclear is whether these channels (which are activated by voltage as well as $[Ca^{2+}]_i$) actually play any role in setting the resting membrane potential. Whilst there is no direct evidence on this point yet, we have investigated the effects of acidosis upon the resting membrane conductance of the rat type-I cell by using voltage ramps over a limited range of potentials (e.g. -90 to -30 mV). The results of these experiments indicate a decrease in resting membrane conductance with the acid-sensitive current components having a reversal potential of around -75mv (see Fig. 4 & Buckler & Vaughan-Jones, 1994). These data are therefore consistent with the depolarisation being due to the inhibition of a K^+-channel (although a parallel involvement of other ion conductance changes is not excluded). Whatever the channel/s responsible for the initial depolarisation, it is possible that modulation of K_{Ca}-channels by acidity play an important role in controlling subsequent electrical activity.

ACID CHEMOTRANSDUCTION BY THE RAT TYPE-I CELL; A MODEL

The preceding considerations of the effects of a hypercapnic acidosis upon pH_i, $[Ca^{2+}]_i$, membrane potential and ionic conductances, permit a reasonably detailed model for acid chemotransduction by the type-I cell. The steps are summarised in Fig. 4 and below.

1) Upon application of a hypercapnic acidosis, CO_2 rapidly enters the type-I cell and is hydrated by carbonic anhydrase to yield H_2CO_3 which dissociates to H^+ and HCO_3^-. This causes a rapid initial fall in pH_i, the magnitude of which is governed by the cell's intrinsic buffering capacity. The accompanying extracellular acidosis modulates cellular pH_i-regulatory mechanisms to ensure that a large intracellular acidosis is maintained throughout the duration of the hypercapnic acidosis.

2) The fall of pH_i inhibits K_{Ca}-channels and decreases resting membrane conductance.

3) The decrease in resting membrane conductance causes membrane depolarisation, (a receptor potential) which, in some cases, leads to the generation of action potentials.

4) The combination of the receptor potential and the action potentials mediate voltage-gated Ca^{2+}-entry.

5) Increased voltage-gated Ca^{2+}-entry causes a rapid initial rise in $[Ca^{2+}]_i$ which then partially adapts.

6) The rise of $[Ca^{2+}]_i$ promotes neurosecretion which excites sensory nerve endings.

7) A rapid increase in carotid sinus nerve afferent discharge ensues.

One major aspect of this model which still requires elucidation is the identity of the excitatory transmitter(s) involved in transmission from type-I cell to nerve ending.

REFERENCES

Aickin, C.C. (1984) Direct measurement of intracellular pH and buffering power in smooth muscle cells of Guinea-pig vas deferens. J. Physiol. (Lond.) 349:571-585.

Aickin, C.C. & Thomas, R.C. (1977) Microelectrode measurement of the intracellular pH and buffering power of mouse soleus muscle fibres. J. Physiol. (Lond.) 267:571-585.

Alper, S.L. (1991). The band 3-related anion exchanger (AE) gene family. Ann. Rev. Physiol. 53:549-64.

Aronson, P. (1985). Kinetic properties of the plasma membrane Na^+/H^+ exchanger. Ann. Rev. Physiol. 47:545-60

Aronson, P., Nee, A. & Suhm, M.A. (1982). Modifier role of internal H^+ in activating the Na^+/H^+ exchanger in renal microvillus membrane vesicles. Nature 299:161-163.

Austin, C. & Wray, S. (1993). Extracellular pH signals affect rat vascular tone by rapid transduction into intracellular pH changes. J. Physiol. (Lond.) 466:1-8.

Biscoe, T.J. & Duchen, M.R. (1990). Responses of type I cells dissociated from the rabbit carotid body to hypoxia. J. Physiol. (Lond.) 428:39-59.

Biscoe, T.J., Duchen, M.R., Eisner, D.A., O'Neil, S.C. & Valdeolmillos, M. (1989). Measurements of intracellular Ca^{2+} in dissociated type-I cells of the rabbit carotid body. J. Physiol. 416:421-434.

Black, A.M.S., McCloskey, D.I. & Torrance, R.W. (1971). The responses of carotid body chemoreceptors in the cat to sudden changes of hypercapnia and hypoxic stimuli. Respir. Physiol. 13:36-49.

Bonanno, J.A. (1991). K^+-H^+ exchange, a fundamental cell acidifier in corneal epithelium. Am. J. Physiol. 260:C618-625.

Buckler, K.J. & Vaughan-Jones, R.D. (1994). Hypercapnia promotes membrane depolarisation and voltage-gated calcium entry in rat carotid body type-I cells. J. Physiol. (Lond) submitted.

Buckler, K.J. & Vaughan-Jones, R.D. (1993). Effects of acidic stimuli on intracellular calcium in isolated type-I cells of the neonatal rat carotid body. Pflugers Arch. (in press)

Buckler, K.J., Vaughan-Jones, R.D., Peers, C., Lagadic-Gossmann, D. & Nye, P.C.G. (1991a). Effects of extracellular pH, P_{CO2} and HCO_3- on intracellular pH in isolated type-I cells of the neonatal rat carotid body. J. Physiol. (Lond) 444:703-721.

Buckler, K.J., Vaughan-Jones, R.D., Peers, C., & Nye, P.C.G. (1991b). Intracellular pH and its regulation in isolated type-I carotid body cells of the neonatal rat. J. Physiol. (Lond) 436:107-129.

Buckler, K.J. & Vaughan-Jones, R.D. (1990). Application of a new pH-sensitive fluoroprobe (carboxy-SNARF-1) for intracellular pH measurements in small isolated cells. Pflugers. Arch. 417:234-239.

Buckler, K.J., Nye, P.C.G, Peers, C. & Vaughan-Jones, R.D. (1990). Effects of simulated respiratory and metabolic acidosis/alkalosis on pH_i in isolated type-I carotid body cells from the neonatal rat. J. Physiol. (Lond) 426:66P.

Counillon, L. & Pouyssegur, J. (1993). Molecular biology and hormonal regulation of vertebrate Na^+/H^+ exchanger isoforms. In "Molecular biology and function of carrier proteins." Soc. Gen. Physiol. Vol 48. L. Reuss, J.M. Russell & M.L. Jennings, ed., Rockerfeller University Press, New York.

Donnelly, D.F. & Kholwadwala, D. (1992). Hypoxia decreases intracellular calcium in adult rat carotid body glomus cells. J. Neurophysiol. 67:1543-1551.

Ellis, D. & Thomas, R.C. (1976) Microelectrode measurement of the intracellular pH of mammalian heart cells. Nature 262:224-225.

Fidone, S., Gonzalez, C., and Yoshizaki, K (1982). Effects of low oxygen on the release of dopamine from the rabbit carotid body in vitro. J. Physiol.(Lond) 333:93-110.

Fonteriz, R.I., Vaughan-Jones, R.D. & Lagadic-Gossmann, D.L. (1993). Hypoxia inhibits acid extrusion from the guinea-pig isolated ventricular myocytes. J. Physiol. (Lond.) 467:277P.

Gonzalez, C., Almarez, L., Obeso, A. & Rigual, R. (1992). Oxygen and acid chemotransduction in the carotid body chemoreceptors. TINS 15:146-153.

Gray, B.A. (1968). Responses of the perfused carotid body to changes in pH and pCO_2. Respir. Physiol. 4:580-584.

Hanson, M.A., Nye, P.C.G. & Torrance, R.W. (1981) The exodus of an extracellular bicarbonate theory of chemoreception and the genesis of an intracellular one. In: "Arterial chemoreceptors". C. Belmonte, D.J. Pallot, H. Acker & S. Fidone. ed. Leicester University Press, Leicester (1981).

He, S.-F., Wei, J.-H. & Eyzaguirre, C. (1991). Intracellular pH and some membrane characteristics of cultured carotid body glomus cells. Brain Res. 547:258-266.

Iturriaga, R. & Lahiri, S. (1991). Carotid body chemoreception in the absence and presence of CO_2-HCO_3^-. Brain Res. 568:253-260.

Lopez-Lopez, J., Gonzalez, C., Urena, J. & Lopez-Barneo, J. (1989). Low pO_2 selectively inhibits K channel activity in chemoreceptor cells of the mammalian carotid body. J. Gen. Physiol. 93:1001-1015.

Peers, C. (1990). Selective effects of extracellular pH on Ca^{2+}-dependent K-currents in type-I cells isolated from the neonatal rat carotid body. J. Physiol.(Lond.) 422:381-395.

Peers, C. & Green, F.K. (1991). Inhibition of Ca^{2+}-activated K^+ currents by intracellular acidosis in isolated type-I cells of the neonatal rat carotid body. J. Physiol.(Lond.) 437:589-602.

Richmond, P. & Vaughan-Jones, R.D. (1993). K^+-H^+ exchange in isolated carotid body type-I cells of the neonatal rat is caused by nigericin contamination. J. Physiol. (Lond.) 467:277P.

Rigual, R., Lopez-Lopez, J.R. & Gonzalez, C. (1991). Release of dopamine and chemoreceptor discharge induced by low pH and high pCO_2 stimulation of the cat carotid body. J. Physiol.(Lond.) 433:519-531.

Rigual, R., Gonzalez, E., Gonzalez, C. & Fidone, S. (1986). Synthesis and release of catecholamines by the cat carotid body in vitro: Effects of hypoxic stimulation. Brain Res. 374:101-109.

Rocher, A., Obeso, A., Gonzalez, C. & Herreros, B. (1991). Ionic mechanisms for the transduction of acidic stimuli in rabbit carotid body glomus cells. J. Physiol. 433:533-548.

Roos, A. & Boron, W.F. (1981). Intracellular pH. Physiol. Rev. 61:296-434.

Stea, A., Alexander,S.A. & Nurse, C.A. (1991). Effects of pH_i and pH_o on membrane currents recorded with the perforated-patch method from cultured chemoreceptors of the rat carotid body. Brain Res. 567:83-90.

Stea, A., & Nurse, C.A. (1989). Chloride channels in cultured glomus cells of the rat carotid body. Am. J. Physiol. 257:C174-C181.

Tolkovsky, A.M. & Richards, C.D. (1987) Na^+/H^+ Exchange is the major mechanism of pH regulation in cultured sympathetic neurones: measurements in single cell bodies and neurites using a fluorescent pH indicator. Neurosci. 22:1093-1102.

Vaughan-Jones, R.D. & Wu, M-L. (1990). Extracellular H^+ inactivation of Na^+/H^+ exchange in the sheep cardiac Purkinje fibre. J. Physiol. 428:441-466

Vaughan-Jones, R.D. (1986) An investigation of chloride-bicarbonate exchange in the sheep cardiac purkinje fibre. J. Physiol. (Lond.) 379:377-406.

Urena, J., Lopez-Lopez, J., Gonzalez, C. & Lopez-Barneo, J. (1989) Ionic currents in dispersed chemoreceptor cells of the mammalian carotid body. J. Gen. Physiol. 93:979-999.

Wilding, T.J., Cheng, B. & Roos, A. (1992). pH regulation in adult rat carotid body glomus cells. J. Gen. Physiol. 100:593-608.

NEUROTRANSMITTERS IN THE CAROTID BODY

Nanduri R. Prabhakar

Department of Medicine,
Case Western Reserve University School of Medicine
Cleveland, Ohio 44106 U.S.A.

INTRODUCTION

One of the most fundamental physiological stimuli is oxygen, or more appropriately the lack of oxygen, i.e., hypoxia. The discovery that the carotid bodies are the principal sensory organs for monitoring the arterial oxygen opened new perspectives in respiratory physiology. The chemoreceptor organ morphologically resembles a miniaturized brain. It is comprised of type I (also called glomus) cells that are of neural crest origin and contain neurotransmitters. Glomus cells are in functional contact with afferent nerve endings; whereas the type II (or sustentacular) cells resemble glia. Currently, it is believed that the type I cells are the initial transducers of the hypoxic stimuli. Transduction mechanism(s) may involve biochemical or biophysical processes (Acker, 1989; Biscoe & Duchen, 1990; Fidone & Gonzalez, 1986). Neurochemical(s), on the other hand, are essential for sensory transmission in the carotid body (Fidone & Gonzalez, 1986; Prabhakar, 1992). The general consensus is that in response to low O_2 glomus cells release neurochemical(s), which act on the nearby afferent nerve ending to increase the sensory discharge (Biscoe & Duchen, 1990; Fidone & Gonzalez, 1986; Prabhakar, 1992). Glomus cells are endowed with several types of chemicals that function as transmitters or modulators else where in the nervous system. These include biogenic amines, neuropeptides and nitric oxide (NO) and carbon monoxide (CO). Some of these neurochemicals co-exist within the same glomus cell (Wang et al., 1992b), and perhaps co-released during hypoxia. In view of this, the notion that hypoxia releases a "single" neurochemical, perhaps is no longer tenable.

In addition to type I cells, some of these chemicals are localized to the nerve fibers that regulate carotid body activity (Fidone & Gonzalez, 1986.) So far, no neurotransmitters have been demonstrated within the type II cells. The purpose of this article is to review the possible roles of neurotransmitters in the initiation and maintenance of carotid body sensory activity by hypoxia.

ACETYLCHOLINE (ACh)

Schweitzer and Wright (1938) were the first to note the stimulatory effects of ACh on

Arterial Chemoreceptors: Cell to System
Edited by R. O'Regan *et al*, Plenum Press, New York, 1994

Subsequently, for more than two decades, i.e., from 1940 to 1970, several studies examined the role of ACh in the carotid body response to hypoxia. Evidence for and against the role of ACh as the mediator of the carotid body response to hypoxia has been reviewed extensively (Fidone & Gonzalez, 1986).

There is little doubt with regards to the presence of ACh in the carotid bodies. Chemoreceptor tissue contains the enzymatic machinery necessary for its synthesis and degradation, and hypoxia may release ACh-like material from mammalian carotid bodies (Fidone & Gonzalez, 1986). Furthermore, the presence of cholinergic receptors (muscarinic and nicotinic types) has been reported in rabbit and cat carotid bodies (Dinger et al., 1985, 1986). The problem with ACh as the mediator of the hypoxic response, however, stems from the following studies. The stimulatory actions of ACh varies with species. For instance, in cats, ACh stimulates, whereas in rabbits, it inhibits, the carotid bodies (Monti-Bloch et al., 1980). Moreover, cholinergic antagonists which block the actions of exogenous ACh have little influence on the chemosensory response to hypoxia (Fidone & Gonzalez, 1986). Species variations and the lack of effect of cholinergic blockers on hypoxic excitation cast serious doubts on its role as the principal mediator of the sensory response to low PO_2.

Recently Fitzgerald and his associates (Fitzgerald & Shirahata, 1992) re-examined the role of ACh in the carotid body. They tested the effects of cocktail of cholinergic receptor blockers (i.e., α-bungarotoxin + atropine + mecamylamine) on the carotid body response to hypoxia in anesthetized cats. This combination of cholinergic blockers attenuated the carotid body response to hypoxia. Based on these findings it was concluded that ACh is an excitatory transmitter that is necessary for the hypoxic response. Interestingly, cholinergic blockers also attenuated the carotid body response to CO_2. Given the possibility that ACh may mediate the ventilatory response to CO_2 acting on the medulla oblongata (Dev & Loescheke, 1979), it is likely that it plays a prominent role in the carotid body response to hypercapnia. If this is true, then the attenuation of hypoxic response by cholinergic blockers could conceivably be secondary to an attenuation of the carotid body response to CO_2. Nonetheless, these studies by Fitzgerald (Fitzgerald & Shirahata, 1992) are not only interesting but also point to the complexity of cholinergic receptors especially the muscarinic (M1, M2, M3) and nicotinic (neuronal and non-neuronal) subtypes. Future studies using specific agonists and antagonists to cholinergic receptor subtypes may provide important information as to the role of ACh in the carotid body.

CATECHOLAMINES

While ACh was the focus of interest between 1940 and 1970, catecholamines, especially dopamine, became the center of attention in the 70's in carotid body research. Lever and Boyd (Lever & Boyd, 1957; Lever et al., 1959) were the first to report catecholamines in rabbit and cat carotid bodies. It is clear from subsequent studies that the chemoreceptor organ resembles chromaffin tissues containing catecholamines. In fact, it has now become a common practice to identify glomus cells by catecholamine fluorescence. There is a good deal of confusion with regard to catecholamine content in mammalian carotid bodies. Much of this is due to (a) different techniques used for measurements of catecholamines and (b) expressing the amine content per carotid body (which varies considerably) without normalizing the data either per milligram of protein or weight of the carotid bodies. Fidone and Gonzalez in their elegant review (Fidone & Gonzalez, 1986), tabulated results from different laboratories including variations in methodological approaches and species differences. It is evident from their review that dopamine (DA) is the major catecholamine in the carotid body in many species, followed by norepinephrine (NE). However, epinephrine (E) content is either negligible or is even absent in some species.

Dopamine (DA)

More than 90% of the glomus cells contain tyrosine hydroxylase (TH), the rate limiting enzyme in catecholamine synthesis, suggesting that type I cells synthesize dopamine. Additionally, TH is also present in nerve endings originating from petrosal and sympathetic ganglia (Fidone & Gonzalez, 1986).

DA is not only the most abundant, but also the most extensively studied catecholamine in the carotid body. Fidone and co-workers (Fidone et al., 1982) were the first to demonstrate release of DA from rabbit carotid bodies during hypoxia. Later studies (Gonzalez et al. 1992) not only confirmed these observations, but further showed that DA release by hypoxia depends on the presence of extracellular calcium and perhaps requires depolarization. In recent years the technique of voltammetry has been used to study the release of catecholamines in the nervous system, the advantage of this technique being that it is possible to monitor DA release along with the neural activity. Using this technique on rat carotid bodies, Donnelly et al. (1993) found no apparent relation between DA release and chemosensory excitation by hypoxia. Buerk and Lahiri (1993), on the other hand, working with cat carotid bodies observed that DA release coincided with the neural response to hypoxia. Whether these discrepancies are due species variations remain to be established. Fishman et al. (1985) reported that hypoxia releases DA from glomus cells dissociated from rat carotid bodies. We recently confirmed the release of DA from isolated glomus cells using differential pulse voltammetry (Prabhakar et al., 1993). Thus far, these studies demonstrate that hypoxia releases DA from the carotid body and much of it comes from glomus cells.

Although it is certain hypoxia releases DA from the carotid body, its significance in chemo-transmission is a much debated topic in carotid body physiology (Fidone & Gonzalez, 1986; Gonzalez et al., 1992). Because of its abundance and the release by hypoxia, it was thought that DA may mediate the augmentation of chemosensory discharge by low PO_2. However, much of the pharmacological data suggest that DA is in fact an inhibitory transmitter in the carotid body. Exogenous administration of DA inhibits carotid body sensory discharge in cats, rabbits, and dogs (Fidone & Gonzalez, 1986). The effects of DA on *in vitro* carotid bodies are more complex and exhibit marked species differences. In *in vitro* preparations DA inhibits the sensory discharge of the cat carotid body, whereas augments the chemosensory activity in rabbits (Monti-Bloch et al., 1980). In human subjects, systemic infusion of DA depresses the hypoxic ventilatory drive (Ward & Nino, 1992), a finding consistent with its inhibitory action observed in experimental animals. Blockade of dopaminergic receptors by haloperidol increases the baseline activity and potentiates the sensory response to hypoxia in experimental animals (Lahiri et al, 1980). However, Zapata (1975) noted that the inhibitory effects were sometimes followed by slowly developing excitation in cat carotid bodies. We found similar biphasic pattern of DA on the rat carotid body (Prabhakar and Runold, unpublished observations). Thus far, studies on experimental animals and humans are consistent with the notion that DA is inhibitory to the carotid body activity.

While its significance in the initiation of hypoxic excitation is debated, there are studies suggesting that DA may be of importance in the maintenance of the sensory response to sustained hypoxia. Ponte and Sadler (1989) examined the effects of haloperidol on the carotid body response to sustained hypoxia in anaesthetized rabbits. These authors found that prior to the blockade of DA receptors, hypoxia augmented the sensory activity and the increased activity was maintained throughout the 15 min of hypoxic challenge. After blockade of DA receptors, excitation in the initial period of hypoxia was unaffected, whereas, the magnitude of excitation in the later phase was significantly attenuated. They concluded that DA may play an important role in the maintenance of hypoxic excitation. Ward and Nino (1992) examined the effects of systemic infusion of DA on ventilatory response to sustained hypoxia in awake human subjects. They found a biphasic hypoxic ventilatory response to a sustained low PO_2 challenge, i.e., initial augmentation followed by a ventilatory "roll off". In response to systemic infusion of DA, the initial increase in ventilation was reduced and the magnitude of subsequent ventilatory roll off was attenuated. Because DA cannot cross the blood brain barrier, these authors attributed the effects of DA to the carotid body. These observations indirectly suggest that DA may have a dual action on the carotid body, namely, an initial inhibitory action that would account for the depression of ventilation, and a subsequent excitatory effect. Taken together, the findings of Ponte and Sadler (1989) in experimental animals and that of Ward and Nino (1992) in humans, it is conceivable that DA may play a role in maintenance of sensory activity during sustained hypoxic challenge. Stimulation of the sinus nerve inhibits the sensory activity (Fidone & Gonzalez, 1986) and this inhibition seems to be mediated by DA (Lahiri et al., 1984).

From the above studies, it is evident the effects of DA on carotid body activity are complex. Depending on species, DA either inhibits or excites the carotid bodies. This complexity could conceivably be due to its actions on multiple dopaminergic receptor subtypes that are now classified as D1, D2, D3, D4. With regards to the carotid body, D2 receptors have been demonstrated both on type I cells (presynaptic) and on afferent nerve endings (post synaptic) (Dinger et al., 1981; Mir et al., 1984). Future studies dealing with the analysis of other dopaminergic subtypes may provide insights as to the significance of DA in carotid body chemotransmission.

Norepinephrine (NE)

Besides dopamine, norepinephrine (NE), is the major catecholamine in the carotid body. Till recently, sympathetic nerve fibers were thought to be the only source of NE in the carotid body. It is now established that type I cells can also synthesize NE (Fidone & Gonzalez, 1986). Moreover, being situated close to the carotid arteries, glomus tissue is continuously being exposed to circulating NE. Thus, NE in the carotid bodies arises from three different sources, namely sympathetic nerves, glomus cells and circulating blood. Reviewed below is the pertinent literature dealing with the effects and significance of NE in carotid body function.

In human subjects, intravenous infusion of NE stimulates breathing, an effect attributed to activation of carotid bodies. However, no obvious relation was found between simultaneous measurements of ventilation and the carotid body sensory activity in response to NE (Bisgard et al., 1979). Thus, it is possible that the respiratory stimulation observed in humans might in part be due to its actions on central neurones involved in regulation of breathing. Direct recordings of the carotid body activity in experimental animals have shown that NE causes inhibition as well as excitation of the chemosensory activity; often inhibition precedes the excitation (Bisgard et al., 1979; Prabhakar et al., 1992). We found that this biphasic pattern in carotid body response to NE depends on (a) mode of administration and (b) the dose of the amine. For instance, in a given experiment NE given as a bolus produced an inhibition followed by excitation; however, infusion of the same dose produced only inhibition (Prabhakar et al., 1992). Analysis of the dose-response showed inhibition of sensory discharge at lower and excitation at higher doses of NE. The fact that similar effects are also seen *in vitro* suggests that the effects of NE in part are due to its direct actions on carotid body (Prabhakar et al., 1992). Milsom and Sadig (1983) reported that NE inhibited some chemoreceptor units in rabbits, whereas, similar doses stimulated other fibers, indicating interfiber variability among different chemoreceptor units.

It is clear from these studies that NE has a dual effect on the carotid body sensory discharge, namely inhibition and excitation. These dual effects of NE on chemosensory activity appears to be due to its action on different adrenoceptor sub-types (α or β subtypes). ß-adrenoceptor agonists stimulate the carotid bodies (Folgering et al., 1982; Lahiri et al., 1981). and their activation is coupled to the cAMP second messenger (Mir et al., 1983). Our recent results suggest that the inhibitory actions of NE in the carotid body are coupled to α_2-adrenoceptors (Kou et al., 1991b). Evidence for the involvement of α_2-adrenoceptors include (a) presence of α_2-adrenoceptor binding sites, (b) inhibition of chemosensory activity by guanabenz, an α_2-agonist, and (c) reversal of the guanabenz and demonstrate that the inhibitory actions of NE in the carotid body are elicited by α_2 receptors and the excitatory effects are mediated by β-adrenoceptors. The distribution of different adrenoceptor subtypes in the chemoreceptor tissue remain to be studied.

Several studies suggest that NE mediates efferent regulation of carotid body activity by sympathetic nerves. Depending on the stimulus variables, electrical stimulation of pre- or post-ganglionic sympathetic nerves either inhibit or stimulate the carotid body and these effects were blocked by adrenoceptor antagonists indicating the involvement of NE (O'Regan, 1981). Hypoxia augments the sympathetic outflow to the carotid body (see Prabhakar & Kou, 1994, for refs.). We recently examined the effects of sympathectomy and assessed the role of NE in carotid body response to sustained hypoxia (Prabhakar & Kou, 1994). The results showed that the magnitude of the carotid body response to hypoxia was greater after sympathectomy, an effect seen seen only at 10 and 20 min of hypoxic challenge, but not during the initial 5 min. These findings suggest that sympathetic outflow has a slowly building inhibitory influence on the chemosensory response. Studies with α_2-adrenergic blockade suggest that part of the inhibitory effects are due to activation of α_2-adrenoceptors by endogenous NE (Prabhakar & Kou, 1994).

Although NE stimulates carotid body activity (Milsom & Sadig, 1983; Folgering et al., 1982) there no compelling evidence for its role in the initiation of chemosensory response to hypoxia. Nonetheless, the studies with sympathetic activation indicate that over excitation of the carotid body activity during sustained hypoxia is regulated by endogenous NE via α_2-adrenoceptors. Such an efferent regulation by sympathetic nerves could be of potential physiological significance during chronic hypoxemia.

INDOLAMINES AND ADENINE NUCLEOSIDES

Carotid bodies contain 5-hydroxy tryptamine (5-HT). Much of the amine comes either from blood (uptake mechanism) or synthesized to some extent within the chemoreceptor tissue. Nishi (1975) reported that exogenous administration of 5-HT results in a brisk augmentation of sensory discharge followed by inhibition. The receptors responsible for 5-HT actions and their significance in the carotid body function has yet to be established. It is well known that hypoxia increases the tissue levels of adenosine (McQueen & Ribiero, 1983; Runold et al., 1990a,b). Consequently, it was thought that adenosine may play an important role in the carotid body response to hypoxia. Exogenous administration of adenosine stimulates the carotid and aortic bodies (McQueen & Ribiero, 1983; Runold et al., 1990a). Stimulatory actions of adenosine were seen in *in vitro* carotid bodies, suggesting some direct action of nucleoside on chemotransmission (Runold et al., 1990b). The effects of adenosine in part are mediated by P_2-receptors (McQueen & Ribiero, 1983). The precise role of adenosine in the carotid body response to hypoxia remain to be established.

NEUROPEPTIDES

Almost three decades ago, Torrance (1968) mentioned the possibility that carotid body may release a polypeptide that may have a role in chemoreception. Nearly the same time, Pearse (1969), a British morphologist, reported that type I cells of the carotid body resemble Amine Precursor Uptake Decarboxylation cell system (APUD), and suggested that they secrete a polypeptide, which was provisionally named as "glomin", that could be of importance in chemoreception. Now it is established that mammalian carotid bodies contain several neuropeptides. Much of the research in the 80's focused on the distribution and physiological significance of peptides in carotid body chemotransmission.

Substance P (SP)

SP is an undecapeptide that belongs to a group of structurally related neuropeptides called tachykinins. In the cat, SP-like immunoreactivity (SP-ir) is localized to many glomus cells and nerve fibers innervating the glomus tissue (Prabhakar et al, 1989b). Chronic ablation of the sinus nerve abolishes SP-ir in nerve fibers but not in the glomus cells, suggesting that these nerve fibers are of petrosal ganglion origin (Prabhakar, 1992). Furthermore, SP-ir seems to be confined only to those glomus cells that are in close opposition to afferent nerve endings (Chen et al., 1986). Type I cells contain mRNA for the pre-protachykinin gene that encodes SP, as evidenced by *in situ* hybridization histochemistry (Prabhakar, 1992), suggesting that glomus cells synthesize SP. Cat carotid body contains neutral endopeptidase, an enzyme that hydrolyses peptides such as SP (Kumar et al. 1992). Thus far, studies on cat carotid body demonstrate that SP is synthesized in glomus cells and the enzymatic machinery responsible for its hydrolysis is also present in the chemoreceptor tissue. Sustained hypoxic challenge for one hour increases SP content (Prabhakar et al., 1989b), whereas in rabbits, intermittent hypoxia decreases SP content of carotid bodies (Hansen et al., 1986).

McQueen (1980) was the first to report that exogenous administration of SP stimulates the carotid body activity in anesthetized cats. Subsequent studies confirmed the excitatory effects of SP on the carotid body activity *in vivo* (Prabkakar, 1992). On the other hand, Monti-Bloch and Eyzaguirre (1985) reported excitatory and inhibitory effects of SP on carotid body activity *in vitro*. Kou et al. (1991a), re-examined the effects of SP on the isolated superfused cat carotid bodies and found that the peptide stimulated the carotid bodies in a dose-dependent manner and no evidence for inhibitory actions were evident *in vitro*. The effects of SP on carotid body sensory discharge of species other than cats have also been examined. SP stimulates the carotid body in rats (Cragg et al., 1994) and rabbits (Gallagher et al., 1985) The studies described thus far suggest that SP stimulates the carotid bodies and its excitatory effects seems to be uniform across the species.

Maxwell et al. (1990) reported that intravenous administration of SP potentiates hypoxic ventilatory drive in conscious human subjects. On the other hand, peptides such as vasoactive intestinal peptide (VIP) were found to have no effect on hypoxic ventilatory drive. These authors attributed the increased hypoxic ventilatory drive by SP to its actions on carotid bodies. We found that phosphoramidon, a peptidase inhibitor significantly potentiated the hypoxic response of cat carotid bodies *in vivo* (Kumar et al., 1990) and *in vitro* (Prabkakar, 1992). It has been known for several years that neonatal administration of capsaicin irreversibly depletes certain neuropeptides, especially SP. DeSanctis et al. (1991) and Cragg et al. (1994), observed a blunted hypoxic ventilatory drive in adult rats that were treated with capsaicin neonatally. Studies on humans and experimental animals suggest that SP is associated with chemosensory excitation by hypoxia.

The availability of peptidyl and non-peptidyl antagonists for SP allowed us to examine further the role of SP in carotid body response to hypoxia. Intracarotid administration of peptidyl SP antagonists (spantide and D-Pro^2,D-Tryp^{7,9} -SP or DPDT-SP), at doses that blocked the excitatory effects of exogenous SP markedly attenuated the chemosensory response to hypoxia in cats (Prabhakar, 1992) and rats (Cragg et al., 1994). However, SP antagonists had no effect on the carotid body response to hypercapnia or other excitatory stimuli (Prabhakar, 1992; Cragg et al., 1994). It should, however, be pointed out that peptidyl SP antagonists were effective only when given as a continuous infusion but not as a bolus. Being peptides, these antagonists are rapidly hydrolyzed by blood proteases when given as a bolus. Recent study has shown that the hypoxic response can be prevented both *in vivo* and *in vitro* cat carotid bodies by a non-peptidyl SP receptor (NK-1) antagonist (Prabhakar et al., 1993d). More importantly, comparable doses of an enantiomer of the SP antagonist has no effect on the chemosensory response to hypoxia (Prabhakar et al., 1993d). These studies provide convincing evidence that endogenous SP by its action on NK-1 receptors is coupled to hypoxic excitation of the carotid body in cats. The localization of NK-1 receptors in carotid bodies remains to be investigated. Furthermore, the role of NKA, another tachykinin peptide that is co-localized with SP in type I cells of the carotid body (Prabhakar et al., 1989b) has received less attention.

The studies described thus far gives a scenario where SP may function as a "classical" neurotransmitter or a modulator in the genesis of the carotid body response to hypoxia. Some of our observations indicate other actions of SP. For instance, SP increases mitochondrial respiration in a dose-dependent manner and the peptide indeed has the ability to cross lipid bilayers as evidenced by partition coefficient analysis (Prabhakar et al. 1989a). These observations indicate that some of the actions of SP could be due to its action on mitochondrial metabolism. Consistent with such a notion is the finding that antimycin A, a blocker of cytochrome oxidase, prevents the chemosensory excitation by SP and hypoxia but not the stimulation by other excitatory stimuli (Prabhakar, 1992). Exogenous SP increases $[Ca^{2+}]_i$ of the glomus cells isolated from adult rat carotid bodies (Bright & Prabhakar unpublished observations), indicating that the peptide may modulate the release of neurochemicals by interfering with calcium channels. Thus, the effects of SP in the carotid body seem to be complex and it cannot be viewed as a classical neurotransmitter that acts only on the afferent nerve endings. Further information on second messenger systems coupled to the SP receptor and the effects of SP on ionic conductances of type I cells would be of great interest in understanding the mechanism(s) of action of SP in the carotid body.

Enkephalins (ENK)

Enkephalins are localized to type I cells and are co-localized with TH (Wang et al., 1992b). Studies by Hansen et al. (1984) indicate that short term exposure to hypoxia may release enkephalins. Exogenous administration of Met-enkephalins inhibits the sensory discharge probably by acting on delta-type of ENK-receptors (McQueen & Ribiero, 1980). Blockade of enkephalin receptors by naloxone has no effect on baseline activity, but potentiates the hypoxic response (Pokorski & Lahiri, 1981). These observations indicate that enkephalins act as inhibitory modulators of chemosensory response to hypoxia. The mechanism(s) of enkephalin action in the carotid body have not yet been examined in detail. Possibly ENK may influence the release of other transmitters in the carotid body as they do elsewhere in the nervous system.

Atrial Natriuretic Peptide (ANP)

In addition to blood gases, the carotid bodies are sensitive to changes in blood osmolarity (Fidone & Gonzalez, 1986). ANP is a hormonal regulator of natriuresis and diuresis. Wang and his co-workers (Wang et al., 1991) have examined the distribution and effects of ANP in the carotid bodies. These authors have demonstrated (a) ANP-like immunoreactivity in type I cells and (b) that the biologically active fragment atriopeptin III inhibits the carotid body response to hypoxia. The effects of ANP are associated with increased levels of cGMP, suggesting that in the carotid body ANP receptors are coupled to membrane bound guanylate cyclase. Since hypoxia may release ANP, it is conceivable that it may be an important modulator of the hypoxic response.

Other Peptides

In addition, chemoreceptor tissue contains several other peptides, including galanin, CGRP (Ichikawa & Helke, 1993) and cholecystokinin-like activity (Kummer et al., 1985). The significance of these peptides has yet to be studied.

GASES AS TRANSMITTERS OR MODULATORS IN THE CAROTID BODY

Until recently, nitric oxide (NO) and carbon monoxide (CO) were thought to be noxious gases that are harmful to the body. It now established that mammalian cells synthesize NO and CO and that they act as chemical messengers in various physiological systems (Snyder, 1992). Reviewed below are the studies that examined the significance of NO and CO in the carotid body function.

Nitric Oxide (NO)

We examined the distribution of nitric oxide synthase (NOS), an enzyme that catalyzes the formation of NO, in cat carotid bodies, and assessed the possible role of NO in carotid body function (Prabhakar et al., 1993b) Many nerve plexuses innervating the chemoreceptor tissue were positive for NOS, indicating that the nerve fibers are the primary source of NO production in the carotid body. Biochemical analysis has shown that NOS activity is dependent on molecular O_2, and the enzyme activity was less at low PO_2 compared to normoxic controls. Inhibition of NOS activity by L-nitro arginine augmented the chemosensory activity, implying that endogenous NO is inhibitory to the carotid body. Moreover, the effects of NOS inhibitors were associated with marked decreases in cGMP levels suggesting that the effects of NO are coupled in part to haem-containing soluble guanylate cyclase activity. Independent studies by Wang et al. (1992a) are consistent with the notion that NO is an inhibitory chemical messenger in the carotid body. Wang et al. (1992a) have further shown that NOS-positive fibers originate from the petrosal ganglion. The fact that the sinus nerve fibers contain NOS and that NO is inhibitory suggests that it may mediate inhibition by sinus nerve efferents. Interestingly, NOS activity was co-localized with SP and not with TH (Wang et al., 1992a). These observations indicate potential interaction of SP-ergic system with NO.

It has been postulated that augmentation of chemosensory activity by hypoxia is due to decreased availability of an inhibitory chemical messenger (see Prabhakar et al., 1993b for refs.). Several neurochemicals inhibit carotid body activity, but they seem to be released by hypoxia. Thus, the identity of putative neurochemical whose availability is decreased during low PO_2 remains elusive. Our observation that low PO_2 decreases NOS activity may be relevant to this idea and suggests that NO could be one of the purported inhibitory chemical messengers. It is possible that low sensory activity during normoxia is due to a constant inhibitory action of NO, whereas increased sensory activity under hypoxia is due to "disinhibition" resulting from reduced production of NO. Interestingly, the levels of PO_2 that reduced the NOS activity are not only modest, but also comparable to those that produce intense stimulation of the carotid body activity (Prabhakar et al. 1993b). Thus, the decreased NO production by low PO_2 might constitute one of the important steps in producing the sensory excitation by hypoxia.

Carbon Monoxide (CO)

Recent studies have shown that CO is synthesized by mammalian cells and may function as transmitter in the nervous system (Snyder, 1992). The enzymes haemoxygenase I and II (HO-I and -II) catalyze the formation of CO and molecular oxygen is required for CO synthesis (Snyder, 1992). HO-II is constitutive and is present predominantly in neuronal tissues. We, in collaboration with Dinerman and Snyder, examined the distribution of HO-II in cat carotid bodies. We found that HO-II is distributed in many type I cells. Furthermore, inhibition of HO-II by Zn-protoporphyrin-9 augmented the sensory activity of the carotid bodies in a dose-dependent manner and maximal doses were found to be 3 to 10 µM. These observations indicate that type I cells of the carotid bodies are capable of producing CO and it is inhibitory to the carotid body activity (Prabhakar et al., 1993c). Consistent with this notion are the recent preliminary studies by Lahiri and his co-workers, who reported that low doses of CO inhibits chemosensory activity of the isolated cat carotid bodies (Lahiri et al., 1993). Future studies may provide insights as to the role of CO in the carotid body function.

SUMMARY

It is amazing that the carotid body, which weighs less than a milligram, contains as many neurotransmitters as the brain tissue. Since the discovery that the carotid body is a sensory organ for detecting arterial oxygen, much attention has been focused in delineating the role of neurochemicals in chemosensory augmentation by hypoxia. Considerable progress has been accomplished in understanding the distribution and the effects of neurochemicals on sensory activity of the carotid body. Being a slowly adapting type of sensory receptor, the increase in chemosensory activity persists during sustained hypoxia. Less attention has been given to the role of neurochemicals in the maintenance of sensory discharge during sustained hypoxia. Such an information will be of physiological significance in understanding the role of carotid bodies in chronic hypoxia. Although it is well recognized that in addition to oxygen, carotid bodies sense CO_2, relatively little information is available as to the role of neurochemicals in carotid body CO_2 chemoreception.

It has long been postulated that heme-containing proteins in the carotid body are important for oxygen-sensing mechanism(s) (Fidone & Gonzalez, 1986). The discovery that gases such as NO and CO can be synthesized by carotid bodies and that they may function as chemical messengers, may be relevant to this idea. The enzymes responsible for the synthesis of NO and CO possess heme moiety and require molecular oxygen. Putative targets of action of NO and CO are the heme-containing enzymes that regulate nucleotide levels and cellular respiration. Future studies with NO and CO may unravel important insights into their hitherto unrecognized roles in oxygen chemoreception.

I am grateful to Dr. Kumar for his critical comments, and to Cheryl Diane Gilliam-Walker for her secretarial assistance. The work reported here was done in collaboration with Drs. Cragg, Kumar, Kou, and Runold. The research is supported by grants from National Institutes of Health: HL-38986; HL-45780; and a Research Career Development Award, HL-02599.

REFERENCES

Acker, H. (1989) PO_2 chemoreception in arterial chemoreceptors. Annu. Rev. Physiol. 51:835-844

Biscoe, T.J. & M.R. Duchen (1990) Monitoring PO_2 by the carotid chemoreceptor. News in Physiol. Sci. 5:229-233

Bisgard, G.E., R.A. Mitchell, & D.A. Herbert (1979) Effects of dopamine, norepinephrine, and 5-hydroxytryptamine on the carotid body of the dog. Respir. Physiol. 37:61-80

Buerk, D.G. & S. Lahiri (1993) Detecting dopamine release in cat carotid body in response to hypoxia using nafion, thin-film coated recessed microelectrodes. FASEB J. 7:3661 .

Chen, I.V., R.D. Yates, & J.T. Hansen (1986) Substance P-like immunoreactivity in rat and cat carotid bodies: Light and electron microscopic studies. Histol. Histopathol. 1:203-212 .

Cragg, P.A., M. Runold, Y.R. Kou & N.R. Prabhakar (1994) Tachykinin antagonists in carotid body responses to hypoxia and substance P in the rat. Respir. Physiol. In press

De Sanctis, G.T., F.H.Y. Green & J.E. Remmers. (1991) Ventilatory responses to hypoxia and hypercapnia in awake rats pretreated with capsaicin. J. Appl. Physiol. 70:1168-1174

Dev, N.B. & H.H. Loescheke (1979) A cholinergic mechanism involved in the respiratory chemosensitivity of the medulla oblongata in the cat. Pflüg. Arch. 379:29-36

Dinger, B., C. Gonzalez, K. Yoshizaki & S. Fidone (1981) [3-H]-spiroperidol binding in normal and denervated carotid bodies. Neurosci. Lett. 21:51-55

Dinger, B., C. Gonzalez, K. Yoshizaki & S. Fidone (1985) Localization and function of cat carotid body nicotinic receptors. Brain Res. 339:295-304

Dinger,B.G., T. Hirano & S.J. Fidone. (1986) Autoradiographic localization of muscarinic receptors in rabbit carotid body. Brain Res. 367:328-331

Donnelly, D.F. & T.P. Doyle (1993) Free tissue catecholamines of rat carotid body, in vitro, during maturation and following chronic hypoxia. Soc. Neuro. Abstract 19:574.1

Fidone, S.J. & C. Gonzalez (1986) Initiation and control of chemoreceptor activity in the carotid body, in: "Handbook of Physiology - Section 3: The Respiratory System," N.S. Cherniack & J.G. Widdicombe, eds., Am. Physiol. Soc., Bethseda, MD

Fidone, S.J., C. Gonzalez & K. Yoshizaki (1982) Effects of low oxygen on the release of dopamine from the rabbit carotid body in vitro. J. Physiol. (London), 333:81-91

Fishman, M.C., W.L. Greene, & D. Platika (1985) Oxygen chemoreception by carotid body cells in culture. Proc. Natl. Acad. Sci. (USA) 82:1448-1450

Fitzgerald, R.S. & M. Shirahata, (1992) Carotid body chemotransduction, in:"Control of Breathing and Its Modelling Perspective," Y. Honda, Y. Miyamoto, K. Konno & J.G. Widdicombe, eds., Plenum Press, New York

Folgering, H., J. Ponte & T. Sadig (1982) Adrenergic mechanisms and chemoreception in the carotid body of the cat and rabbit. J. Physiol. (London) 325:1-21

Gallagher, P.J., G. Paxinos & S.W. White (1985) The role of substance P in arterial chemoreflex control of ventilation. J. Auton. Nerv. System. 12:195-210

Gonzalez, C., L. Almaraz, A. Obeso & R. Rigual (1992) Oxygen and acid chemoreception in the carotid body chemoreceptors. TINS 15:146-153

Hansen, G., L. Jones & S. Fidone (1986) Physiological chemoreceptor stimulation decreases enkephalin and substance P in the cat carotid body. Peptides 7:767-769

Ichikawa, H. & C.J. Helke, (1993) Distribution, origin and plasticity of galanin immunoreactivity in the rat carotid body. Neurosci. 52:757-767

Kou, Y.R., G.K. Kumar & N.R. Prabhakar (1991a) Importance of substance P in the chemoreception of the carotid body in vitro. FASEB J. 5:A1118

Kou, Y.R., P. Ernsberger, P.A. Cragg, N.S. Cherniack &N.R. Prabhakar, (1991b) Role of a_2-adrenergic receptors in the carotid body response to isocapnic hypoxia. Respir. Physiol. 83:353-364

Kumar, G.K., M. Runold, R.D. Ghai, N.S. Cherniack & N.R. Prabhakar (1990) Occurrence of neutral endopeptidase activity in the cat carotid body and its significance in chemoreception. Brain Res. 517:341-343

Kummer, W., K. Addicks, M. Henkel & C. Heym (1985) Cholecystokinin-like immunoreactivity in cat extra-adrenal paraganglia. Neurosci. Lett. 55:207-210

Lahiri, S., T. Nishino, A. Mokashi & E. Mulligan (1980) Interaction of dopamine and haloperidol with O_2 and CO_2 chemoreception in carotid body. J. Appl. Physiol. 49:45-51

Lahiri, S., M. Pokorski & R.O. Davies (1981) Augmentation of carotid body chemoreceptor responses by isoproterenol in the cat. Respir. Physiol. 44:351-364

Lahiri, S., N. Smatresk, M. Pokorski, P. Barnard, A. Mokashi & K.H. McGregor (1984) Dopaminergic efferent inhibition of carotid body chemoreceptors in chronically hypoxic cats. Am. J. Physiol. 247:R24-R28

Lahiri, S., R. Iturriaga, A. Mokashi, D.K. Ray & D. Chugh (1993) CO-binding heme pigments participate in O_2 chemoreception in the carotid body. FASEB J. 7:2649

Lever, J.D. & J.D. Boyd (1957) Osmiophilic granules in glomus cells of the rabbitcarotid body. Nature 179:1082-1083

Lever, J.D., P.R. Lewis & J.D. Boyd (1959) Observations on the fine structure and histochemistry of the carotid body in the cat and rabbit. J. Anat. 93:478-490

Maxwell, D.L., R.W. Fuller, C.M.S. Dixon, F.M.C. Cuss, & P.J. Barnes (1990) Ventilatory effects of substance P, vasoactive intestinal peptide, and nitroprusside in humans. J. Appl. Physiol. 68:295-301.

McQueen, D. S. (1980) Effects of substance P on carotid chemoreceptor activity in cats, J. Physiol. (London) 302:31-47

McQueen, D.S., & J.A. Ribeiro, (1980) Inhibitory actions of methionine-enkephalin and morphine on the cat carotid chemoreceptors. Br. J. Pharmacol. 71:297-305

McQueen, D.S. & J.A. Ribeiro, (1983) On the specificity and type of receptor involved in carotid body chemoreceptor activation by adenosine in the cat. Br. J. Pharmacol. 80:347-354

Milsom, W. K. & T. Sadig (1983) Interaction between norepinephrine and hypoxia on carotid body chemoreception in rabbits. J. Appl. Physiol. 55:1893-1898

Mir, A.K., D.J. Pallot & S.R. Nahorski (1983) Biogenic amine stimulated cyclic adenosine-3', 5'-monophosphate formation in the rat carotid body. J. Neurochem. 41:663-669

Mir, A.K, D.S. McQueen, D.J. Pallot & S.R. Nahorski (1984) Direct biochemical and neuropharmacological identification of dopamine D-2 receptors in the rabbit carotid body Brain Res. 291:273-283

Monti-Bloch, L. & C. Eyzaguirre (1980) A comparative physiological and pharmacological study of cat and rabbit carotid body chemoreceptors. Brain Res. 193:449-470

Monti-Bloch, L. & C. Eyzaguirre (1985) Effects of methionine-enkephalin and substance P on the chemosensory discharge of the cat carotid body. Brain Res. 338:297-307

Nishi, K. (1975) The action of 5-hydroxytryptamine on chemoreceptor discharges of the cat's carotid body. Br. J. Pharmacol. 55:27-40

O'Regan, .R.G. (1981) Responses of carotid body chemosensory activity and blood flow to stimulation of sympathetic nerves in the cat. J. Physiol. (London) 315:81-88

Pearse, A.G.E. (1969) The cytochemistry and ultrastructure of polypeptide hormone-producing cells of the APUD series and the embryologic, physiologic and pathologic implications of the concept. J. Histochem. Cytochem. 17:303-313

Pokorski, M., & S. Lahiri (1981) Effects of naloxone on carotid body chemoreception and ventilation in the cat. J. Appl. Physiol. 51:1533-1538

Ponte, J. & C.L. Sadler (1989) Interactions between hypoxia, acetylcholine and dopamine in the carotid body of rabbit and cat. J. Physiol. (London) 410:595-610

Prabhakar, N.R., M. Runold, G.K. Kumar, N.S. Cherniack, & A. Scarpa (1989a) Substance P and mitochondrial oxygen consumption: Evidence for a direct intracellular role for the peptide. Peptides. 10:1003-1006

Prabhakar, N.R., S.C. Landis, G.K. Kumar, D.M. Kilpatrick, N.S. Cherniack & S.E. Leeman (1989b) Substance P and neurokinin-A in the cat carotid body: Localization, exogenous effects and changes in content in response to arterial PO_2. Brain Res. 481:205-214.

Prabhakar, N.R. (1992) Significance of excitatory and inhibitory neurochemicals in hypoxic chemotransmission of the carotid body. In: "Control of Breathing and Its Modelling Perspective." Y. Honda, Y. Miyamoto, K. Konno & J.G. Widdicombe. eds., Plenum Press, New York.

Prabhakar, N.R.. Y-R. Kou, P.A. Cragg & N.S. Cherniack (1992) Effect of arterial chemoreceptor stimulation: Role of norepinephrine in hypoxic chemotransmission. in: "Neurobiology and Cell Physiology of Chemoreception," P.G. Data, S. Lahiri & H. Acker, eds., Plenum Press, New York, In press .

Prabhakar, N.R., R. Sharma, F. Agani & M. Gratzl (1993a) Detection ofneurochemical release induced by chemical stimulants and hypoxia from PC-12 and carotid body cells with microvoltammetry. FASEB J. 7:2302

Prabhakar, N.R., G.K. Kumar, C.H. Chang, F.H. Agani & M.A. Haxhiu (1993b) Nitric oxide in the sensory function of the carotid body. Brain Res. 625:16-22

Prabhakar, N.R., F.H. Agani, J.L. Dinerman & S.H. Snyder (1993c) Endogenous carbon monoxide (CO) and carotid body sensory activity. Soc. Neurosci. 19:574.3

Prabhakar, N.R., H. Cao, J.A. Lowe, III & R.M. Snider (1993d) Selective inhibition of the carotid body sensory response to hypoxia by the substance P receptor antagonist CP-96,345. Proc. Natl. Acad. Sci. (USA) In press

Prabhakar, N.R. & Y.R. Kou, (1994) Inhibitory sympathetic action on the carotid body responses to sustained hypoxia. Respir. Physiol., In press

Runold, M., N.S. Cherniack & N.R. Prabhakar (1990a) Effect of adenosine on chemosensory activity of the cat aortic body. Res. Physiol. 80:299-306

Runold, M., N.S. Cherniack & N.R. Prabhakar (1990b) Effect of adenosine on isolated and superfused cat carotid body activity. Neurosci. Lett. 113:111-114 .

Schweitzer A. & S. Wright (1938) Action of prostigmin and acetylcholine on respiration. Q. J. Exp. Physiol. 28:33-47

Snyder, S.H. (1992) Nitric oxide: First in a new class of neurotransmitters. Science 257:494-496

Torrance, R.W. (1968) Prolegomena. In: "Arterial Chemoreceptors," R.W.Torrance, ed., Blackwell, Oxford

Wang, Z.-Z., L. He, L.J. Stensaas, B.G. Dinger & S.J. Fidone (1991) Localization and in vitro action of atrial natriuretic peptide in the cat carotid body. J. Appl. Physiol. 70:942-946

Wang, Z.-Z., D.S. Berdt, S.H. Snyder, S.J. Fidone & L.J. Stensaas (1992a) Nitric oxide synthase in the carotid body. Soc. Neurosci. 18:1197

Wang, Z.-Z., L.J. Stensaas, B. Dinger & S.J. Fidone (1992b) Coexistence of biogenic amines and neuropeptide in type I cells of the cat carotid body. Neurosci. 47:473-480

Ward, D.S. & M. Nino (1992) The effects of dopamine on the ventilatory response to sustained hypoxia in humans. In: "Control of Breathing and its Modelling Perspectives," Y. Honda, Y. Miyamoto, K. Konno & J.G. Widdicombe, eds., Plenum Press, New York

Zapata, P. (1975) Effects of dopamine on carotid chemo-and baroreceptors in vitro. J. Physiol. (Lond) 244:235-251

REFLEXES ARISING FROM THE ARTERIAL CHEMORECEPTORS

David J. Paterson and Piers C. G. Nye

University Laboratory of Physiology, Parks Road,
Oxford, UK. OX1 3PT

This short review gives a general survey of the reflex effects of the excitation of the arterial chemoreceptors. It focuses on responses that increase minute ventilation and those that determine the distribution of blood flow within the cardiovascular system, but also touches on influences that occur alongside these. Particular emphasis is given to discussion of the role of the carotid bodies in the generation of exercise hyperpnoea. More comprehensive coverage of this material may be found in reviews by O'Regan and Majcherczyk (1982), Eyzaguirre et al. (1983), Daly (1984), Fitzgerald & Lahiri (1986), and Cunningham (1987). The role of the carotid body in acclimatization to high altitude is covered by Bisgard's chapter in this book.

THE DRIVE TO BREATHE FROM ARTERIAL CHEMORECEPTORS

It is easy to arrange for the arterial chemoreceptors to be the sole source of the drive to breathe. This can be done by allowing an anaesthetized, hypoxic animal to hyperventilate so that its arterial PCO_2 is lowered to a value below the threshold for the reflex ventilatory effects of the central chemoreceptors. The results of such an experiment are shown in Fig. 1 where the discharge of a single chemoreceptor fibre in a hypoxic, hypocapnic cat is displayed above the pneumotachogram before and after a breath of 100% oxygen. After a 4s lung-to-carotid body circulation delay the chemoreceptor is silenced, the ongoing inspiration is terminated, and apnoea continues until the combined drive from central and peripheral chemoreceptors has risen sufficiently for breathing to return. This demonstration that the arterial chemoreceptors can assume complete responsibility for the drive to breathe requires that conditions be rigged in their favour i.e. that the animal is hypocapnic and that its 'wakefulness' drive is abolished by anaesthesia, but such conditions are not beyond the bounds met in clinical situations. Furthermore they emphasize that the primary reflex role of the carotid body is to sustain ventilation in hypoxia. They also emphasize the value of the Dejours test, the abrupt surreptitious silencing of arterial chemoreceptor discharge by one or two breaths of 100% oxygen. This is the most satisfactory way of assessing the reflex power of the arterial chemoreceptors at any given moment because it pre-empts the excitatory input from the central chemoreceptors that intervenes to replace it (Perret, 1960)

Such pre-emption is important because a rise of only 1 or 2 Torr in medullary PCO_2 can excite the more slowly responding central chemoreceptors to contribute an extra drive equal to the entire resting ventilation. It is hard to measure a rise in PCO_2 as small as this from the end-tidal or even from arterial blood gases, so longer term experiments, in which central PCO_2 has been given time to rise, often do not satisfactorily assess arterial chemoreceptor drive. Experiments in which the carotid bodies are removed surgically, or silenced by the *continuous* breathing of a hyperoxic gas mixture fall into this category. Another, more complicated technique for estimating the contribution that the arterial chemoreceptors make to the resting drive to breathe involves vascular isolation of the central and peripheral chemoreceptors so that the gas tensions of the blood perfusing them can be controlled independently (Berkenbosch et al., 1979a). These elegant and technically demanding experiments suggest that in the anaesthetized cat about 40% of the euoxic drive to breathe comes from the carotid bodies. The rat may rely on its peripheral chemoreceptors for as much as 50% of its resting drive (Cardenas & Zapata, 1983), and this includes a small contribution from aortic and abdominal chemoreceptors (Martin-Body et al., 1985; Marshall, 1987).

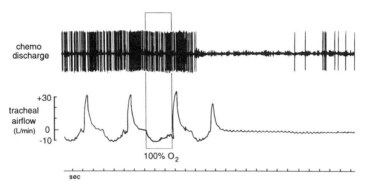

Figure 1. Chemoreceptor discharge and tracheal airflow responses to inspiration of 100% oxygen in an anaesthetized hypoxic, hypocapnic cat. Traces from top down: chemoreceptor discharge, tracheal airflow and time scale. The shaded box marks a single breath of 100% oxygen. Four to five seconds later arterial chemoreceptor discharge is silenced and apnoea starts.

The arterial chemoreceptors are the only source of the extra ventilatory drive in hypoxia. In man the carotid body alone contributes essentially all the hypoxic ventilatory drive, and this is shown in Fig. 2 where intact subjects double their isocapnic ventilation in response to a reduction of alveolar PO_2 to 50 Torr, while subjects whose carotid bodies have been removed, but whose aortic bodies are intact, do not respond to the same challenge. The dog receives a small ventilatory drive from its aortic bodies (Daly & Ungar, 1966; Hopp et al., 1991) but this amounts only to about one seventh of the combined drive from both sets of arterial chemoreceptors.

CARDIOVASCULAR ADJUSTMENTS TO HYPOXIA

The aortic bodies are widely thought to be more important than the carotid bodies in the reflex control of the circulation (Comroe & Mortimer, 1965; Daly & Ungar, 1966). They elicit reflex vasoconstriction which redistributes blood flow away from robust tissues such as the kidney, gut and resting muscle, towards the heart and brain, organs which cannot survive without a continuous supply of oxygen. A major component of this reflex redistribution of blood flow during stimulation of the arterial chemoreceptors is illustrated in Fig. 3 where the injection of sodium cyanide, which powerfully stimulates their discharge, halves femoral blood flow to hind limb skeletal muscle while it transiently stimulates breathing. The coincident bradycardia, which spares the oxygen needs of the heart, is modest in this panel but if breathing is inhibited by stimulation of the superior laryngeal nerve, or by passing water over the nasopharynx (Fig. 3B), the bradycardia can become extreme. This powerful reflex inhibition of heart rate, which occurs by the excitation of vagal motoneurones innervating the sino-atrial node, is appropriate when chemoreceptor excitation fails to bring more oxygen into the lungs and may be viewed as a last ditch attempt to conserve the tissue PO_2 of the heart. It is very pronounced during diving in animals such as the seal (e.g. Elsner et al., 1977; Daly, 1984) where it has been shown to depend upon the excitation of peripheral chemoreceptors by experiments in which normal heart rate is restored during a dive by reoxygenation of the carotid body. This 'diving reflex', which is also seen in man and which can be dramatic in some individuals (Fig. 4), is facilitated by concurrent stimulation by cold water of facial receptors running with the trigeminal nerve. The widespread peripheral vasoconstriction combined with bradycardia epitomise the underlying effects of chemoreceptor stimulation upon the cardiovascular system. This combination of responses forces most tissues to resort to anaerobic metabolism while it allows the heart and brain to draw on the substantial oxygen stores of venous blood. The overriding of bradycardia (and to some extent vasoconstriction) by breathing efforts demonstrates that gating of the reflex effects of peripheral chemoreceptor stimulation adjusts the vascular response to the immediate conditions. So long as breathing movements continue to ventilate the lungs, vagal bradycardia is blocked by synaptic inhibition arising from central respiratory neurones. The activity of pulmonary stretch receptors excited by inflation of the lungs also contributes to the gating of vagal activity (James & Daly, 1969; Daly, 1991).

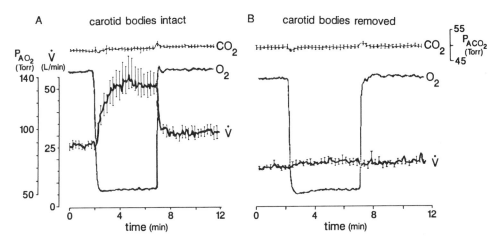

Figure 2. Ventilatory response to hypoxia with CO_2 held constant at 50 Torr in normal subjects and in subjects whose carotid bodies have been surgically removed. Both panels show P_ACO_2, P_AO_2 and ventilation (V). Ventilation is doubled by hypoxia in the intact subjects (panel A), but it does not change in subjects lacking carotid bodies (panel B). (Modified with permission from Ward & Robbins, 1987.)

The gate that controls the reflex autonomic pathway from arterial chemoreceptors is closed during inspiration, the active part of the respiratory cycle, and this contributes to sinus arrhythmia in which heart rate is slowed only during expiration. The abrupt falls in arterial blood pressure in Fig. 7 show how opening the gate by the cessation of breathing in response to Dejours tests, can dramatically reduce arterial blood pressure. A related gate occludes the reflex slowing of heart rate that results from tonic excitation of baroreceptor activity but in this case the gate is closed only by central inspiratory activity and not by the discharge of pulmonary stretch receptors (Daly et al., 1986). It too contributes to the generation of sinus arrhythmia. The reflex increase in systemic vascular resistance that diverts blood away from robust tissues is attenuated, though not abolished, by inspiratory efforts (James & Daly, 1969). This component is not observable on a breath-by-breath basis because the sympathetic influences responsible for it are mediated by second messenger systems that have slow time constants. It is interesting to note that other sensory inputs that elicit bradycardia are not gated out by inspiration. For example the reflex inhibition of heart rate which occurs in concert with rapid shallow breathing when pulmonary C-fibres are excited by drugs such as veratridine or phenylbiguanide is unaffected by inspiration (Daly, 1991; Daly & Kirkman, 1989), and similarly the reflex effects of cardiac receptors also bypass the gate (Daly & Kirkman, 1989).

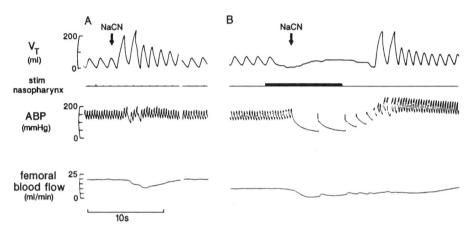

Figure 3. A. Intracarotid injection of sodium cyanide (NaCN) in a macaque monkey reflexly increases tidal volume (V_T), reduces femoral blood flow and has little effect on heart rate. B. When breathing is inhibited by passing water over the nasopharynx (solid marker) the same dose of cyanide causes a marked bradycardia which reduces arterial blood pressure in spite of the raised peripheral resistance that is indicated by the reduction in femoral blood flow. (Modified with permission from Daly et al., 1978.)

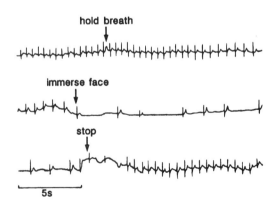

Figure 4. ECG showing the 'diving reflex' in an exercising man. Breath hold alone has little effect on heart rate, but immersion of the face in water promptly causes a pronounced bradycardia. The traces are continuous. (Modified with permission from Stromme & Blix, 1976.)

The diversion of blood flow towards the heart and brain does not depend solely on vasoconstriction in robust tissues and the relief of cardiac work by bradycardia. The redistribution of flow to the heart and brain is reinforced by reflex vasodilatation of both coronary and cerebral blood vessels and this depends at least in part on the parasympathetic nervous system (Ito & Feigl, 1985; Ponte & Purves, 1974; Hackett et al., 1972). Coronary vasodilatation is complemented by reduced ventricular contractility caused by reduced sympathetic tone, and possibly by increased vagal tone, to the ventricular myocardium (Hainsworth et al., 1979). These responses vividly illustrate that the classical dogma in which the autonomic nervous system seesaws between either parasympathetic or sympathetic activation does not always hold, for parts of both autonomic divisions are activated by chemoreceptor excitation, sympathetic vasoconstriction being combined with vagal bradycardia. The simultaneous activation of both autonomic divisions may even be directed at a single target, the sino-atrial node, for O'Donnell and Bower (1992) have shown that when the cat's carotid body is excited by hypoxia, vagal blockade by atropine can turn a parasympathetically mediated 56 beat per minute reduction in heart rate into a sympathetically mediated 28 beat per minute increase. Qualitatively similar results have been published by Little and Oberg (1975).

INTERACTION OF CHEMORECEPTOR AND BARORECEPTOR REFLEXES

The cardiovascular components of the arterial chemoreflex can have complex effects on arterial blood pressure. This is because the rapidly activated slowing of heart rate tends to reduce blood pressure while the more slowly activated peripheral vasoconstriction raises it. It is therefore normal to see a rise in arterial blood pressure when breathing efforts are preferentially gating out the bradycardia, but a fall when the powerful bradycardia of the apnoeic diving reflex is given free rein. These changes inevitably elicit substantial changes in the discharge of arterial baroreceptors, so it is not surprising to discover that the reflex effects arising from chemoreceptors are modulated by those from baroreceptors which compete for the same efferent limbs. Mancia et al. (1976) showed that severely raised baroreceptor discharge can completely override the vascular responses to chemoreceptor stimulation. Baroreceptor activation also reduces ventilatory stimulation (Attinger et al., 1976). This effect can be thought of in terms of the matching of overall ventilation and perfusion, for a raised blood pressure can signify an unnecessarily high cardiac output and a reduced need for oxygen transport within both the cardiovascular system and the lungs. (e.g. Wright, 1930; Bishop, 1974; Heistad et al., 1975; Attinger et al., 1976). In man the rise in arterial blood pressure which reflects the increase in total peripheral resistance almost invariably associated with hypoxia appears to be mediated entirely by the carotid body. This is shown by the absence of a rise in carotid body resected subjects (Honda, 1992).

OTHER REFLEX EFFECTS FROM ARTERIAL CHEMORECEPTORS

The excitation of arterial chemoreceptors has reflex effects on variables that are often overlooked in discussions of cardiovascular and ventilatory control. These include a threefold increase in the rate of tracheal secretion (Davis et al., 1982) which counters the drying influence of increased ventilation, and bronchoconstriction which is normally blocked by reflex bronchial dilatation arising from pulmonary stretch receptors. Chemoreflex bronchoconstriction may only be apparent when the airways are sensitized by the inspiration of bronchoconstrictors such as methacholine or by asthma (Denjean et al., 1991). There has also been the suggestion that oxygen's partner in metabolism, glucose, is made more available by release from the liver in response to excitation of the carotid body (Alvarez-Buylla & de Alvarez-Buylla, 1988). This harks back to the now largely forgotten condition of asphyxial hyperglycaemia known to Bernard in the nineteenth century, and studied before the discovery of the arterial chemoreceptors by Macleod (1909). The reflex effects of arterial chemoreceptor discharge on renal function are complicated by competing reflexes excited by changes in arterial and atrial pressure and by the direct effects of hypoxia on the kidney. Further complication is added by the many components of the renal response that are available for alteration. These include glomerular filtration rate, filtration fraction, and electrolyte and water reabsorption, each of which may change to give different urine flows and concentrations. Complicated influences give complicated responses, reflected by reports that hypoxia may either increase or decrease urine flow and the reabsorption of sodium. The results of experiments on anaesthetized animals are matched by those on subjects at altitude, for both diuresis and anuresis are reported (Ward et al., 1989). Honig's group (Honig, 1989) have emphasized the tendency of hypoxia to raise haematocrit rapidly by a natriuretic increase in urine flow, increased reabsorption of plasma in systemic tissues, and reduced thirst. The increased excretion of sodium survives denervation of the kidney but not denervation of the carotid body (Karim et al., 1987) so although it originates in the carotid body it has a humoral component and is therefore not strictly a reflex response. The purely reflex effects of carotid body stimulation on renal function recorded at constant arterial blood pressure and without systemic hypoxia act by increasing the discharge of the renal sympathetic nerves. This preferentially constricts the afferent arterioles, reducing glomerular filtration rate and filtration fraction as well as renal blood flow. There is also a concurrent reduction in sodium excretion and urine flow (Karim et al., 1987). It seems therefore that, in the short term, the reflex effects of the carotid body on renal function complement those on the circulations of skeletal muscle, intestine and other splanchnic organs. They are primarily concerned with the diversion of blood flow away from the kidney (Al-Obaidi & Karim, 1992), a response that almost inevitably reduces urine flow. Humoral influences tending to increase urine flow may become more important when hypoxia is sustained for hours rather than minutes. Like their effects on other vascular beds, the arterial baro- and chemoreflexes compete for control of renal function. Activation of the former reduces sympathetic tone while activation of the latter increases it. If baroreceptor activity is intense it can reveal underlying responses to chemoreceptor activation that are of the opposite sign to those normally expressed, i.e. excitation of the chemoreceptors now increases urine flow and sodium excretion (Karim & Al-Obaidi, 1993). Raised plasma osmolality has been reported to inhibit the discharge of arterial chemoreceptors in the intact cat (Gallego & Belmonte, 1979). This inhibition contrasts with the excitation reported in isolated carotid bodies (Gallego et al., 1979) and it presumably results from reduction in the resistance of the vessels perfusing the organ. The effect requires a physiologically large (5%) change in osmolality before any change in discharge is observed.

OSCILLATIONS OF DISCHARGE AND THE DRIVE TO BREATHE

Gating of the reflex effects of chemoreceptor discharge by the respiratory cycle is not confined to cardiovascular responses. It can also be seen in the pattern of breathing. Here the behaviour of the gate differs from that of its cardiovascular counterpart because instead of closing in inspiration it opens, allowing excitation to have its maximal effect on ventilation during this phase (Black & Torrance, 1971; Eldridge, 1972). Much has been made of the possible significance that this phase-dependent excitation of ventilation by chemoreceptor discharge may have in exercise because it may select parts of the natural oscillation of chemoreceptor discharge that occurs with each breath. For example it is possible that, with a four second respiratory cycle and a four or five second lung-to-carotid body circulation delay, the open gate would allow only the troughs of the oscillating chemoreceptor discharge to pass at rest, while the altered respiratory cycle duration and circulation delay of exercise might result in passage of the peaks. There is little direct evidence for such an arrangement but if it exists it would enhance the effective mean discharge of chemoreceptors even in the absence of a rise in the true mean level of either discharge or arterial gas tensions (see Cunningham, 1975).

INTERACTION OF VENTILATORY INFLUENCES FROM PERIPHERAL AND CENTRAL CHEMORECEPTORS

The effects of hypoxia and carbon dioxide on chemoreceptor discharge are not simply additive. They multiply, giving a fan of response lines, with sensitivity to CO_2 increasing in hypoxia (Fig. 5). This fan is similar to that observed when ventilation is plotted against P_ACO_2, and it is reasonable to ask whether the former can account entirely for the latter or whether there is further interaction in the brainstem between peripheral and central chemoreceptor input. The supposition that it may take more than just the fan of discharge to give the fan of ventilation is given substance by the observation that the point at which the CO_2-response lines converge is close to 20 Torr for discharge (in the cat, Fitzgerald & Parks, 1971; Lahiri & Delaney, 1975; Nye & Painter, 1989) and close to 40 Torr for ventilation (in man, Lloyd & Cunningham, 1963). The question is not easily resolved in man because chemoreceptor discharge cannot be recorded, but it appears that in the cat, which has a low resting P_ACO_2, the point of convergence of the ventilatory lines is close to that of discharge (DeGoede et al., 1981) and the fan is generated entirely by the peripheral chemoreceptors (Berkenbosch et al., 1979b). In this species the ventilatory responses to excitation of peripheral and central chemoreceptor inputs are therefore purely additive (Heeringa et al., 1979; Berkenbosch et al., 1984). However, the situation may not be so simple in man because, as pointed out by Robbins (1989), although ventilation is insensitive to CO_2 in hypocapnia, giving the 'dogleg' of Fig. 5, it is nevertheless excited by hypoxia in this range. This suggests that in man the peripheral chemoreceptors are active in hypocapnia below the point at which the ventilatory lines converge i.e. below the threshold at which the reflex effects of the central chemoreceptors appear. The cat is, appropriately, reported by some (Berkenbosch et al., 1984) to lack a dog-leg, though Grunstein et al. (1975) do show one.

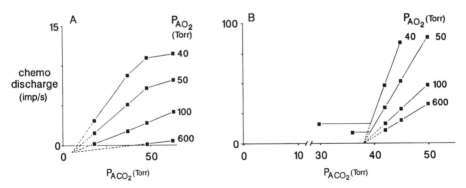

Figure 5. Hypoxic enhancement of CO_2-sensitivity of carotid body discharge (A) and of ventilation (B) giving similar fans. Discharge was recorded in the cat (Nye & Painter, 1989) and ventilation was recorded in man (Lloyd & Cunningham, 1963). B shows the 'dog-legs' that occur below ca. 40 Torr PCO_2. Here hypoxia has little or no effect on ventilatory sensitivity to CO_2 but it does increase ventilation.

THE ARTERIAL CHEMOREFLEX IN EXERCISE

During exercise, ventilation (V_E) increases in direct proportion to CO_2 production (VCO_2) until the intensity of exercise is greater than approximately 60% of maximum achievable work rate. At this point V_E increases disproportionately to increases in VCO_2. This point is known as the 'ventilatory threshold' or 'anaerobic threshold' because it coincides with the reduction in arterial pH caused by the release of lactic acid from anaerobic metabolism. The arterial chemoreceptors are shown to be responsible for this threshold as subjects without carotid bodies (Wasserman et al., 1975) and subjects lacking respiratory chemoreception (Shea et al., 1993) fail to compensate for the build-up of metabolites by hyperventilating - they lack an anaerobic threshold. It is now well established that exercise increases the 'hypoxic sensitivity' of the arterial chemoreflex in direct proportion to the rise in VCO_2 (Douglas et al., 1913; Cunningham et al., 1966; Weil et al., 1972) and that this increased sensitivity determines the position of the anaerobic threshold. This concept is illustrated in Fig. 6 which shows observations made by Douglas at the turn of the century. In these the slope of the V_E/VCO_2 relationship in exercise was steeper at altitude ($P_{A}O_2$ ca. 60 Torr) than it was at sea level. However, the mechanisms that regulate the increased hypoxic gain of the arterial chemoreflex in exercise have not been fully resolved.

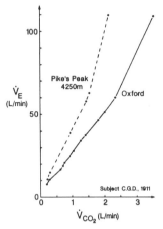

Figure 6. The ventilatory response of C.G. Douglas to several intensities of exercise near sea level (Oxford, 55 m) and at an altitude of 4250 m (Pike's Peak, Colorado, ca. 60 Torr $P_{A}O_2$). Note that the ventilatory response to exercise is markedly increased by hypoxia.

EXERCISE BELOW THE ANAEROBIC THRESHOLD

It is still widely believed that light exercise causes little change in the sensitivity of the arterial chemoreflex, however Cunningham et al. (1966) observed that light exercise can potentiate the sensitivity of the carotid bodies, noting that the ventilatory response to two breaths of hypoxia was greater in exercise than at rest. This idea was further developed and quantified by Weil et al. (1972) who showed that very mild exercise enhances the hypoxic ventilatory drive, an effect that increases in proportion to the intensity of exercise (Fig. 7). If a two or three breaths of 100% oxygen (the Dejours test) are given during light steady-state exercise, below the anaerobic threshold so there is no lactic acid to excite the arterial chemoreceptors, ventilation is reduced within a few seconds (Perret, 1960; Dejours, 1962). This shows that the absolute contribution that the arterial chemoreceptors make to ventilatory drive increases progressively as ventilation rises towards its new steady state (Cunningham et al., 1968). The progressively increasing role of the carotid bodies during this rise is underlined by the observation that the rate of rise is slower in hyperoxia (Griffiths et al., 1986) and after surgical removal of the carotid bodies (Wasserman et al., 1975). Furthermore hypoxia increases the time constant of the transient. The transient is also slowed by beta adrenergic blockade and this has led some workers to propose that the slowed ventilatory response is caused by a reduced cardiac output - cardiodynamic hyperpnoea (Petersen et al., 1983). However, beta blockade markedly reduces carotid body discharge and its sensitivity to both hypoxia (Folgering et al., 1982) and potassium (Paterson & Nye, 1988), so it is likely that the slower rise in ventilation results from direct inhibition of the carotid body rather than from a lack of excitation acting indirectly via the heart.

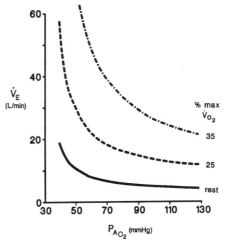

Figure 7. Ventilatory response to hypoxia during mild to moderate levels of exercise in man. Sensitivity to hypoxia is increased markedly at levels of oxygen consumption that are not associated with excitatory changes in the pH, PCO_2 or PO_2 of arterial blood (Reproduced with permission from Weil et al. 1972)

Interestingly, subjects with congenital central hypoventilation syndrome who have no functional peripheral or central chemosensitivity have a normal ventilatory response in aerobic exercise (Shea et al., 1993): they maintain isocapnic buffering without chemical feedback. This shows that respiratory chemoreception is not essential for the control of ventilation during aerobic exercise, an observation which highlights the redundancy that nature has built into the respiratory control system.

EXERCISE ABOVE THE ANAEROBIC THRESHOLD

It is generally accepted that the increase in ventilatory sensitivity to VCO_2 above the anaerobic threshold is mediated by the carotid bodies (Wasserman et al., 1975), an idea supported by the observation that subjects whose carotid bodies have been removed, and subjects born insensitive to changes in arterial blood gas tensions (Shea et al., 1993), do not have an anaerobic threshold. Acidosis is traditionally regarded as the prime signal that stimulates the carotid bodies to cause this extra increase in ventilation. However, many studies now cast doubt on whether acid is the only, or indeed the mandatory stimulus for this response. For example, patients with McArdle's syndrome cannot produce acid during exercise yet they still have the well established threshold (Hagberg et al., 1982) and subjects who have undergone glycogen depletion to reduce the amount of substrate available for lactic acid production also have an anaerobic threshold that is independent of changes in arterial pH (Heigenhauser et al., 1983; Busse et al., 1991). Using the Dejours test to assess ventilatory drive from the arterial chemoreflex during air-breathing ramp increases in work rate presents a paradox, because it results in very little reduction in ventilation even at exercise intensities that result in substantial increases in lactic acid concentration (unpublished observations by Burleigh and Robbins from our Laboratory). This suggests that either the carotid bodies are not involved in the unsteady-state ventilatory response to exercise, that hyperoxia does not silence their activity during incremental exercise, or that other inputs can very quickly assume the role of the carotid body. However, when the Dejours test is given in heavy steady-state, air-breathing exercise there is an abrupt and large reduction in ventilation before there are any significant changes in the concentration of lactic acid (Asmussen & Nielsen, 1946).

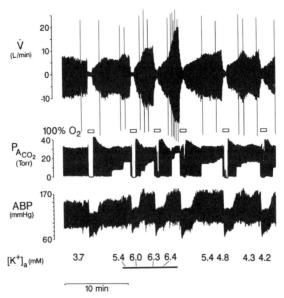

Figure 8. Ventilatory response of a hypoxic (P_aO_2 39 Torr) rhesus monkey to abrupt switches of 100% oxygen (hollow boxes) before, during and after a KCl infusion (horizontal bar). Traces from the top down: tracheal airflow, alveolar PCO_2 and arterial blood pressure (ABP). CO_2 was added to the inspirate to keep P_ACO_2 constant when ventilation rose. A switch to 100% O2 virtually abolished the excitation of ventilation by hyperkalaemia. When the KCl was stopped, ventilation decreased with the fall in $[K^+]_a$. (Reproduced with permission from Paterson et al., 1992).

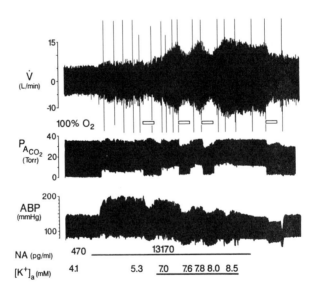

Figure 9. Ventilatory response of a euoxic (P_aO_2 100 Torr) monkey to abrupt switches of 100% oxygen (hollow boxes) during concurrent infusions of noradrenaline (NA) and KCl (horizontal bars). Traces from the top down: tracheal airflow, alveolar PCO_2, arterial blood pressure (ABP). Note that NA caused a small increase in ventilation and that hyperoxia had little effect on ventilation during the NA infusion. When KCl was added in the presence of the NA infusion, there was a marked increase in ventilation which was reduced by hyperoxia. (Reproduced with permission from Paterson et al., 1992).

This led to the idea that a chemical released from working muscle, an 'anaerobic work substance', excites the carotid bodies. The short latency of the ventilatory response to the Dejours test was accounted for by assuming that the substance was rapidly inactivated by high oxygen.

Recent work has suggested that exercise-induced hyperkalaemia fulfils many of the criteria of the anaerobic work substance. Potassium is released from contracting muscle in direct proportion to VCO_2. It is well correlated with V_E in normal subjects (Paterson et al., 1989; Busse et al., 1991), in patients with McArdle's syndrome (Paterson et al., 1990) and in glycogen-depleted subjects (Busse et al., 1991). Band et al. (1985) first showed that physiological levels of hyperkalaemia excite ventilation by direct excitation of the arterial chemoreceptors in the anaesthetized cat. The effect of potassium on chemoreceptor discharge is markedly sensitive to oxygen, being much greater in hypoxia and almost absent in high oxygen (Burger et al., 1988). This makes it behave as if, like the hypothetical anaerobic work substance, it is rapidly inactivated by a rise in arterial oxygen. In the decerebrate cat (Paterson & Nye, 1991) and sedated rhesus monkey (Paterson et al., 1992) hyperkalaemia markedly increases ventilation during hypoxia and the Dejours test essentially abolishes its stimulatory effect (Fig. 8). Raised plasma noradrenaline also increases ventilation in euoxia, an effect enhanced in the monkey by hyperkalaemia (Fig. 9). We have recently observed that the excitation of the cat's carotid body discharge by noradrenaline and hyperkalaemia interact additively (unpublished observation from this laboratory). McLoughlin et al. (1992) also report that lactic acid potentiates the discharge of the arterial chemoreflex in hyperkalaemia.

THE MECHANISM RESPONSIBLE FOR ENHANCEMENT OF THE ARTERIAL CHEMOREFLEX IN EXERCISE

Several candidates have been considered to be possible contributors to the enhanced role of the carotid body in exercise. For example potassium increases the sensitivity of the arterial chemoreflex and interacts multiplicatively with hypoxia to provide a powerful drive to breathe. Qayyum et al. (1994) observed that modestly raising the concentration of arterial plasma potassium (by ca. 1mM), by drinking 64 mmoles of KCl, significantly increases hypoxic ventilation both at rest and in light exercise. This provided the first direct evidence that modest rises in plasma potassium can modulate the sensitivity of the arterial chemoreceptor reflex in conscious man.

Potassium is not the only chemical factor that can enhance the sensitivity of the ventilatory reflex. Both acidosis and raised catecholamines increase chemoreceptor discharge and ventilation (McLoughlin et al., 1992; Cunningham et al., 1963; O'Regan & Majcherczyk, 1982) and the effects of these stimuli are also increased in hypoxia and markedly reduced in high oxygen. Thus it would not be surprising to find a three-way interaction among exercise-induced changes in potassium, acid and catecholamines that enhances the sensitivity of the peripheral chemoreflex, the efficacy of this response being modulated by oxygen. In addition the peripheral chemoreceptor reflex loop may be enhanced by descending pathways from hypothalamic and cortical projections (Eldridge et al., 1981).

Finally, the contribution that the arterial chemoreflex makes to the control of exercise hyperpnoea is far from settled. There are clear species differences that show little role for this reflex in exercise in some animals (e.g. pony, Forster et al., 1983). However, the Dejours test reveals that, at least in man, the carotid bodies play an important role in the matching of ventilation to metabolic rate in exercise, and that the by-products of heavy exercise modulate the sensitivity of the arterial chemoreflex.

We gratefully acknowledge discussion with and help from Dr Rosie Painter in preparing and reviewing both the text and figures.

REFERENCES

Al-Obaidi, M., & Karim, F. (1992). Primary effects of carotid chemoreceptor stimulation on gracilis muscle and renal blood flow and renal function in dogs. J. Physiol. 455:73-88.

Alvarez-Buylla, R., & de Alvarez-Buylla, E.R. (1988). Carotid sinus receptors participate in glucose homeostasis. Respir. Physiol. 72:347-359.

Asmussen, E., & Nielsen, M. (1946). Studies on the regulation of respiration in heavy work. Acta Physiol. Scand. 12:171-188.

Attinger, F.M., Attinger, E.O., Cooperson, D., & Gottschalk, W. (1976). Interactions between carotid sinus mechanoreceptor and chemoreceptor reflex loops. Pflugers Arch. 363:255-261.

Band, D.M., Linton, R.A.F., Kent, R., & Kurer, F.L. (1985). The effect of peripheral chemodenervation on the ventilatory response to potassium. Respir. Physiol. 60:217-225.

Berkenbosch, A., Heeringa, J., Olievier, C.N., & Kruyt, E.W. (1979a). Artificial perfusion of the ponto-medullary region of cats. A method for separation of central and peripheral effects of chemical stimulation of ventilation. Respir. Physiol. 37:347-364.

Berkenbosch, A., Van Dissel, J., Olievier, C.N., DeGoede, J., & Heeringa, J. (1979b). The contribution of the peripheral chemoreceptors to the ventilatory response to CO2 in anaesthetized cats during hyperoxia. Respir. Physiol. 37:381-390.

Berkenbosch, A., Van Beek, J.H.G.M., Olievier, C.N., DeGoede, J., & Quanjer, P.H.H. (1984). Central respiratory CO2 sensitivity at extreme hypocapnia. Respir. Physiol. 55:95-102.

Bishop, B. (1974). Carotid baroreceptor modulation of diaphragm and abdominal muscle activity in the cat. J. Appl. Physiol. 36:12-19.

Black, A.M.S., & Torrance, R.W. (1971). Respiratory oscillations in chemoreceptor discharge in the control of breathing. Respir. Physiol. 13:221-237.

Burger, R.E., Estavillo, J.A., Kumar, P., Nye, P.C.G., & Paterson, D.J. (1988). Effects of potassium, oxygen and carbon dioxide on the steady-state discharge of cat carotid body chemoreceptors. J. Physiol. 401:519-531.

Busse, M.W., Maassen, N., & Konrad, H. (1991). Relation between plasma K+ and ventilation during incremental exercise after glycogen depletion and repletion in man. J. Physiol. 443:469-476.

Cardenas, H., & Zapata, P. (1983). Ventilatory reflexes originated from carotid and extracarotid chemoreceptors in rats. Am. J. Physiol. 244:R119-R125.

Comroe, J.H., & Mortimer, L. (1965). The respiratory and cardiovascular responses of temporally separated aortic and carotid bodies to cyanide, nicotine, phenyldiguanide and serotonin. J. Pharmac. Exp. Ther. 146:33-41.

Cunningham, D.J.C. (1975). A model illustrating the importance of timing in the regulation of breathing. Nature. 253:440-442.

Cunningham, D.J.C. (1987). Studies on arterial chemoreceptors in man. J. Physiol. 384:1-26.

Cunningham, D.J.C., Hey, E.N., Patrick, J.M., & Lloyd, B.B. (1963). The effect of noradrenaline infusion on the relation between pulmonary ventilation and the alveolar PO2 and PCO2 in man. Ann. NY Acad. Sci. 109:756-771.

Cunningham, D.J.C., Lloyd, B.B., & Spurr, D. (1966). Doubts about the 'anaerobic work substance' as a stimulus to breathing in exercise. J. Physiol. 186:110-111.

Cunningham, D.J.C., Spurr, D., & Lloyd, B.B. (1968). The drive to ventilation from arterial chemoreceptors in hypoxic exercise. In "Arterial Chemoreceptors." R.W. Torrance, ed., Blackwell, Oxford pp. 301-323.

Daly, M.deB. (1984). Breath-hold diving: mechanisms of cardiovascular adjustments in the mammal. In "Recent Advances in Physiology." vol 10. P.F. Baker., ed., Churchill Livingstone, pp. 201-245.

Daly, M.deB. (1991). Some reflex cardioinhibitory responses in the cat and their modulation by central inspiratory neuronal activity. J. Physiol. 439:559-577.

Daly, M.deB., & Ungar, A. (1966). Comparison of the reflex responses elicited by stimulation of the separately perfused carotid and aortic body chemoreceptors in the dog. J. Physiol. 182:379-403.

Daly, M.deB., Korner, P.I., Angell James, J.E., & Oliver, J.R. (1978). Cardiovascular-respiratory reflex interactions between carotid bodies and upper-airways receptors in the monkey. Am. J. Physiol. 234:H293-H299.

Daly, M.deB., Ward, J., & Wood, L.M. (1986). Modification by lung inflation of the vascular responses from the carotid body chemoreceptors and other receptors in dogs. J. Physiol. 378:13-30.

Daly, M.deB., & Kirkman, E. (1989). Differential modulation by pulmonary stretch afferents of some reflex cardioinhibitory responses in the cat. J. Physiol. 417:323-341.

Davis, B., Chinn, R., Gold, J., Popovac, D., Widdicombe, J.G., & Nadel, J.A. (1982). Hypoxemia reflexly increases secretion from tracheal submucosal glands in dogs. J. Appl. Physiol. 52:1416-1419.

DeGoede, J., Berkenbosch, A., Olievier, C.N. & Quanjer, P.H.H. (1981). Ventilatory response to carbon dioxide and apnoeic thresholds. Respir. Physiol. 45:185-199.

Dejours, P. (1962). Chemoreflexes in breathing. Physiol. Rev. 42:335-358.

Denjean, A., Canet, E., Praud, J.P., Gaultier, C., Bureau, M., & Gagne, B. (1991). Hypoxia-induced bronchial responsiveness in awake sheep: Role of carotid chemoreceptors. Respir. Physiol. 83:201-210.

Douglas, C.G., Haldane, J.S., Henderson, Y., & Schneider, E.C. (1913). Physiological observations made on Pike's Peak, Colorado, with special reference to adaptation to low barometric pressures. Phil. Trans. Roy. Soc. B 203:185-318.

Eldridge, F.L. (1972). The importance of timing on the respiratory effects of intermittent carotid body stimulation. J. Physiol. 222:319-333.

Eldridge, F.L., Millhorn, D.E., & Waldrop, T.G. (1981). Exercise hyperpnea and locomotion: parallel activation from the hypothalamus. Science. 211:844-846.

Elsner, R., Angell James, J.E., & Daly, M.deB. (1977). Carotid body chemoreceptor reflexes and their interactions in the seal. Am. J. Physiol. 232:H517-H525.

Eyzaguirre, C., Fitzgerald, R.S., Lahiri, S. & Zapata, P. (1983). Arterial Chemoreceptors. In "Handbook of Physiology. The Cardiovascular System." vol III. American Physiological Society. Bethesda Maryland, pp. 557-621.

Fitzgerald, R.S., & Parks, D.C. (1971). Effect of hypoxia on carotid chemoreceptor response to carbon dioxide in cats. Respir. Physiol. 12:218-229.

Fitzgerald, R.S. & Lahiri, S. (1986). Reflex Responses to Chemoreceptor Stimulation. In "Handbook of Physiology. The Respiratory System." vol II pt 1. American Physiological Society. Bethesda Maryland, pp. 313-362.

Forster, H.V., Pan, L.G., Bisgard, G.E., Kaminski, R.P., Dorsey, S.M., & Busch, M.A. (1983). Hyperpnea of exercise at various PIO2 in normal and carotid body-denervated ponies. J. Appl. Physiol. 54:1387-1393.

Gallego, R., & Belmonte, C. (1979). The effects of blood osmolality changes on cat carotid body chemoreceptors in vivo. Pflugers Arch. 380:53-58.

Gallego, R., Eyzaguirre, C., & Monti-Bloch, L. (1979). Thermal and osmotic responses of arterial receptors. J. Neurophysiol. 42:665-680.

Griffiths, T.L., Henson, L.C., & Whipp, B.J. (1986). Influence of inspired oxygen concentration on the dynamics of the exercise hyperpnoea in man. J. Physiol. 380:387-403.

Grunstein, M.M., Derenne, J.P. & Milic-Emili, J. (1975). Control of depth and frequency of breathing during baroreceptor stimulation in cats. J. Appl. Physiol. 39:395-404.

Guazzi, M., Baccelli, G., & Zanchetti, A. (1968). Reflex chemoceptive regulation of arterial pressure during natural sleep in the cat. Am. J. Physiol. 214:969-978.

Hackett, J.G., Abboud, F.M., Mark, A.L., Schmid, P.G., & Heistad, D.D. (1972). Coronary vascular responses to stimulation of chemoreceptors and baroreceptors: evidence for reflex activation of vagal cholinergic innervation. Circ. Res. 31:8-17.

Hagberg, J.M., Coyle, E.F., Carroll, J.E., Miller, J.M., Martin, W.H., & Brooke, M.H. (1982). Exercise hyperventilation in patients with McArdle's disease. J. Appl. Physiol. 52(4):991-994.

Hainsworth, R., Karim, F., & Sofola, O.A. (1979). Left ventricular inotropic responses to stimulation of carotid body chemoreceptors in anaesthetized dogs. J. Physiol. 287:455-466.

Heeringa, J., Berkenbosch, A., DeGoede, J., & Olievier, C.N. (1979). Relative contribution of central and peripheral chemoreceptors to the ventilatory response to CO2 during hyperoxia. Respir. Physiol. 37:365-379.

Heigenhauser, G.J.F., Sutton, J.R., & Jones, N.L. (1983). Effect of glycogen depletion on the ventilatory response to exercise. J. Appl. Physiol. 54(2):470-474.

Heistad, D., Abboud, F.M., Mark, A.L., & Schmid, P.G. (1975). Effect of baroreceptor activity on ventilatory response to chemoreceptor stimulation. J. Appl. Physiol. 39:411-416.

Honda, Y. (1992). Respiratory and circulatory activities in carotid body-resected humans. J. Appl. Physiol. 73:1-8.

Honig, A. (1989). Peripheral arterial chemoreceptors and reflex control of sodium and water homeostasis. Am. J. Physiol. 257:R1282-R1302.

Hopp, F.A., Seagard, J.L., Bajic, J., & Zuperku, E.J. (1991). Respiratory responses to aortic and carotid chemoreceptor activation in the dog. J. Appl. Physiol. 70:2539-2550.

Ito, B.R., & Feigl, E.O. (1985). Carotid chemoreceptor reflex parasympathetic coronary vasodilation in the dog. Am. J. Physiol. 249:H1167-H1175.

James, J.E., & Daly, M.deB. (1969). Cardiovascular responses in apnoeic asphyxia: role of arterial chemoreceptors and the modification of their effects by a pulmonary vagal inflation reflex. J. Physiol. 201:87-104.

Karim, F., Poucher, S.M., & Summerill, R.A. (1987). The effects of stimulating carotid chemoreceptors on renal haemodynamics and function in dogs. J. Physiol. 392:451-462.

Karim, F., & Al-Obaidi, M. (1993). Modification of carotid chemoreceptor-induced changes in renal haemodynamics and function by carotid baroreflex in dogs. J. Physiol. 466:599-610.

Lahiri, S., & Delaney, R.G. (1975). Stimulus interaction in the responses of carotid body chemoreceptor single afferent fibres. Resp. Physiol. 24:249-266.

Little, R., & Oberg, B. (1975). Circulatory responses to stimulation of the carotid body chemoreceptors in the cat. Acta Physiol. Scand. 93:34-50.

Lloyd, B.B., & Cunningham, D.J.C. (1963). A quantitative approach to the regulation of human respiration. In "The Regulation of Human Respiration." D.J.C. Cunningham & B.B. Lloyd, eds., Blackwell,Oxford, pp. 331-349.

Macleod, J.J.R. (1909). Studies in experimental glycosuria: IV. The cause of hyperglycaemia produced by asphyxia. Am. J. Physiol. 23:278-302.

Mancia, G., Shepherd, J.T., & Donald, D.E. (1976). Interplay among carotid sinus, cardiopulmonary, and carotid body reflexes in dogs. Am. J. Physiol. 230:19-24.

Marshall, J.M. (1987). Analysis of cardiovascular responses evoked following changes in peripheral chemoreceptor activity in the rat. J. Physiol. 394:393-414.

Martin-Body, R.L., Robson, R.J., & Sinclair, J.D. (1985). Respiratory effects of sectioning the carotid sinus glossopharyngeal and abdominal vagal nerves in the awake rat. J. Physiol. 361:35-45.

McLoughlin, P., Linton, R.A.F., & Band, D.M. (1992). The effect of intravenous infusions of KCl and lactic acid on ventilation in anaesthetised cats. J. Physiol. 446:426P.

Nye, P.C.G., & Painter, R. (1989). Quantifying the steady-state discharge of the carotid body of the anaesthetized cat. J. Physiol. 417:172P.

O'Donnell, C.P., & Bower, E.A. (1992). Heart rate changes evoked by hypoxia in the anaesthetized, artificially ventilated cat. Exp. Physiol. 77:271-283.

O'Regan, R.G., & Majcherczyk, S. (1982). Role of peripheral chemoreceptors and central chemosensitivity in the regulation of respiration and circulation. J. Exp. Biol. 100:23-40.

Paterson, D.J., & Nye, P.C.G. (1988). The effect of beta adrenergic blockade on the carotid body response to hyperkalaemia in the cat. Respir. Physiol. 74:229-238.

Paterson, D.J., Robbins, P.A., & Conway, J. (1989). Changes in arterial plasma potassium and ventilation during exercise in man. Respir. Physiol. 78:323-330.

Paterson, D.J., Friedland, J.S., Bascom, D.A., Clement, I.D., Cunningham, D. A., Painter, R., & Robbins, P.A. (1990). Changes in arterial K+ and ventilation during exercise in normal subjects and subjects with McArdle's syndrome. J. Physiol. 429:339-348.

Paterson, D.J., & Nye, P.C.G. (1991). Effect of oxygen on potassium-excited ventilation in the decerebrate cat. Respir. Physiol. 84:223-230.

Paterson, D.J., Dorrington, K.L., Bergel, D.H., Kerr, G., Miall, R.C., Stein, J.F., & Nye, P.C.G. (1992). Effect of potassium on ventilation in the rhesus monkey. Exp. Physiol. 77(1):217-220.

Perret, C. (1960). Hyperoxie et regulation de la ventilation durant l'exercice musculaire. Helv. Physiol. et Pharmacol. Acta. 18:72-97.

Petersen, E.S., Whipp, B.J., Davis, J.A., Huntsman, D.J., Brown, H.V., & Wasserman, K. (1983). Effects of beta-adrenergic blockade on ventilation and gas exchange during exercise in humans. J. Appl. Physiol. 54:1306-1313.

Ponte, J., & Purves, M.J. (1974). The role of the carotid body chemoreceptors and carotid sinus baroreceptors in the control of cerebral blood vessels. J. Physiol. 237:315-340.

Qayyum, M.S., Barlow, C.W., Paterson, D.J., & Robbins, P.A. (1993). Increased ventilatory sensitivity to hypoxia with raised arterial potassium concentration at rest and during exercise in man. J. Physiol. (in press).

Robbins, P.A. (1989). Design and analysis of experiments for studying hypoxia-hypercapnia interactions in respiratory control. In "Modeling and parameter estimation in respiratory control." M.C.K. Khoo, ed., Plenum,New York, pp.83-89.

Shea, S.A., Andres, L.P., Shannon, D.C., & Banzett, R.B. (1993). Ventilatory responses to exercise in humans lacking ventilatory chemosensitivity. J. Physiol. 468:623-640.

Stromme, S.B., & Blix, A.S. (1976). Indirect evidence for arterial chemoreceptor reflex facilitation by face immersion in man. Aviat. Space Environ. Med. 47:597-599.

Ward, M.P., Milledge, J.S., & West, J.B. (1989). Acute Mountain Sickness. In "High Altitude Medicine and Physiology." University of Pennsylvania Press, pp. 369-379.

Ward, S.A., & Robbins, P.A. (1987). The ventilatory response to hypoxia. In "The Control of Breathing in Man." B.J. Whipp, ed., Manchester University Press, pp. 29-44.

Wasserman, K., Whipp, B.J., Koyal, S.N., & Cleary, M.G. (1975). Effect of carotid body resection on ventilatory and acid-base control during exercise. J. Appl. Physiol. 39:354-358.

Weil, J.V., Byrne-Quinn, E., Sodal, I.E., Kline, J.S., McCullough, R.E., & Filley, G.F. (1972). Augmentation of chemosensitivity during mild exercise in normal man. J. Appl. Physiol. 33(6):813-819.

Wright, S. (1930). Action of adrenaline and related substances on respiration. J. Physiol. 69:493-499.

CENTRAL INTEGRATION OF CHEMORECEPTOR AFFERENT ACTIVITY

David Jordan

Department of Physiology, Royal Free Hospital School of Medicine,
Rowland Hill Street, London, NW3 2PF

There is an abundance of literature concerning the possible transduction mechanisms and neurotransmitters that act within the carotid body, the activity of carotid chemoreceptor afferents to various stimulants, and the reflex effects produced by altering chemoreceptor afferent discharge. However, relatively little information is available regarding the mechanisms which intervene between the activity in the afferent nerve fibres and the alterations evoked in motor outflow. In this short review I will summarise what is known regarding the sites of termination of arterial chemoreceptor afferents and the integration of these afferents with other afferent inputs, respiration, and higher centres at the second and higher order neurones. In addition, these will be compared to the pathways underlying the responses evoked by a second set of chemoreceptor afferents, those arising from the pulmonary chemoreceptor afferents variously termed "J-receptors", "pulmonary C-fibre afferents" or "pulmonary chemoreceptor afferents". When activated these afferents evoke a marked vagal bradycardia, a depressor response and either rapid shallow breathing or apnoea. These afferents are of interest since the bradycardia they evoke is unaffected by respiratory gating (Daly & Kirkman, 1989; Daly, 1991) whereas the bradycardia evoked by arterial chemoreceptor or baroreceptor afferents is powerfully gated both by the central respiratory cycle and lung inflation (Daly, 1986; Davidson et al., 1976). This may suggest that the central mechanisms underlying the two chemoreceptor reflexes are fundamentally different. Hence, it is worth comparing the pathways responsible for both reflexes. The effects of these two types of afferent on the relevant motor neuronal pools has been discussed elsewhere in this volume (Jones et al., 1994) and will not be discussed in detail here.

BRAINSTEM TERMINATIONS OF CHEMORECEPTOR AFFERENTS

Afferent fibres travelling in the carotid sinus and vagus nerves terminate almost entirely within the dorsomedial medulla, in the nucleus tractus solitarius (NTS), with a few terminating in the area postrema and trigeminal nucleus. These terminations were first demonstrated by anatomical techniques utilising degeneration techniques (Cottle, 1964). However, they have been visualised recently with more sensitive techniques utilising anterograde transport of tracer substances such as tritiated amino acids or horseradish peroxidase (HRP) and its conjugates. These tracers are taken up from the cut ends of nerves or following injection into tissues and then transported anterogradely to the terminations of the afferent fibres where they can be visualised histologically. Much of the earlier data has been reviewed in full (Jordan & Spyer, 1986) so only a summary will be provided here. The NTS is a longitudinal nucleus spanning the length of the medulla oblongata. It has been divided into several subnuclei based both on cytoarchitectonic features, and on the basis of the inputs and outputs of the various subnuclei (Loewy & Burton, 1978). Following application of HRP to the central cut ends of the IXth and Xth nerves (Ciriello et al, 1981b) reaction product was localised ipsilaterally in most of the NTS subnuclei, although the relative density of terminations varied. In addition, there was an innervation of the contralateral medial and commissural subnuclei. These terminations will include all the vagal and glossopharyngeal afferents.

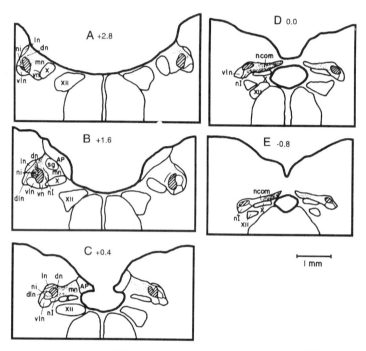

Figure 1. Schematic representations of the cat dorsomedial medulla showing the NTS and its subnuclei. Sections are ordered in mm relative to obex (D) from rostral (A) to caudal (E). They illustrate the location of WGA-HRP labelled terminals (fine dots) in relation to the tractus solitarius (hatched) after injecting the tracer into the left carotid body. Reproduced with permission from Claps and Torrealba (1988).

When considering afferents of particular functions, other studies have been more specific. HRP has been applied to the cut end of the carotid sinus nerve (Panneton & Loewy, 1980; Ciriello et al, 1981a). From these studies it appears that the medial, dorsomedial, lateral and commissural regions of the ipsilateral NTS receive the densest innervation from carotid sinus afferent fibres. In addition, some afferents cross the midline and terminate in the contralateral commissural and medial subnuclei.

Of course, these carotid sinus nerve afferent fibres will include those originating from both the carotid body chemoreceptors and the carotid sinus baroreceptors and it is not necessarily the case that both functional groups will terminate in the same brainstem regions. Claps and Torrealba (1988) attempted to answer this problem in cats by restricting their injections of WGA-HRP to the region of the carotid body. With these restricted injections, terminal labelling was localised in the NTS from about 1.2 mm rostral to the obex to about 2.8 mm caudal to it. Rostral to the obex the greatest ipsilateral projection sites were in the dorsal subnucleus and lateral to the tractus, in the interstitial subnucleus. There is also some terminal labelling medial to the tractus (Fig.1). At obex and more caudally, many terminals were found in the medial subnucleus but the densest terminations were within the commissural nucleus. Some fibres were seen to cross the midline caudal to the obex and terminate within the contralateral commissural and medial subnuclei. A similar pattern of labelling has also been reported following injections of WGA-HRP into the carotid bodies of rats (Finley & Katz, 1992).

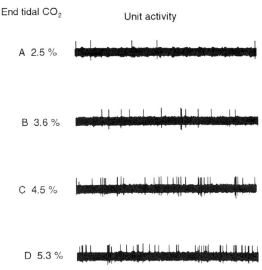

Figure 2. Activity of a single unmyelinated carotid chemoreceptor afferent fibre. Recordings of the ongoing activity of a chemoreceptor afferent in the petrosal ganglion. End-tidal CO_2 was adjusted from the resting state (B) by hyperventilating (A) or hypoventilating (C, D) the animal.

Whilst these anatomical techniques are of importance in delineating the overall areas of termination of any particular set of afferent fibres, they cannot provide very detailed information regarding the terminations of afferents with a particular function. Nor can they distinguish between afferents with myelinated and unmyelinated axons. This is of particular interest since both the vagus and carotid sinus nerves contain different functional groups of afferents. Even the same functional type of afferent e.g. baroreceptor or chemoreceptor may be either myelinated or unmyelinated and these may have different reflex effects.

To address this problem various neurophysiological techniques have been used. In particular, the use of 'antidromic mapping' has proved useful in localising the regions of termination of functionally identified afferent fibres travelling in the carotid sinus nerve, the vagus and its various branches. Essentially, this technique entails recording ongoing and evoked activity in sensory ganglion cells. By studying and manipulating this activity the function of the afferent can be determined. For example, when recording from sensory neurones in the petrosal ganglion, apart from the obvious difference in their background firing pattern, the activity of arterial baroreceptor and chemoreceptor afferents can be distinguished by their response to carotid occlusion. Baroreceptor afferents are silenced whilst the irregular discharge of chemoreceptor afferents is increased by the ensuing hypoxia (Donoghue et al., 1984). In addition, arterial chemoreceptor afferents respond to changes in arterial carbon dioxide (Fig. 2) as monitored by changes in end-tidal CO_2. The brainstem is then stimulated in a serial manner to determine sites from which this afferent fibre can be

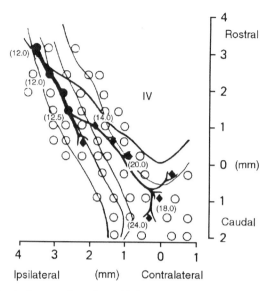

Figure 3. Projection of a single unmyelinated carotid chemoreceptor afferent fibre. A schematic view of the dorsal surface of the cat medulla oblongata showing the fourth ventricle. Superimposed on this is the medial and lateral extent of the tractus solitarius and its nucleus. Scales indicate distances in mm from the obex. Sites of stimulating electrode penetrations are indicated classed according to the type of depth-threshold profile obtained, i.e. axonal (●), terminal field (♦) or no response (O). Figures in parentheses indicate the antidromic latency. Modified and reproduced with permission from Donoghue et al. (1984).

activated by low threshold stimuli. Reconstructions of the histological sections allows a representation of the terminal fields of the afferent to be determined (Fig. 3).

Using this technique, carotid chemoreceptor afferents were found to branch and terminate in the dorsomedial and medial subnuclei of the NTS and occasionally in the lateral parts of the nucleus. In addition, the commissural nucleus at the level of, and caudal to the obex was also found to receive a major bilateral innervation from chemoreceptor afferents (Donoghue et al., 1984). This projection of arterial chemoreceptors is distinct from that of carotid sinus baroreceptor afferents. Arterial baroreceptor afferents project predominantly to the dorsal and lateral divisions of the NTS at levels rostral to the obex, with lesser input to the medial and commissural regions (Donoghue et al., 1984).

The same technique has also been employed to localise the terminations of slowly- (Donoghue et al., 1982) and rapidly- (Davies & Kubin, 1986) adapting pulmonary stretch receptor afferents, and of unmyelinated afferents accessible from the pulmonary and bronchial circulations (Kubin et al., 1991). The NTS sites of termination of different afferent inputs is summarised in a gross manner in Fig. 4. If the areas of major projection are studied (shaded areas) it can be seen that functionally different afferents terminate in distinct regions of the NTS, although there is some overlap.

Arterial baroreceptors, whether from the carotid sinus or aortic arch, project primarily to the lateral and dorsal regions of the NTS. Terminations of chemoreceptor afferents are found mainly in the dorsomedial and medial regions both rostral and caudal to the obex, with little input to the lateral parts of the nucleus. Lung stretch afferents project predominantly to the medial NTS rostral to the obex, but whereas the slowly adapting afferents are found primarily in this region, those from rapidly adapting receptors also terminate caudal to the obex in the medial subnucleus and the commissural nucleus. Finally, the terminations of both pulmonary and bronchial unmyelinated afferents is not dissimilar to the projections of arterial chemoreceptors with a projection to the medial subnucleus rostral to the obex and the commissural nucleus caudal to the obex.

Whilst this technique of antidromic activation has been useful in determining the regions of termination of different groups of afferents, ultimately, the pattern of termination is an inference from the depth-threshold profiles. There are therefore limitations when details of the fine terminals are required. Recently, the pattern of termination of identified afferent fibres has been visualised directly in experiments in which intracellular recordings have been made from identified single afferent fibres in the brainstem. Subsequent intra-axonal injection

Receptor Type	Divisions of the NTS		
	Medial	Commissural	Lateral
myelinated carotid baroreceptor (2)	● ● ●	●	● ● ● ● ● ● ● ●
unmyelinated carotid baroreceptor (2)	● ● ●	●	● ● ● ●
unmyelinated carotid chemoreceptor (2)	● ● ● ○ ● ● ●	● ● ● ○ ● ● ○	● ●
myelinated lung SAR (1)	● ● ● ● ● ●		● ●
myelinated lung RAR (3)	● ● ○ ● ● ○ ○	● ● ● ○ ● ● ○ ○	● ●
unmyelinated bronchial receptor (4)	● ● ● ○ ● ● ●	● ● ● ○ ● ● ○	
unmyelinated pulmonary receptor (4)	● ● ● ○ ● ●	● ● ○ ● ●	

Figure 4. A summary of the major regions of termination within the NTS of the cat of cardiovascular and pulmonary afferents as determined by antidromic mapping studies. The relative densities of ipsilateral (●) and contralateral (○) regions of termination is denoted by the number of dots and the most extensive regions of termination are shaded. Based on data from 1) Donoghue et al., (1982), 2) Donoghue et al., (1984), 3) Davies & Kubin (1986) 4) Kubin et al., (1991).

of HRP allowed direct visualisation of the terminations. This technique has been successfully performed for slowly- and rapidly-adapting lung stretch afferents (Kalia & Richter, 1985, 1988) and afferents travelling in the superior laryngeal nerve (Bellingham & Lipski, 1992) but the terminations of arterial chemoreceptors has not yet been described using this technique.

THE NUCLEUS TRACTUS SOLITARIUS AS A SITE OF INTEGRATION

There are now well documented accounts of the interactions which occur when different reflex afferents are stimulated in concert, and of the effects of respiration on the efficacy of reflex actions (Daly, 1986). The arterial chemoreceptor reflex is of particular interest as it evokes alterations in both cardiovascular and respiratory effectors simultaneously. Brief stimulation of the arterial chemoreceptors only slows the heart when given during expiration, the same stimulus given in inspiration is without effect (Davidson et al., 1976). In addition, similar brief chemoreceptor stimuli have different respiratory effects depending on the respiratory phase in which they are applied (Black & Torrance, 1971; Eldridge, 1972). This respiratory modulation of the effectiveness of chemoreceptor inputs is so extreme that with longer stimuli the resultant effect on heart rate is entirely dependent on the magnitude of the simultaneously evoked increase in respiration. When respiratory effects are small or respiration is controlled then chemoreceptor stimulation evokes the primary slowing of the heart. However, with larger respiratory efforts the bradycardia is reversed to a tachycardia (Daly & Scott, 1962). There are several sites at which such interactions may occur. The NTS was postulated as one such site. Although it is clear that afferents with different function terminate in distinct regions of the NTS, there is also a certain amount of overlap between their terminal fields (Fig. 4). By analogy with the dorsal horn of the spinal cord, it was suggested that afferent inputs arriving at the NTS may be modulated by presynaptic mechanisms acting on the afferent terminals themselves, or that postsynaptic interactions on NTS neurones may occur. This possibility has previously been reviewed in detail for the whole range of afferent input into the NTS (Jordan & Spyer, 1986) and so the present discussion will focus on the possible modulation of arterial chemoreceptor and pulmonary C-fibre inputs to the NTS.

In cats and rabbits Jordan & Spyer (1979) could find no evidence that the presynaptic terminals of carotid sinus afferents were modified during the respiratory cycle suggesting that if the respiratory 'gating' of chemoreceptor reflexes was occurring within the NTS it must be acting at postsynaptic sites, at the second or higher order neurones.

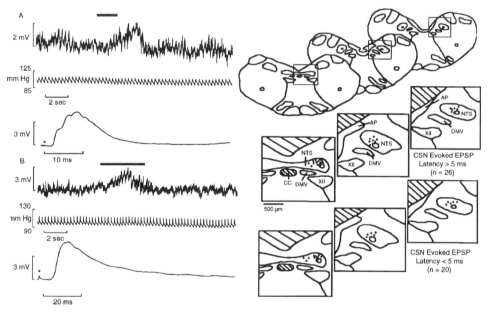

Figure 5. Activity and location of NTS neurones responsive to carotid chemoreceptor stimulation.
Left: Responses of two neurones in which carotid sinus nerve stimulation evoked EPSP's at latencies <5 ms (A) and >5 ms (B). Panels are arranged so that top traces are slow speed records of membrane potential and arterial blood pressure showing the response to activation of the chemoreceptors during the bar. The bottom sweeps in A & B are averages of responses to 25 sinus nerve stimuli given at the dot. Right: Reconstruction of the sites of recording chemoreceptor-sensitive neurones separated into those excited by sinus nerve stimulation with latencies less than or greater than 5 ms. Modified and reproduced with permission from Mifflin (1992).

The properties and location of the second order neurones in the chemoreceptor pathway have been described recently in cats (Mifflin, 1992, 1993; Spyer et al., 1990). In those studies intracellular recordings were made from neurones in the NTS which received excitatory input (EPSP's) from electrical stimulation of the carotid sinus nerve and which were excited by chemoreceptor stimuli such as CO_2-saturated bicarbonate solution injected into the lingual artery. Some of these cells received input at very short latencies leaving little doubt that they were second order neurones (Fig. 5) whereas others had longer latencies which might indicate a monosynaptic input from slower conducting afferents or a polysynaptic input. Whatever, these two groups were indistinguishable on the basis of their responses to chemoreceptor input or location (Fig. 5). All were found between 1 mm caudal and 2 mm rostral to the obex, in the dorsal and medial NTS and commissural nucleus. These are the same regions in which terminations were localised by antidromic mapping (Donoghue et al., 1984).

One interaction of the chemoreceptor reflex that has been of interest to physiologists is that with the baroreceptor reflex. These two reflex inputs have opposite effects on arterial blood pressure and respiration, whilst both evoke a primary bradycardia. Several authors have attempted to determine the location of neurones receiving convergent input from the arterial baroreceptors and chemoreceptors. Within the confines of the NTS this has proven remarkably difficult. None of the chemoreceptor responsive neurones recorded by Mifflin (1992) could be demonstrated to receive an inhibitory input from the arterial baroreceptors though some cells received excitatory inputs from both afferent inputs. A similar excitatory convergence was previously demonstrated by Lipski et al. (1976) in neurones located just ventral to the NTS. In neither study did it appear that the neurones were second order neurones. Cells with this pattern of input would be consistent with relay neurones projecting to the cardiac vagal motor outflow. However, since no cells have been identified which have opposing convergent inputs from these two groups of afferents, the question remains as to the site of the interactions regulating sympathetic outflow and respiration.

The possibility that the NTS is the site of the respiratory modulation of the effectiveness of the chemoreceptor input (Daly, 1986) has also been studied recently. Neither the phase of the central respiratory cycle, nor of lung inflation could be shown to alter the carotid sinus nerve evoked EPSP in chemoreceptor-sensitive neurones in the NTS (Mifflin, 1993; Spyer et al., 1990). This lack of effect mirrors the lack of influence of respiration on NTS baroreceptor-sensitive cells reported earlier (Mifflin et al., 1988a). The question then arises as to where these interactions are occurring. At least some of the effects of central respiratory drive appear to be imposed at the level of the vagal preganglionic neurones themselves (Gilbey et al., 1984) though the effects of lung inflation are probably imposed elsewhere (Jordan & Spyer, 1987). Similarly, it is possible that the modulatory effects of respiration on the sympathetic outflow is imposed at the level of the 'presympathetic' neurones in the rostral ventrolateral medulla or the sympathetic preganglionic neurones since both groups of neurones show respiratory modulation of their discharge (McAllen, 1987; Boczek-Funke et al., 1992).

The localisation of groups of neurones responsible for transmitting the afferent information through the NTS has also been attempted in a series of studies in which synaptic transmission has been impaired permanently by lesions or temporarily by pharmacological means. Housley & Sinclair (1988) lesioned small areas of the NTS in rats by injecting the neurotoxin kainic acid. Lesions of the caudal NTS involving the commissural nucleus markedly attenuated the ventilatory response to hypoxia whereas lesions rostral to the obex involving the lateral and dorsolateral subnuclei were ineffective.

Synaptic transmission in this commissural region of the NTS appears to involve excitatory amino acids. Microinjections of the glutamate antagonists l-glutamic acid diethyl ester (GDEE) or kynurenic acid into this region blocks hypoxic hyperventilation (Brew et al., 1990). In addition, simultaneous blockade of NMDA and non-NMDA receptors by microinjections of the appropriate antagonists blocks the effects of stimulating the carotid body chemoreceptors with CO_2-saturated saline (Vardhan et al., 1993). Interestingly, injections of either NMDA or non-NMDA antagonists alone was without effect. This blockade of the chemoreceptor response by amino acid antagonists could be mimicked by application of inhibitory amino acid agonists such as muscimol. This was not due to a generalised depression of activity in the central respiratory and cardiovascular reflex pathways as these same injections left the pulmonary chemoreflex intact. In fact, it is necessary to block synaptic transmission in a more caudal region of the commissural nucleus in order to attenuate the pulmonary chemoreflex (Bonham & Joad, 1991). Although injections of cobalt into this region blocked the rapid shallow breathing and bradycardic effects evoked by injections of phenylbiguanide into the pulmonary circulation, the depressor response was unaffected suggesting that the sympathetic and vagal limbs of the reflex had already separated at this early stage in the reflex pathway. Similar cobalt microinjections into the commissural nucleus lateral to the "chemoreceptor area" attenuate the Hering-Breuer apnoea evoked by lung inflation (Bonham & McCrimmon, 1990).

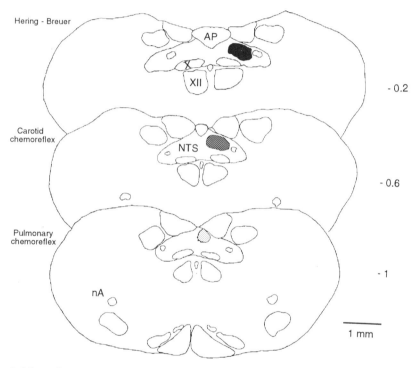

Figure 6. Schematic representation of the sites within the rat brainstem from which cobalt microinjections abolished phenylbiguanide-evoked rapid shallow breathing or lung inflation-evoked apnoea. In addition the sites where chemoreceptor-evoked hyperventilations were abolished by kainate lesions or micoinjections of excitatory amino acid antagonists are also shown. Based on data from Bonham & Joad (1991), Bonham & McCrimmon (1990), Brew et al. (1990), Housley & Sinclair (1988) and Vardhan et al. (1993) respectively.

HYPOTHALAMIC MODULATION OF CHEMORECEPTOR REFLEXES

Stimulation of the "hypothalamic defence area" evokes a pattern of autonomic, behavioural and endocrine changes known as the "defence response". These include pupillary dilatation, piloerection, behavioural alerting, tachypnoea, a marked pressor response and tachycardia (see Jordan, 1990 for review). The tachycardia evoked during the defence response is unexpected since similar rises in arterial pressure evoked by other means are buffered by the arterial baroreceptors and result in bradycardia. It is now clear that during such stimulation the arterial baroreceptor reflex is inhibited (Coote et al., 1979). At least part of this inhibition occurs at the level of the NTS. Hypothalamic stimulation hyperpolarises baroreceptor-sensitive NTS cells, making them less excitable (Mifflin et al., 1988b) and this is mediated by $GABA_A$ receptors in the NTS (Jordan et al., 1988). In addition to an inhibition of the baroreceptor reflex, Hilton & Joels (1965) suggested that the pressor response evoked during the defence response was in part due to a facilitation of the arterial chemoreceptor reflex. Intracellular recordings from NTS neurones have now confirmed this (Silva-Carvalho et al., 1993). In this study some neurones were hyperpolarised as described by Mifflin et al. (1988b) and these were excited by inflation of the carotid sinus but unaffected by carotid chemoreceptor stimulation. In addition, however, another group of neurones were recorded which received short latency excitatory inputs from the defence area which facilitated sinus nerve-evoked inputs to the cells. These neurones were unaffected by baroreceptor stimuli but were excited by chemoreceptor stimulation (Fig. 7).

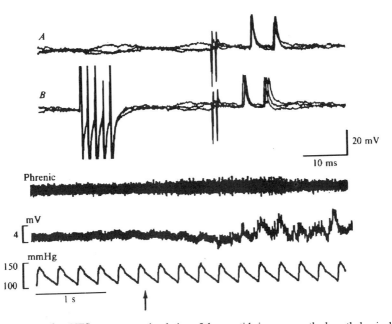

Figure 7. Response of an NTS neurone to stimulation of the carotid sinus nerve, the hypothalamic defence area and carotid arterial chemoreceptors. Upper traces: Responses evoked by 2 stimuli applied to the sinus nerve alone (A) and preceded 30 ms by stimulation of the defence area (B). Lower traces: Phrenic nerve activity, neuronal membrane potential and arterial blood pressure monitored during injection of CO_2-saturated saline at the arrow. Reproduced with permission from Silva-Carvalho et al. (1993).

Since defence area stimulation has been shown to inhibit arterial baroreceptor reflexes but facilitate arterial chemoreceptor reflexes, the question arises as to its effects on other chemoreceptor responses. Is the pulmonary chemoreflex also augmented during the defence response? In recent studies in cats we have demonstrated that stimulation of the hypothalamic defence area markedly attenuates the bradycardia evoked by injecting phenylbiguanide into the pulmonary circulation and similarly reduces the excitatory input from such stimuli to neurones in the NTS (D. Jordan, Y. Wang & J.F.X. Jones, unpublished observations). Clearly then, in this respect, the pulmonary chemoreflex is more like the arterial baroreceptor reflex than the arterial chemoreceptor reflex.

SUMMARY

The sites of termination within the dorsal medulla of afferents arising from the arterial chemoreceptors and pulmonary C-fibre afferents has been summarised and the effect of stimulating these afferents on second order neurones in the NTS described. The extent of our knowledge concerning the interactions of these reflex inputs within the NTS has been discussed. Clearly, further experimental work is required to fully elucidate the neural pathways underlying these, and other, reflex pathways.

The financial support of the Medical Research Council and Wellcome Trust is gratefully acknowledged.

REFERENCES

Bellingham, M.C. & Lipski, J. (1992) Morphology and electrophysiology of superior laryngeal nerve afferents and postsynaptic neurons in the medulla oblongata of the cat. Neurosci. 48: 205-216.

Black, A.M.S. & Torrance, R.W. (1971) Respiratory oscillations in chemoreceptor discharge in the control of breathing. Respir. Physiol. 13: 221-237.

Boczek-Funke, A., Dembowsky, K., Häbler, H. -J., Jänig, W. & Michaelis, M. (1992) Respiratory-related activity patterns in preganglionic neurones projecting into the cat cervical sympathetic trunk. J. Physiol. (Lond.) 457: 277-296.

Bonham, A.C. & Joad, J.P. (1991) Neurones in commissural nucleus tractus solitarii required for full expression of the pulmonary C fibre reflex in rat. J. Physiol. (Lond.) 441: 95-112.

Bonham, A.C. & McCrimmon, D.R. (1990) Neurones in a discrete region of the nucleus tractus solitarius are required for the Breuer-Hering reflex in rat. J. Physiol. (Lond.) 427: 261-280.

Brew, S., de Castro, D., Housley, G.D. & Sinclair, J.D. (1990) The role of glutamate in the transmission of the hypoxic input to respiration through the nucleus of the tractus solitarius. In "Chemoreceptors and Chemoreceptor Reflexes." H. Acker, A. Trzebski & R. G. O'Regan eds., Plenum Press, New York. pp 331-338.

Ciriello, J., Hrycyshyn, A.W. & Calaresu, F.R. (1981a) Horseradish peroxidase study of brainstem projections of carotid sinus and aortic depressor nerves in the cat. J. Autonom. Nerv. Syst. 4: 43-61.

Ciriello, J., Hrycyshyn, A.W. & Calaresu, F.R. (1981b) Glossopharyngeal and vagal afferent projections to the brainstem of the cat: a horseradish peroxidase. J. Autonom. Nerv. Syst. 4: 63-79.

Claps, A. & Torrealba, F. (1988) Carotid body connections: A WGA-HRP study in the cat. Brain Res. 455: 123-133.

Coote, J.H., Hilton, S.M. & Perez-Gonzalez, J.F. (1979) Inhibition of the baroreceptor reflex on stimulation in the brainstem defence centre. J. Physiol. (Lond.) 288: 549-560.

Cottle, M.K. (1964) Degeneration studies of primary afferents of IXth and Xth cranial nerves in the cat. J. Comp. Neurol. 122: 329-343.

Daly, M. de B. (1986) Interactions between respiration and circulation. In "Handbook of Physiology . Section 3, The Respiratory System. Vol. 2, Control of Breathing, Part II." N.S. Cherniack & J.G. Widdicombe, eds., American Physiological Society, Bethesda. pp 529-594.

Daly, M. de B. (1991) Some reflex cardioinhibitory responses in the cat and their modulation by central inspiratory neuronal activity. J. Physiol. (Lond.) 439: 559-577.

Daly, M. de B. & Kirkman, E. (1989) Differential modulation by pulmonary stretch afferents of some reflex cardioinhibitory responses in the cat. J. Physiol. (Lond.) 417: 323-341.

Daly, M. de B. & Scott, M.J. (1962) An analysis of the primary cardiovascular reflex effects of stimulation of the carotid body chemoreceptors in the dog. J. Physiol. (Lond.) 162: 555-573.

Davidson, N.S., Goldner, S. & McCloskey, D.I. (1976) Respiratory modulation of baroreceptor and chemoreceptor reflexes affecting heart rate and cardiac vagal efferent nerve activity. J. Physiol. (Lond.) 259: 523-530.

Davies, R.O. & Kubin, L. (1986) Projection of pulmonary rapidly adapting receptors to the medulla of the cat: an antidromic mapping study. J. Physiol. (Lond.) 373: 63-86.

Donoghue, S., Garcia, M., Jordan, D. & Spyer, K.M. (1982) The brainstem projections of pulmonary stretch afferent neurones in cats and rabbits. J. Physiol. (Lond.) 322: 353-363.

Donoghue, S., Felder, R.B.., Jordan, D. & Spyer, K.M. (1984) The central projections of carotid baroreceptors and chemoreceptors in the cat: a neurophysiological study. J. Physiol. (Lond.) 347: 397-409.

Eldridge, F.L. (1972) The importance of timing on the respiratory effects of intermittent carotid sinus nerve stimulation. J. Physiol. (Lond.) 222: 319-333.

Finley, J.C.W. & Katz, D.M. (1992) The central organization of carotid body afferent projections to the brainstem of the rat. Brain Res. 572: 108-116.

Gilbey, M.P., Jordan, D., Richter, D.W. & Spyer, K.M. (1984) Synaptic mechanisms involved in the inspiratory control of vagal cardio-inhibitory neurones in the cat. J.Physiol. (Lond.) 356: 65-78.

Hilton, S.M. & Joels, N. (1965) Facilitation of chemoreceptor reflexes during the defence reaction. J. Physiol. (Lond.) 176: 20-21P.

Housley, G.D. & Sinclair, J.D. (1988) Localization by kainic acid lesions of neurones transmitting the carotid chemoreceptor stimulus for respiration in the rat. J. Physiol. (Lond.) 406: 99-114.

Jones, J.F.X., Wang, Y. & Jordan, D. (1994) Activity of cardiac vagal motoneurones during the pulmonary chemoreflex in the anaesthetized cat., this volume

Jordan, D. (1990) Autonomic changes in affective behavior. In "Central Regulation of Autonomic Functions." A.D. Loewy & K.M. Spyer, eds., Oxford University Press, New York. pp. 349-366.

Jordan, D., Mifflin, S.W. & Spyer, K.M. (1988) Hypothalamic inhibition of neurones in the nucleus tractus solitarius in the cat is GABA mediated. J. Physiol. (Lond.) 399: 389-404.

Jordan, D. & Spyer, K.M. (1979) Studies on the excitability of sinus nerve afferent terminals. J. Physiol. (Lond.) 297: 123-134.

Jordan, D. & Spyer, K.M. (1986) Brainstem integration of cardiovascular and pulmonary afferent activity. Prog. Brain Res. 67: 295-314.

Jordan, D. & Spyer, K.M. (1987) Central neural mechanisms mediating respiratory-cardiovascular interactions. In "Neurobiology of the Cardiorespiratory System." E.W. Taylor, ed., Manchester University Press, Manchester. pp 322-341.

Kalia, M. & Richter, D.W. (1985) Morphology of physiologically identified slowly adapting lung stretch receptor afferents stained with intra-axonal horseradish peroxidase in the nucleus of the tractus solitarius of the cat. I. A light microscopic analysis. J. Comp. Neurol. 241: 503-520.

Kalia, M. & Richter, D.W. (1988) Rapidly adapting pulmonary receptor afferents: I. Arborization in the nucleus of the tractus solitarius. J. Comp. Neurol. 274: 560-573.

Kubin, L., Kimura, H. & Davies, R.O. (1991) The medullary projections of afferent bronchopulmonary C fibres in the cat as shown by antidromic mapping. J. Physiol. (Lond.) 435: 207-228.

Lipski, J., McAllen, R.M. & Trzebski, A. (1976) Carotid baroreceptor and chemoreceptor inputs onto single medullary neurones. Brain Res. 107: 132-136.

Loewy, A.D. & Burton, H. (1978) Nuclei of the solitary tract: efferent projections to the lower brainstem and spinal cord of the cat. J. Comp. Neurol. 181: 421-450.

McAllen, R.M. (1987) Central respiratory modulation of subretrofacial bulbospinal neurones in the cat. J. Physiol. (Lond.) 388:533-545.

Mifflin, S.W. (1992) Arterial chemoreceptor input to the nucleus tractus solitarius. Am. J. Physiol., 263: R368-R375.

Mifflin, S.W. (1993) Absence of respiratory modulation of carotid sinus nerve inputs to nucleus tractus solitarius neurons receiving arterial chemoreceptor inputs. J. Autonom. Nerv. Syst. 42: 191-200.

Mifflin, S.W. & Felder, R.B. (1988) An intracellular study of time-dependent cardiovascular afferent interactions in nucleus tractus solitarius. J. Neurophysiol. 59: 1798-1813.

Mifflin, S.W., Spyer, K.M. & Withington-Wray, D.J. (1988a) Baroreceptor inputs to the nucleus tractus solitarius in the cat: Postsynaptic actions and the influence of respiration. J. Physiol. (Lond.) 399: 349-367.

Mifflin, S.W., Spyer, K.M. & Withington-Wray, D.J. (1988b) Baroreceptor inputs to the nucleus tractus solitarius in the cat: modulation by the hypothalamus. J. Physiol. (Lond.) 399: 369-387.

Panneton, W.M. & Loewy, A.D. (1980) Projections of carotid sinus nerve to the nucleus of the solitary tract in the cat. Brain Res. 191: 239-244.

Spyer, K.M., Izzo, P.N., Lin, R.J., Paton, J.F.R., Silva-Carvalho, L.F. & Richter, D.W. (1990) The central nervous organization of the carotid body reflex. 317-321.

Silva-Carvalho, L., Dawid-Milner, M.S., Goldsmith, G.E. & Spyer, K.M. (1993) Hypothalamic-evoked effects in cat nucleus tractus solitarius facilitating chemoreceptor reflexes. Exp. Physiol. 78: 425-428.

Vardhan, A., Kachrooo, A. & Sapru, H.N. (1993) Excitatory amino acid receptors in commissural nucleus of the NTS mediate carotid chemoreceptor responses. Am. J. Physiol. 264: R41-R50.

CHEMORECEPTOR FUNCTION IN THE FETUS AND NEONATE

Mark Hanson[1] and Prem Kumar[2]

[1]Department of Obstetrics and Gynaecology, UCL Medical School, 86-96 Chenies Mews, London WC1E 6HX; [2]Department of Physiology, University of Birmingham Medical School, Birmingham B15 2TT

INTRODUCTION

The last 15 years has seen an enormous increase in our understanding of arterial chemoreceptor function in fetal and neonatal life. This is of obvious clinical significance: both the identification of fetuses which are not adapting adequately to hypoxia *in utero* and the appropriate care of newborn, especially preterm, infants demands a thorough knowledge of the integrated chemoreflexes which the fetus and neonate mount. In this chapter, we review knowledge of arterial chemoreceptor responses to natural stimuli during development and the chemoreflexes which ensue. We then note the possible effects of pathophysiological processes (especially chronic hypoxaemia) on chemoreceptor function. Finally, we consider the implications of new knowledge on chemoreceptor function over the period for studies on the transduction mechanisms of arterial chemoreceptors.

FETAL CHEMORECEPTOR RESPONSES

Knowledge of chemoreceptor afferent responses in fetal life comes exclusively from sheep. In this species, direct recordings from the carotid sinus (Blanco et al., 1984a) or aortic nerves (Blanco et al., 1982) show that the chemoreceptors are spontaneously active and respond to reductions in P_aO_2 or increases in P_aCO_2 from about 90 days (term = 147 days). Fetal P_aO_2 is normally about 25 mm Hg in late gestation. At this P_aO_2 fetal chemoreceptor discharge is basal and only increases markedly when P_aO_2 is reduced below about 15 mm Hg. Thus, the chemoreceptor hypoxic response curve is displaced to the left compared to that of the adult. In these studies, basal chemoreceptor discharge was high relative to that of the adult basal level in normoxaemia. We do not know if this is a feature of resting chemoreceptor discharge in the fetus *in utero*, or whether it is the result of the high P_aCO_2 and low pH_a resulting from the exteriorization and anaesthesia necessary for performing these studies. Nor have the responses of fetal chemoreceptors to pharmacological stimuli been studied systematically - preliminary evidence suggests that they are relatively less sensitive to cyanide (Blanco et al .,1984a).

In contrast to the response of the chemoreceptors to hypoxia, much less is known of their response to CO_2. In the studies to date, close-arterial injections of CO_2-saturated saline have demonstrated that the fetal carotid body can respond to CO_2. However, no CO_2 response curves have, as yet, been published.

FETAL CHEMOREFLEXES

In contrast to the neonate or adult, stimulation of fetal chemoreceptors by hypoxaemia does not stimulate fetal breathing movements (FBM) (Boddy et al., 1974). This is because brain stem descending inhibitory processes operate to inhibit FBM in hypoxaemia: their importance can be shown by the stimulation of FBM in hypoxia after making lesions in the upper pons (Gluckman et al., 1987). Recent findings show that this stimulation does depend on intact arterial chemoreceptor function (Koos et al., 1992; Johnston et al., in press). Thus the picture emerges of a balance of facilitatory (chemoreceptor-driven) and inhibitory (perhaps pontine) mechanisms operating to regulate the incidence of FBM. In hypoxia the latter predominate. It has frequently been proposed (see for example Johnston, 1991) that this constitutes evidence for a chemosensitive structure, stimulated by hypoxia, in the fetal brain. Its exact site and nature are unknown, although in this regard it is interesting that almitrine also causes FBM to cease in normoxaemia (Moore et al., 1989), an effect independent of the arterial chemoreceptors, but abolished by lesioning in the upper pons (Johnston et al., 1990). Unlike hypoxaemia, raising P_aCO_2 or lowering pH_a stimulates FBM (Boddy et al., 1974), an effect mediated by both peripheral and central chemoreceptors (Hohimer et al., 1983). The stimulation of FBM by CO_2 or acidity is over-ridden by the inhibitory effects of hypoxaemia and also when fetal behavioural state switches to high voltage ECoG.

The predominant effects of fetal chemoreflexes are on the circulation (Hanson, 1989; Jensen & Berger, 1991). In hypoxaemia there is a transient bradycardia and a vasoconstriction in the skin, muscle, and gut (Rudolph, 1984). The initial cardiovascular responses are reflex and the carotid chemoreceptors provide the afferent limb of this reflex. The fall in heart rate is vagally mediated and the peripheral vasoconstriction is partly α-adrenergic (Giussani et al., 1993a). The latter elevates arterial blood pressure in the late gestation fetal sheep. In addition to neural pathways, the vasoconstriction is mediated by catecholamines released from the adrenal medulla, in part in response to direct effects of hypoxia on the gland (Jones et al., 1988). Pulmonary blood flow, which is low in the fetus, and renal blood flow decrease in hypoxaemia and again these processes have a rapid chemoreflex component (Moore & Hanson, 1991).

Hypoxaemia induces a plethora of endocrine changes in the fetus, e.g. increased ACTH, cortisol, AVP, angiotensin II, and endothelin (Wood, 1993). These factors are responsible for components of the vasoconstriction and may interact positively, e.g. the rise in cortisol may potentiate the vasoconstrictor effects of angiotensin II. We investigated the extent to which these changes are chemoreflexly mediated. Chemodenervation delays the rise in cortisol but does not affect the early rise in ACTH (Giussani et al., 1993b). Chemodenervation does not affect the rise in AVP (Giussani et al., 1993c). Its effects on angiotensin II in the fetal sheep are not known. Chemodenervation also delays the rise in catecholamines occurring during severe asphyxia (Jensen & Hanson, 1993). It therefore appears that many of these endocrine changes are responsible for maintaining a redistribution of combined ventricular output over a longer period of time, after the initial chemoreflex changes. They may also be important in reducing urine output and lung liquid secretion in hypoxaemia (Brace, 1993).

NEONATAL CHEMORECEPTOR RESETTING

The rise in P_aO_2 at birth effectively silences the arterial chemoreceptors. Direct recordings have shown that arterial chemoreceptor sensitivity is re-set in early neonatal life (Blanco et al., 1984a; Hanson et al., 1986; Kumar & Hanson, 1989; Mulligan, 1991). This results in moving the stimulus-response curve to hypoxia to the right and therefore increases its slope at any PO_2. A variety of indirect methods have been used to show that chemoreceptor resetting produces an increase in the reflex ventilatory response to hypoxia. These include step reductions (Eden & Hanson, 1987a) or increases (Hertzberg & Lagercrantz, 1987) in F_IO_2. The variability of neonatal breathing however can make results from the single step changes difficult to interpret. We have therefore preferred to use breath-by-breath alternations of F_IO_2 between air and hypoxia over a number of breaths, as this permits the averaging and quantification of the ventilatory response to rapid alternations in chemoreceptor input, over and above the naturally-occurring variation in breathing. Using this method, we found that the magnitude of the response (in terms of the number of respiratory variables alternating as a result of the stimulus and the size of the alternations produced) increased in neonatal life in kittens (Hanson et al., 1989), lambs (Williams & Hanson, 1990) and human infants (Williams et al., 1991). The precise timing of this resetting differed between species. It appears to occur over the first two postnatal weeks in kittens and lambs but may be faster in human babies in whom there is little increase in response after about 48 hours (Calder et al., 1993). It should be noted that the rightward shift in the stimulus response curve itself produces a greater change in chemoreceptor discharge for any change in P_aO_2, without necessarily changing the sensitivity of the chemoreceptor response to PO_2 .

This resetting is defined in terms of P_aO_2. The tissue PO_2 in the carotid body may be higher than in other organs since the blood flow to it is so large. However, it is conceivable that, if there were a large reduction in blood flow to chemoreceptive elements of the carotid body postnatally, it might account for the change in sensitivity to P_aO_2 over this period (Acker, Degner & Hilsman, 1991). However, quantitative measurements of carotid body capillary and large vessel density, made in the lamb over the time when resetting occurs, do not support this idea (Moore et al., 1991a). It therefore appears that the resetting occurs at the level of the chemoreceptors themselves and indeed it has been found that it occurs *in vitro* (Kholwadwala & Donnelly, 1992). In the sheep, the process of resetting at birth is initiated by the rise in P_aO_2, as raising fetal P_aO_2 by ventilating the fetal lungs while the fetus remains *in utero* starts the process (Blanco et al., 1988).

If the postnatal increase of hypoxic sensitivity takes the form of a manipulation of the carotid body's hypoxia sensing mechanism, then the postnatal increase of hypoxic sensitivity will produce an increase in chemoreceptor steady state responses to CO_2. However, as the transient carotid body response to CO_2 is independent of the level of hypoxia (Torrance et al., 1992), the resetting of chemoreceptor sensitivity to hypoxia would not be expected to produce a change in the chemoreceptor response to rapid changes in P_aCO_2. Thus, we predict that there would be a pronounced sensitivity to rapid changes of CO_2 even at a time when the hypoxic sensitivity is weak. Reflex studies confirm this idea in the piglet (Wolsink et al., 1991), kitten (Watanabe et al., 1993), rat (Elnazir & Kumar, 1993), neonatal infant (Cohen & Henderson-Smart, 1990) and lamb (Jansen et al., 1992). However, this needs to be confirmed by direct recordings from chemoreceptor afferent fibres. In the lamb the previous study (Blanco et al., 1984a) used only CO_2-saturated saline to test the responses and in the kitten Marchal et al. (1992), tested dynamic sensitivity with a system which altered inspired CO_2 with a relatively long time constant of 4 seconds.

NEONATAL CHEMOREFLEXES

It is well established that the ventilatory response of the neonate is 'biphasic', an initial increase in ventilation being followed by a fall to, or to below, pre-hypoxia control levels (Hanson, 1986a,b). This response changes over the first few days-weeks in all animals examined including man in two respects; the initial increase in ventilation becomes relatively larger and the secondary fall in ventilation becomes smaller so that a ventilatory hyperpnoea is maintained. The increase in the magnitude of the first phase is explicable in terms of the resetting of chemoreceptor hypoxic sensitivity discussed above. The processes underlying the secondary fall are still debated. The fall is not due to a failure of the peripheral chemoreceptors during hypoxia (Blanco et al., 1984b; Schwieler, 1968).

The biphasic response can be seen in unanaesthetized or anaesthetized animals. The mechanisms producing the response may not be the same under both conditions. Halothane anaesthesia appears to produce a fall in chemoreceptor discharge in hypoxia (Morray et al., 1992). In unanaesthetized neonatal animals and infants, metabolism falls rapidly in hypoxia (Cross et al., 1958; Hill, 1959; Blanco et al., 1984c) and this would be expected to reduce the 'feed-forward' drive to breathe. The mechanism of this rapid reduction in VO_2 is likely to involve brown adipose tissue, and indeed we have shown that the fall is less in neonatal rats genetically deficient in brown adipose tissue (Hanson & Williams, 1987). Thus it is possible that the fall in ventilation does involve some component of a reduction in the stimulus to arterial chemoreceptors.

The other aspect of the biphasic response which has received a great deal of attention is the idea that the secondary fall in ventilation involves the operation of a brain stem inhibitory mechanism similar to that which operates in the fetus (see above). There are several lines of evidence to support this. First, transection of the brain stem through the upper pons or placement of lesions in the pons abolishes the fall in ventilation (Williams & Hanson, 1989; Martin-Body & Johnston, 1988). Support for the operation of such a mechanism comes from the work using reversible cooling of the upper pons, which abolishes the fall in ventilation during the secondary phase although the fall returns when the area is re-warmed (Moore et al., 1991b). Whatever the mechanism involved, it appears to act in hypoxia to 'gate out' the incoming chemoreceptor input and thus to prevent a resultant stimulation of ventilation. The inhibitory process does not constitute a blanket suppression of the effects of all afferent inputs, for stimulation of somatic afferents still produces respiratory effects, even at a time during the secondary phase when the effects of transient chemoreceptor stimulation have been blocked (see Ackland et al., this volume).

PATHOLOGICAL CHANGES IN PERINATAL CHEMORECEPTOR FUNCTION

Perhaps the most important pathophysiological effect on peripheral chemoreceptor function is that of chronic hypoxia. The blunting of ventilatory responses to hypoxia in residents of high altitude is well known and it has been reported (Lahiri et al., 1978) that this is seen in newborns. Other conditions producing chronic hypoxia in children are also reported to reduce respiratory responses to acute episodes of hypoxia (Sorensen & Severinghaus, 1968). The extent to which the blunting is due to effects on the carotid body, as opposed for example the brain stem, is not known. However, such effects are seen in chronically hypoxic neonatal kittens (Hanson et al., 1989) and rats (Eden & Hanson, 1987b). The effect might be due to reduced or delayed chemoreceptor resetting, for example if an adequate rise in P_aO_2 at birth did not occur. In the kitten, chronic hypoxia from birth appears to flatten carotid chemoreceptor the hypoxic response curve (Hanson et al., 1991) although in the rat, whole nerve recordings did not show such a change (Eden & Hanson, 1987b) so further work is needed. If the effect is via a change in the resetting of hypoxia sensitivity, then it should not affect the response to rapid changes in CO_2 (see above); however if the effect were at the brain stem, then reflex effects of both CO_2 and hypoxia should be reduced. Current evidence favours the former as the response to CO_2 was not reduced in high altitude infants. (Lahiri et al., 1978) and Kumar et al. (J. Physiol., in press) found that the response to alternate breaths of high and low CO_2 gas were present in chronically hypoxic rats with a weak ventilatory response to hypoxia. Hertzberg et al (1992) have begun to investigate the mechanisms at the carotid body, showing that the dopamine turn-over rate in chronically hypoxic rats is increased. They propose that the weak chemoreflex is brought about by a higher release of dopamine from the organ. Nurse et al. (this volume) have reported that there are changes in Na^+ channel density in the carotid bodies of chronically hypoxic rats. It will be important to understand these mechanisms more clearly as the pathological changes may be of clinical importance, e.g. in babies suffering hypoxaemia postnatally. In this connection it is interesting that Calder et al. (1994) reported finding absent responses to alternate breaths of hypoxia and air in preterm infants who had suffered respiratory distress syndrome and developed bronchopulmonary dysplasia. Such infants are at an increased risk of sudden infant death syndrome.

Finally, the question of whether chronic hypoxia prenatally, for example from placental insufficiency, can alter chemoreceptor function needs to be addressed. Much evidence now points to intra-uterine mechanisms operating in a substantial proportion of infants suffering 'birth asphyxia', but whether this is due to perturbed chemoreflex defences secondary to hypoxaemia in utero is not known. Animals studies aimed at addressing this problem are now under way (see Bennet & Hanson, 1993).

CHEMOTRANSDUCTION

Recent hypotheses of chemotransduction assume the carotid body type I cell to be the primary transducer element in a composite receptor system with the, closely apposed afferent sinus nerve ending as its post-synaptic element. Physiological stimulation may act to depolarise the type I cell leading to an increase in its $[Ca^{2+}]_i$ which triggers the release of a neurotransmitter substance and gives rise to the generation of action potentials in the afferent neurone. However, the details of the process have not been fully established. In particular, the nature of the channel(s) responsible for cell depolarization and the source(s) of the rise in $[Ca^{2+}]_i$ need further elucidation. Further, no developmental studies have been reported.

The results from reflex studies in the neonate can be taken to suggest that different mechanisms of transduction exist for the carotid body detection of hypoxia and hypercapnia and that these may be affected independently by chronic hypoxaemia from birth. That two transduction mechanisms exist also appears increasingly apparent from much recent work on isolated chemoreceptor cells.

The carotid body type I cell has been shown to be excitable, exhibiting a number of voltage-sensitive, ionic conductances, including those for Na^+, K^+ and Ca^{2+}. Of these much interest has focused upon K^+ currents that are reversibly inhibited by hypoxia, leading to cell depolarization, as a postulated first step in chemotransduction. Interestingly, in view of the post-natal re-setting of hypoxic chemosensitivity, the details of these currents differ depending upon the age of the cells studied. Thus in the adult rabbit (Lopez-Barneo et al., 1988; Duchen et al., 1988; Lopez-Lopez et al., 1989) the K^+ current is voltage-gated, being activated at depolarized potentials and has a Ca^{2+}-independent component that appears to be hypoxically-sensitive, whereas the neonatal rat exhibits a voltage-sensitive, but in this case, Ca^{2+}-dependent, K^+ current that is inactivated by hypoxia (Peers, 1990a). Unfortunately, the possibility of a species difference cannot yet be ruled out. The nature of the K^+ current in fetal cells has not been fully characterized but studies using fetal rabbit cells demonstrate an active K^+ current at resting membrane potentials (Hescheler et al., 1989; Delpiano & Hescheler, 1989).

A major problem with the concept of hypoxic-inactivation of K^+ currents revolves around the finding that current inhibition is not simply correlated to the physiological PO_2 at which the carotid body is believed to operate *in vivo*. Nor has the quantitative contribution of these channels to the resting membrane potential been adequately described. However, evidence for the unique ability of the carotid body type I cell mitochondria to respond to hypoxia over its natural physiological range has been described (Duchen & Biscoe, 1992a,b). In this schema much of the increased $[Ca^{2+}]_i$ during hypoxia arises from intracellular stores, primarily mitochondrial, and these authors provide theoretical reasoning to demonstrate that elevation of $[Ca^{2+}]_i$ from mitochondria alone would provide enough stimulation for transmitter release. The concept of some mitochondrial specialization in the carotid body which confers it with chemosensitivity is not a new one and the link between oxygen sensitivity and cell metabolism, particularly the potential role of a low-affinity cytochrome oxidase (Mills & Jobsis, 1970) has been a keystone to much chemoreceptor physiology.

However, the calculations and interpretations of this hypothesis are questioned by other authors and a role for carotid body mitochondrial Ca^{2+} stores remains to be established. The post-natal maturation of type I cell mitochondrial responses to hypoxia has not been reported.

Carbonic anhydrase inhibitors have been used (Hanson, Nye & Torrance, 1981; Rigual, Lopez-Lopez & Gonzalez, 1991) to show that intracellular pH is the parameter sensed by the carotid body to an hypercapnic stimulus is (pH_i). Since then a number of mechanisms whereby carotid body Type I cells can regulate their pH_i have been characterised. Whilst other cell types may also exhibit similar, transmembrane mechanisms, the carotid body's uniqueness appears to lie in the exquisite sensitivity of its pH_i upon extracellular acidification by hypercapnia (Buckler et al., 1991a,b). As current views on chemotransduction implicate Ca^{2+}-dependent, chemical transmission between Type I cells and their afferent nerve endings, a link between elevations in pH_i and $[Ca^{2+}]_i$ was sought. In view of the finding that post-natal CO_2-sensitivity changes little after birth it is perhaps surprising that an acid sensitive, Ca^{2+}-dependent, K^+ current has been found in neonates (Peers, 1990b; Peers & Green, 1991) but not in adults (see Gonzalez et al., 1992). Such a current presumably acts similarly to the one described for hypoxia, i.e. voltage-dependent Ca^{2+} entry subsequently occurring as a consequence of membrane depolarization. However, as it has also been found that Ca^{2+}-dependent dopamine release by Type I cells is not dihydropyridine sensitive (Obeso et al., 1992), an alternative means of Ca^{2+} entry following intracellular acidification has also been proposed (Rocher et al., 1991). In this model intracellular acidification causes the removal of hydrogen ions via a Na^+-H^+ exchanger and the consequent elevation of intracellular Na^+ leads to an influx of Ca^{2+} following reversal of a Na^+-Ca^{2+} antiporter. At present it is not known whether any of these mechanisms are age-dependent.

REFERENCES

Acker, H., Degner, F. & Hilsmann, J. (1991). Local blood flow velocities in the carotid body of fetal sheep and newborn lambs. J. Comp. Physiol., B, Biochem. System. Env. Physiol. 161:73-79.

Bennet, L. & Hanson, M.A. (1994). Intra-uterine compromise - Physiological consequences. In "Early Fetal Growth and Development". R.H.T. Ward, C.K.Smith & D. Donnai, eds. In press.

Blanco, C.E., Dawes, G.S., Hanson, M.A. & McCooke, H.B. (1982). The arterial chemoreceptors in fetal sheep and newborn lambs. J. Physiol. 330:38P

Blanco, C.E., Dawes, G.S., Hanson, M.A. & McCooke, H. B. (1984). The response to hypoxia of arterial chemoreceptors in fetal sheep and new-born lambs. J. Physiol. 351:25-37.

Blanco, C.E., Hanson, M.A., Johnson, P. & Rigatto, H. (1984b). Breathing pattern of kittens during hypoxia. J. Appl. Physiol. 56(1):12-17.

Blanco, C.E., Hanson, M.A. & McCooke, H.B. (1988). Effects on carotid chemoreceptor resetting of pulmonary ventilation in the fetal lamb in utero. J. Dev. Physiol. 10:167-174.

Boddy, K., Dawes, G.S., Fisher, R., Pinter, S. & Robinson, J.S. (1974). Foetal respiratory movements, electrocortical and cardiovascular responses to hypoxemia and hypercapnia in sheep.
J. Physiol. 243:599-618.

Brace, R. A. (1993). Regulation of blood volume in utero. In "Fetus and Neonate: Volume One: Circulation", M.A. Hanson, J.A.D. Spencer & C.H. Rodeck, eds., pp. 75-98. CambridgeUniversity Press: Cambridge.

Buckler, K.J., Vaughan-Jones, R.D., Peers, C. & Nye, P.C.G. (1991a). Intracellular pH and its regulation in isolated Type I carotid body cells of the neonatal rat. J. Physiol. 436:107-129.

Buckler, K.J., Vaughan-Jones, R.D., Peers, C., Lagadic-Grossman, D. & Nye, P.C.G. (1991b). Effects of extracellular pH, PCO_2 and HCO_3^- on intracellular pH in isolated type-I cells of the neonatal rat carotid body. J. Physiol. 444:703-721.

Calder, N.A., Williams, B.A., Kumar, P. & Hanson, M.A. (1993). The respiratory response of healthy term infants to breath-by-breath alternations in inspired oxygen at two postnatal ages. Pediatr. Res., In press.

Calder, N.A., Williams, B.A., Smyth, J., Boon, A.W., Kumar, P. & Hanson, M.A. (1994). Absence of ventilatory responses to alternating breaths of mild hypoxia and air in infants who have suffered bronchopulmonary dysplasia: implications for the risk of sudden infant death. Pediatr. Res., In press.

Cohen, G. & Henderson-Smart, D.J. (1990). A modified rebreathing method to study the ventilatory response of the newborn to carbon dioxide. J. Dev. Physiol. 14:295-301

Cross, K.W., Tizard, J.P.M. & Trythall, D.A.H. (1958). The gaseous metabolism of the newborn infant breathing 15% O_2. Acta Paed. Scand. 47:217-237.

Delpiano, M.A. & Hescheler, J. (1989). Evidence for a PO_2-sensitive K^+ channel in the type-I cell of the rabbit carotid body. FEBS Lett. 249:195-198.

Duchen, M.R., Caddy, K.W.T., Kirby, G.C., Patterson, D.L., Ponte, J. & Biscoe, T.J. (1988). Biophysical studies of the cellular elements of the rabbit carotid body. Neurosci. 26, 291-311.

Duchen, M.R. & Biscoe, T.J. (1992a). Mitochondrial function in Type I cells isolated from rabbit arterial chemoreceptors. J. Physiol. 450:13-31.

Duchen, M.R. & Biscoe, T.J. (1992b). Relative mitochondrial membrane potential and $[Ca^{2+}]$ in Type I cells isolated from the rabbit carotid body. J. Physiol. 450:33-61.

Eden, G.J. & Hanson, M.A. (1987a). Maturation of the respiratory response to acute hypoxia in the newborn rat. J. Physiol. 392:1-9.

Eden, G.J. & Hanson, M.A. (1987b). Effects of chronic hypoxia from birth on the ventilatory response to acute hypoxia in the newborn rat. J. Physiol. 392:11-19.

Elnazir, B.K. & Kumar, P. (1993). Maturation of the initial ventilatory responses to CO_2 and O_2 in conscious, newborn rats. J. Physiol. 459:337P

Elnazir, B.K., Pepper, D.R. & Kumar, P. (1993). The effect of chronic hypoxia from birth upon the initial ventilatory responses to CO_2 and O_2 in conscious, newborn rats. J. Physiol., In press.

Giussani, D.A., Spencer, J.A.D., Moore, P.J., Bennet, L. & Hanson, M.A. (1993a). Afferent and efferent components of the cardiovascular reflex responses to acute hypoxia in term fetal sheep. J. Physiol. 461:431-449.

Giussani, D.A., McGarrigle, H.H.G., Bennet, L., Moore, P.J., Spencer, J.A.D. & Hanson, M.A. (1993b). Carotid sinus nerve section affects ACTH and cortisol responses to acute isocapnic hypoxia in term fetal sheep. J. Physiol., In press.

Giussani, D.A., McGarrigle, H.H.G., Spencer, J.A.D., Moore, P.J., Bennet, L. & Hanson, M.A. (1993c). Carotid denervation does not affect plasma vasopressin levels during active hypoxia in the late gestation sheep fetus. J. Physiol., In press.

Gluckman, P.D. & Johnston, B.M. (1987). Lesions in the upper lateral pons abolish the hypoxic depression of breathing in unanaesthetized fetal lambs in utero. J. Physiol. 382:373-383.

Gonzalez, C., Almaraz, L., Obeso, A. & Rigual, R. (1992). Oxygen and acid chemoreception in the carotid body chemoreceptors. Trends in Neurosciences 15:146-153.

Hanson, M.A. (1986a). Peripheral chemoreceptor function before and after birth. In "Respiratory control and lung development in the fetus and newborn", B.M. Johnston & P.D. Gluckman, eds. pp. 311-330. Perinatology Press, New York.

Hanson, M.A. (1986b). Maturation of peripheral chemoreceptors and central nervous components of respiratory control in perinatal life. In "Neurobiology of the Control of Breathing"., C.V. Euler & H. Lagercrantz ,eds. pp. 59-65. Raven Press: New York.

Hanson, M.A., Kumar, P. & McCooke, H.B. (1986). Post-natal re-setting of carotid chemoreceptor sensitivity in the lamb. J. Physiol. 382:57P

Hanson, M.A., Nye, P.C.G. & Torrance, R.W. (1981). The exodus of an extracellular bicarbonate theory of chemoreception and the genesis of an intracellular one. In "Arterial chemoreceptors", C. Belmonte, D.J. Pallot, H. Acker & S. Fidone, eds. pp. 403-416. Leicester University Press: Leicester.

Hanson, M.A. & Williams, B.A. (1987). A role for brown adipose tissue in the biphasic ventilatory response of the newborn rat to hypoxia. J. Physiol. 386:70P

Hanson, M.A., Kumar, P. & Williams, B.A. (1989). The effect of chronic hypoxia upon the development of respiratory chemoreflexes in the newborn kitten. J. Physiol. 411:563-574.

Hanson, M.A., Eden, G.J., Nijhuis, J.G. & Moore, P.J. (1989). Peripheral chemoreceptors and other O2 sensors in the fetus and newborn. In "Chemoreceptors and Reflexes in Breathing, A.I. Pack, ed. pp. 113-120. Oxford University Press: New York.

Hanson, M.A. (1989). The importance of baro- and chemoreflexes in the control of the fetal cardiovascular system. J. Dev. Physiol. 10:491-511.

Hertzberg, T. & Lagercrantz, H. (1987). Postnatal sensitivity of the peripheral chemoreceptors in newborn infants.. Arch. Dis. Child. 62:1238-1241.

Hertzberg, T., Hellstrom, S., Holgert, H., Lagercrantz, H. & Pequignot, J.M. (1992). Ventilatory response to hyperoxia in newborn rats born in hypoxia - possible relationship to carotid body dopamine. J. Physiol. 456:645-654.

Hescheler, J., Delpiano, M.A., Acker, H. & Pietruschka, F. (1989). Ionic currents on Type I cells of the rabbit carotid body measured by voltage clamp experiments and the effect of hypoxia. Brain Res. 486:79-88.

Hill, J. R. (1959). The oxygen consumption of newborn and adult mammals.Its dependence on the oxygen tension in the inspired air and on the enviromental temperature. J. Physiol. 149:346-373.

Hohimer, A.R., Bissonnette, J.M., Richardson, B.S. & Machida, C.M. (1983). Central chemical regulation of breathing movements in fetal lambs. Respir. Physiol. 52:88-111.

Jansen, A.O., Ioffe, S. & Chernick, V. (1992). Maturation of steady-state CO_2 sensitivity in vagotomized anaesthetized lambs. J. Appl. Physiol. 72(4):1255-1260.

Jensen, A. & Berger, R. (1991). Fetal circulatory responses to oxygen lack. J. Dev. Physiol. 16:181-207.

Jensen, A. & Hanson, M.A. (1993). Circulatory responses to acute asphyxia in intact and chemodenervated fetal sheep near term. J. Dev. Physiol.. In press.

Johnston, B.M., Moore, P.J., Bennet, L., Hanson, M.A. & Gluckman, P.D. (1990). Almitrine mimics hypoxia in fetal sheep with lateral pontine lesions. J. Appl. Physiol. 69:1330-1335.

Johnston, B. M. (1991). Brain stem inhibitory mechanisms in the control of fetal breathing movements. In "The Fetal and Neonatal Brain Stem", M.A. Hanson, ed. pp. 21-47. Cambridge University Press, Cambridge.

Jones, C.T., Roebuck, M.M., Walker, D.W. & JohstonN, B. M. (1988). The role of the adrenal medulla and peripheral sympathetic nerves in the physiological responses of the fetal sheep to hypoxia. J. Dev. Physiol. 10:17-36.

Kholwadwala, D. & Donnelly, D.F. (1992). Maturation of carotid chemoreceptor sensitivity to hypoxia: in vitro studies in the newborn rat. J. Physiol. 453:461-473.

Koos, B.J., Chao, A. & Doany, W. (1992). Adenosine stimulates breathing in fetal sheep with brain stem section. J. Appl. Physiol. 72:94-99.

Kumar, P. & Hanson, M.A. (1989). Re-setting of the hypoxic sensitivity of aortic chemoreceptors in the newborn lamb. J. Dev. Physiol. 11(4):199-206.

Lahiri, S., Brody, J.S., Motoyama, E.K. & Velasquez, T.M. (1978). Regulation of breathing in newborns at high altitude. J. Appl. Physiol. 44:673-678.

Lopez-Barneo, J., Lopez-Lopez, J.R., Urena, J. & Gonzalez, C. (1988). Chemotransduction in the carotid body: K^+ current modulated by PO_2 in type I chemoreceptor cells. Science 241:580-582.

Lopez-Lopez, J.R., Gonzalez, C., Urena, J. & Lopez-Barneo, J. (1989). Low pO_2 selectively inhibits K channel activity in chemoreceptor cells of the mammalian carotid body. J. Gen. Physiol. 93:1001-1015.

Marchal, F., Bairam, A., Haouzi, P., Crance, J.P., di Giulio, C., Vert, P. & Lahiri, S. (1992). Carotid chemoreceptor response to natural stimuli in the newborn kitten. Respir. Physiol. 87:183-193.

Martin-Body, R.L. & Johnston, B.M. (1988). Central origin of the hypoxic depression of breathing in the newborn.. Respir.Physiol. 71:25-32.

Mills, E. & Jobsis, F.F. (1970). Simultaneous measurement of cytochrome aa3 reduction and chemoreceptor afferent activity in the carotid body. Nature 225:1147-1149.

Moore, P.J., Hanson, M.A. & Parkes, M.J. (1989). Almitrine inhibits breathing movements in fetal sheep. J. Dev. Physiol. 11(5):277-281.

Moore, P.J. & Hanson, M.A. (1991). The role of peripheral chemoreceptors in the rapid response of the pulmonary vasculature of the late gestation fetus to changes in PaO2. J. Dev. Physiol. 16:133-138.

Moore, P.J., Clarke, J.A., Hanson, M.A., Daly, M.D. & Ead, H.W. (1991a). Quantitative studies of the vasculature of the carotid body in fetal and newborn sheep. J. Dev. Physiol. 15:211-214.

Moore, P.J., Parkes, M.J., Noble, R. & Hanson, M.A. (1991b). Reversible blockade of the secondary fall of ventilation during hypoxia in anaesthetized newborn sheep by focal cooling in the brain stem. J. Physiol. 438:242P

Morray, J., Bennet, L., Noble, R. & Hanson, M.A. (1992). Effect of halothane on the carotid chemoreceptor response to hypoxia in anaesthetized kittens. J. Physiol. 446:425P

Mulligan, E.M. (1991). Discharge properties of carotid bodies. Developmental aspects. In "Developmental Neurobiology of Breathing". Haddad, G.G. & Farber, J.P., eds. pp 321-340. Marcel Dekker, New York.

Obeso, A., Rocher, A., Fidone, S. & Gonzalez, C. (1992). The role of dihydropyridine-sensitive Ca^{2+} channels in stimulus-evoked catecholamine release from chemoreceptor cells of the carotid body. Neurosci. 47:463-472.

Peers, C. (1990a). Hypoxic supression of K^+ currents in Type I carotid body cells: Selective effect on the Ca^{2+}-activated K^+ current. Neurosci. Lett. 119:253-256.

Peers, C. (1990b). Effect of lowered extracellular pH on Ca^{2+}-dependent K^+ currents in type I cells from the neonatal rat carotid body. J. Physiol. 422:381-395.

Peers, C. & Green, F.K. (1991). Inhibition of Ca^{2+}-activated K^+ currents by intracellular acidosis in isolated Type I cells of the neonatal rat carotid body. J. Physiol. 422:381-395.

Rigual, R., Lopez-Lopez, J.R. & Gonzalez, C. (1991). Release of dopamine and chemoreceptor discharge induced by low ph and high PCO_2 stimulation of the cat carotid body. J. Physiol. 433:519-531.

Rocher, A. , Obeso, A., Gonzalez, C. & Herreros, B. (1991). Ionic mechanisms for the transduction of acidic stimuli in rabbit carotid body glomus cells. J. Physiol. 433:533-548.

Rudolph, A.M. (1984). The fetal circulation and its response to stress. J. Dev. Physiol. 6:11-19.

Schwieler, G.H. (1968). Respiratory regulation during postnatal development in cats and rabbits and some if its morphological substrate.. Acta. Physiol. Scand. 72, Suppl. 304:1-123.

Sorensen, S.C. & Severinghaus, J.W. (1968). Respiratory insensitivity to acute hypoxia persisting after correction of tetralogy of Fallot. J. Appl. Physiol. 25:221-223.

Torrance, R.W., Bartels, E.M. & McLaren,A. (1993). Update on the bicarbonate hypothesis.. In: "Neurobiology and Cell Physiology of Chemoreception," P.G. Data, S. Lahiri & H. Acker, eds., Plenum Press, New York, In press .

Watanabe, T., Kumar, P. & Hanson, M.A. (1993). Comparison of respiratory responses to CO2 and hypoxia in neonatal kittens. J. Physiol. 459:141P

Williams, B.A. & Hanson, M.A. (1989). The effect of decerebration and brain-stem transection on the ventilatory response to acute hypoxia in normoxic and chronically hypoxic newborn rats. J. Physiol. 414:25P

Williams, B.A. & Hanson, M.A. (1990). Role of the carotid chemoreceptors in the respiratory response of newborn lambs to alternate pairs of breaths of air and a hypoxic gas. J. Dev. Physiol. 13:157-164.

Williams, B.A., Smyth, J., Boon, A.W., Hanson, M.A., Kumar, P. & Blanco, C.E. (1991). Development of respiratory chemoreflexes in response to alternations of fractional inspired oxygen in the newborn infant. J. Physiol. 442:81-90.

Wolsink, J.G., Berkenbosch, A., Degoede, J. & Olievier, N. (1991). Ventilatory sensitivities of peripheral and central chemoreceptors of young piglets to inhalation of CO_2 in air. Pediatr. Res. 30:491-495.

Wood, C. E. (1993). Local and endocrine factors in the control of the circulation. In "Fetus and Neonate; Volume One: Circulation", M.A.Hanson, J.A.D. Spencer & C.H. Rodeck, eds. pp. 100-115. Cambridge University Press; Cambridge

THE ROLE OF ARTERIAL CHEMORECEPTORS IN VENTILATORY ACCLIMATIZATION TO HYPOXIA

Gerald E. Bisgard

Department of Comparative Biosciences
University of Wisconsin
Madison, Wisconsin 53706, USA

INTRODUCTION

Mechanisms of ventilatory control responsible for increased breathing on ascent to altitude have been the object of great interest to respiratory physiologists for many generations (cf. Kellogg, 1977). On exposure to a hypoxic environment there is a time-dependent progressive rise in ventilation which is commonly termed ventilatory acclimatization to hypoxia (VAH). This paper will explore findings associated with VAH, but will not deal with mechanisms of ventilatory control in very long-term residents or natives of high altitude. Previously there was a strong focus on central medullary chemoreceptors as the source for increased ventilatory drive during VAH, but evidence (to be briefly reviewed below) has failed to support this view. Increasing evidence has accumulated suggesting that peripheral chemoreceptors constitute a primary site of ventilatory drive in VAH. The research findings relevant to the role of the peripheral chemoreceptors (carotid body) will be the focus of this chapter. The reader is referred to another recent review of this topic (Weil, 1991).

The characteristics of VAH include a time-dependent rise in ventilation and a fall in alveolar or arterial PCO_2. The time course of VAH varies proportional to the severity of hypoxia (magnitude of altitude exposure). In humans VAH on exposure to approximately 4,300 m requires about 10 days for maximal hyperventilation to be achieved (Forster et al., 1975). Whereas, with exposure to great heights as on expeditions to above 8,000 m on Mt. Everest full VAH is estimated to require more than 30 days (West, 1991). Hyperventilation on completion of acclimatization to 4,300 m is to a P_aCO_2 of 25 Torr (Forster et al., 1975), while the measured P_ACO_2 is 7.5 Torr at the summit of Mt. Everest (West et al., 1983). The ability to hyperventilate at extreme altitude may be advantageous to the ability to climb to great heights as many successful lowlander climbers to these altitudes have very high ventilatory responses to acute hypoxia (Schoene et al., 1984; West, 1991). This infers the importance of the peripheral arterial chemoreflex in altitude acclimatization.

Non-human mammals (referred to as animals in this chapter), generally acclimatize much more rapidly than humans to altitude, except for the rat, which has a time course similar to humans (Olson & Dempsey, 1978; Dempsey & Forster, 1982). Goats complete VAH in 4 to 6 hours (Smith et al., 1986; Engwall & Bisgard, 1990). Cats are known to show significant acclimatization after 48 hours at 4600 m (Vizek et al., 1987).

In this chapter there will be a brief review of mechanisms of VAH with concentration on the role of the peripheral arterial chemoreceptors in VAH. Mostly the focus will be on the carotid body (CB) chemoreceptors as there is little evidence that aortic bodies play a significant role in VAH.

CENTRAL CHEMORECEPTOR MECHANISMS OF ACCLIMATIZATION

The reader is referred to an excellent review of this topic by Dempsey & Forster (1982). Historically, when it became apparent that arterial blood gases showed diminishing stimuli (falling P_aCO_2, alkalosis and rising P_aO_2) during VAH, physiologists turned away from the arterial chemoreceptors as a cause for increasing ventilatory drive during VAH (cf. Kellogg, 1977). They looked to the medullary chemoreceptors as a possible cause for hyperventilation. This seemed to be the correct path when Severinghaus and his colleagues (1963) found that cerebrospinal fluid (CSF) pH was corrected toward normal during VAH. It was thought that CSF pH would accurately reflect the stimulus level at the medullary chemoreceptor and its acidification would provide for increased ventilatory drive, or at least, less damping of input from peripheral chemoreceptors and increased ventilatory drive. The Severinghaus finding was not confirmed in a large series of studies in which the CSF was found to be alkalotic during VAH (Forster et al., 1975, 1976; Dempsey et al., 1974, 1979; Bouverot & Bureau, 1975; Orr et al., 1975; Weiskopf et al., 1976) suggesting that either the bulk CSF did not reflect the stimulus at the central chemoreceptor or that another mechanism was responsible for VAH.

Others attempted to show that calculated pH at the central chemoreceptor was acidified, most likely by lactic acidosis, even though bulk CSF was not acidified (Davies, 1978; Fencl, 1979). However, Musch et al. (1983) could not show a correlation between lactic acid production and change in ventilatory drive at altitude in rats. Recently Xu et al. (1991, 1992) showed that CSF pH near the ventral surface of the medulla did not correlate with ventilatory drive during hypoxia. They postulated that central chemoreceptors responded to membrane gradients rather than local extracellular pH.

In addition to failure of brain lactic acid to correlate with ventilation (Musch et al., 1983), the evidence against a significant central chemoreceptor role in VAH has accumulated in other ways. One of the most important of these are the studies to be described below showing that VAH is greatly diminished in CB denervated animals and that brain hypoxia and acid-base change are not required for acclimatization to proceed. In addition, direct evidence for increased carotid chemoreceptor sensitivity to hypoxia during VAH has accumulated in recent studies.

Acclimatization was postulated to be dependent on a fall in arterial PCO_2; thus, if the change in PCO_2 could be prevented, then acclimatization would not occur. This postulate was pursued in two human subject experiments (Eger et al., 1968 and Cruz et al., 1980). The goal was to maintain eucapnia and thereby prevent acid-base compensation at the central chemoreceptor and therefore diminish the central chemoreceptor stimulus. Unfortunately, inadequate control of PCO_2 and lack of clear cut results prevented precise interpretation of the data from these studies. It is very difficult to perform such experiments in human subjects because of their slow acclimatization period requiring prolonged hypoxic exposure and the difficulty in controlling P_ACO_2 with sufficient precision under these conditions.

Such is not the case in goats in which good control of blood gases is possible with constant monitoring of end-tidal PCO_2 and frequent arterial blood gas analysis. In addition, the rapid acclimatization rate (4 hours) facilitates maintaining eucapnia. In two such studies acclimatization occurred while eucapnia was maintained (Engwall & Bisgard, 1990; Ryan et al., 1993a) (Fig. 1).

The results of these studies further diminish the view that central chemoreceptors are critical to VAH. This is clear in the goat, but one cannot entirely rule out some role for central chemoreceptors in other species, though there is no compelling evidence for such a mechanism. Rather, it appears changes at the central chemoreceptor are likely secondary to the hyperventilation originating from other sources (Dempsey & Forster, 1982)

ALTERNATIVE CNS MECHANISMS OF ACCLIMATIZATION

CNS stimulation as the result of either prolonged peripheral chemoreceptor input or by direct effects of CNS hypoxia have also been proposed as a possible mechanisms of acclimatization. Forster & Dempsey (1981) postulated that CNS hyperexcitability could be an important source of increased ventilatory drive, based on finding of increased ventilatory responses to a variety of stimuli at high altitude, including exercise, acute hypoxia, hypercapnia and doxapram infusion (Dempsey et al., 1972; Forster et al., 1971, 1974). Increased CNS activity was found in EEG studies which supported their view that CNS mechanisms may contribute to VAH in humans (Forster et al., 1975; Schmeling, 1977). There is little evidence to refute these findings and some animal studies indicate the potential for CNS mechanisms to contribute to VAH. Ou et al. (1983) using intact and decerebrate cats exposed to 5500 m found evidence that suprapontine structures can exert a facilitatory activity contributing to VAH. But, VAH could be initiated in the absence of these structures.

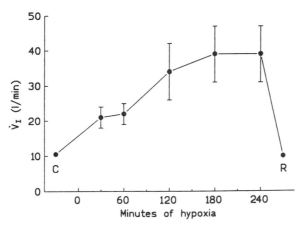

Figure 1. Time-dependent increase in ventilation in 6 goats during isocapnic hypoxia (P_aO_2 near 40 Torr). C is control normoxic ventilation, R is ventilation on return to normoxic conditions. Data redrawn from Engwall & Bisgard (1990).

Gallman and Millhorn (1988) have demonstrated a long-term facilitation of ventilation after ten minutes of hypoxia in peripheral chemoreceptor denervated cats. This was associated with the diencephalon as established by sectioning experiments. Such a finding would support the postulated increased CNS facilitation of Forster and Dempsey (1981).

Millhorn et al. (1980a, 1980b) have shown that repeated stimulation of the carotid sinus nerve results in long-term-facilitation of ventilation in anesthetized or decerebrate cats by a serotoninergic mechanism. A similar long-term-facilitation of ventilation has been demonstrated in awake dogs after repeated short hypoxic exposures (Cao et al., 1992). Thus, there is the potential for repeated CB stimulation to result in persisting hyperventilation, a common finding on return to normoxia after VAH.

CNS monaminergic metabolism is modified during chronic hypoxia; however, any potential relationship of these changes to VAH have not been established (Olson et al., 1983; Olson, 1987).

The above animal and human results suggest the possibility of CNS facilitation in VAH; however, studies in goats do not find an important role for a CNS contribution to VAH (see below).

HYPOXIC VENTILATORY DECLINE AND ACCLIMATIZATION

In humans on acute exposure to hypoxia there is a fall in ventilation after the initial few minutes of hyperventilation termed roll-off or hypoxic ventilatory decline (HVD) (Easton et al., 1986; 1988a). This may slow the onset of VAH on exposure to chronic hypoxia (Huang et al., 1984). HVD may result from either an adaptation at the peripheral chemoreceptors (Bascom et al., 1990), or be due to central ventilatory depression (Easton, 1988a; Berkenbosch et al., 1992). Most workers favor the latter view, and relate it to inhibitory CNS neurochemicals such as GABA, adenosine or dopamine (Easton et al., 1988b; Tatsumi et al., 1992; Eldridge et al., 1985). It appears that whatever the mechanism of HVD, it must subside with time in humans who reside for the week or more it takes for VAH to develop. Indeed, reversal of HVD may contribute to VAH in man. There are insufficient data from animals to make any statements relevant to the role of CNS depression of ventilation on ascent to altitude. The cat is the only known animal model which clearly shows HVD with acute hypoxia (Tatsumi et al., 1992a), but the possible role of HVD in VAH has not been studied in cats.

ROLE OF CAROTID BODIES IN ACCLIMATIZATION TO HYPOXIA

Well controlled studies of VAH in animals following CB denervation have shown that VAH is significantly attenuated in the denervated vs. intact animals showing the importance of the CB in VAH (Bouverot & Bureau, 1975; Fordyce & Tenney, 1984; Forster et al., 1976, 1981; Olson et al., 1988; Smith et al., 1986). These findings by themselves indicate an important role for the carotid bodies in VAH, but do not define their role.

In order to better understand the relationship of CNS vs. CB interaction in VAH, a CB perfusion model was developed which allows separation of the CB circulation from the systemic arterial circulation (including the CNS) in the awake goat (Busch et al., 1985). In this model surgical ligation of vessels cranial to one CB are carried out so that blood perfusing one CB does not reach the brain (Fig. 2). Blood serving the perfused CB is passed through an extracorporeal circulation system which can control blood gases to the CB. The opposite CB is denervated and the primary brain blood supply is via the common carotid artery on the denervated side. The systemic arterial blood gases are controlled by the concentrations of inspired gases and ventilation. It has been established that ventilatory responses to acute and prolonged hypoxia are normal after unilateral CB denervation in the goat (Busch et al, 1983). Using this model several studies have been completed relevant to VAH as outlined below.

The first question addressed with the CB perfusion model was: is brain hypoxia essential for VAH to be induced? To answer this question the CB PO_2 was maintained at near 40 Torr for six hours while the systemic circulation (including CNS) was maintained normoxic (Busch et al., 1985). In these studies systemic arterial blood gas measurements, (primarily P_aCO_2) were used to quantify changes in ventilation. It was found that isolated CB hypoxia produced the typical progressive fall in P_aCO_2 and rise in P_aO_2 that occurs during VAH in intact goats showing that brain hypoxia was not a required element needed to produce VAH (Fig. 3).

A similar study showed that isolated CB hypoxia could produce VAH during eucapnic systemic normoxia (Bisgard et al., 1986b). Maintaining eucapnia prevented the well known respiratory alkalosis which is typical of VAH. This provided evidence that respiratory alkalosis produced by CB stimulation did not cause some modification in central chemosensitivity which could induce VAH, making a strong case against central chemoreceptors having a role in VAH.

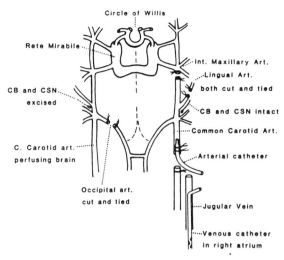

Figure 2. Diagram of goat cerebral circulation and ligations allowing isolated perfusion of the intact carotid body with an extracorporeal circuit. From Busch et al. (1985).

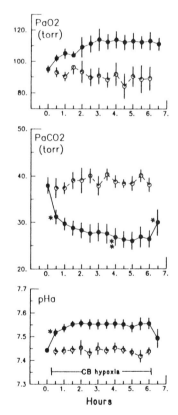

Figure 3. Changes in systemic arterial blood gases and pH in 6 awake goats as a result of perfusion of the carotid body with hypoxic blood (perfusion PO_2 near 40 Torr) (closed symbols). Open symbols indicate hyperoxic control carotid body perfusion in 3 goats. All values are mean (SEM). * indicates significant different from control, time 0. ** indicates significantly different from acute carotid body hypoxia (0.5 h). From Busch et al. (1985).

In another CB perfusion study the mode of CB stimulation was changed from hypoxia to hypercapnia (Bisgard et al., 1986a). The rationale behind this was to determine the specificity of the CB stimulation mode in producing VAH. Four hours of normoxic-hypercapnia was induced at the CB in awake goats and again the systemic circulation was maintained normoxic. Steady-state CB hypercapnia (mean CB PCO_2 78 Torr) caused steady hyperventilation but no progressive, time-dependent hyperventilation typical of VAH (Fig. 4). These findings strongly indicated that CB hypoxia was the essential element in inducing VAH in goats. Furthermore, the data suggested that it was not CNS conditioning by CB afferent activity that produced VAH as the same sinus nerve chemoreceptor afferents are known to be stimulated by hypoxia and hypercapnia.

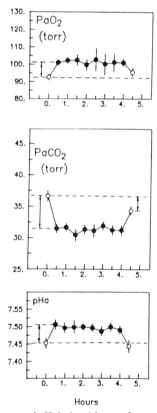

Hours

Figure 4. Systemic arterial blood gases and pH during 4 hours of normoxic-hypercapnic carotid body perfusion in 6 awake goats (perfusion PCO_2 78 Torr) (closed symbols). Control normocapnic perfusion is also illustrared (open symbols). From Bisgard et al. (1986a).

The last relevant CB perfusion study carried out sought to determine if prolonged (four hours) brain hypoxia could modulate the input from the CB and further tested the role of brain hypoxia in VAH in the awake goat (Weizhen et al., 1992). In this study the CB was maintained normoxic and systemic (including brain) hypoxia was induced by inhalation of hypoxic gas sufficient to attain a P_aO_2 of 40 Torr. The animals were maintained eucapnic throughout the studies and only those found to have minimal response to aortic body stimulation were selected for study. These experiments showed that systemic (CNS) hypoxia produced mild hyperventilation which was maximal after 30 min of hypoxia. After 30 min the hyperventilation was sustained for the remaining 3.5 hours of brain hypoxia, but there was no time-dependent progressive increase in ventilation typical of VAH. Indeed, ventilation was increased only about 4 liters/min above the control value as compared to 30 liters/min after four hours of CB hypoxia with systemic eucapnia in awake goats or during whole body hypoxia (Bisgard et al., 1986b; Engwall & Bisgard, 1990; Ryan et al., 1993a). Thus, brain hypoxia appears to play little role in VAH in the goat. Other findings in this study included lack of any change in the ventilatory response to acute CB hypoxia (during brain normoxia) after return to normoxic conditions, and lack of change in the response to inhaled CO_2 (with CB held normoxic) after the four hours of brain hypoxia (Weizhen et al., 1992). Both these findings indicate that prolonged eucapnic brain hypoxia (P_aO_2 40 Torr) does not modify the central controller response to either central (medullary chemoreceptors) or peripheral (CB) stimuli in awake goats.

The results from the awake goat were extended to include studies of chemoreceptor discharge from single carotid sinus afferents in chloralose anesthetized goats during up to four hours of hypoxic or hypercapnic stimulation (Nielsen et al., 1988; Engwall et al., 1988). These studies showed that eucapnic hypoxia caused a time-dependent rise in CB afferent discharge frequency beginning after one hour of hypoxia (P_aO_2 40 Torr)(Nielsen et al., 1988) (Fig. 5). Normoxic hypercapnia (mean P_aCO_2 85 Torr) caused a sustained elevated CB afferent discharge frequency but no time-dependent trend to elevate frequency as with hypoxia (Engwall et al., 1988). These studies were compatible with findings from awake CB perfused or normal CB intact animals during prolonged hypoxia or normoxic hypercapnia (Bisgard et al., 1986a,1986b; Engwall & Bisgard, 1990; Ryan et al., 1993a).

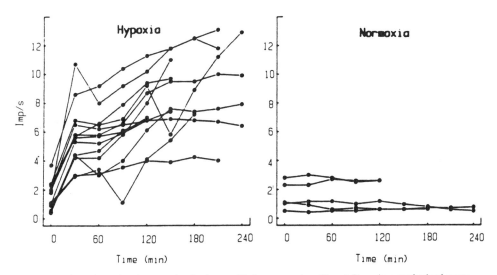

Figure 5. Time-dependent increase in single carotid chemoreceptor afferent fibers in anesthetized goats maintained in steady-state hypoxia (left) or normoxia (right) for up to 4 hours. From Nielsen et al. (1988).

The above studies indicate that increased CB sensitivity to hypoxia is the primary source for increased ventilatory drive during VAH in goats and that brain hypoxia does not play a significant role in VAH at the arterial or CB perfusion PO_2 used (near 40 Torr in all studies).

Compatible with results from the goat, Vizek et al. (1987) have shown that the cat has both an increased ventilatory response as well as increased CB afferent discharge response to acute hypoxia after two days of VAH.

VENTILATORY RESPONSE TO ACUTE HYPOXIA ASSOCIATED WITH ACCLIMATIZATION

In earlier studies ventilatory responses to hypoxia were not consistently found to change in association with VAH (cf. Forster, 1974). This trend has changed in more recent studies indicating that elevated ventilatory responses to acute hypoxia are commonly observed during and after acclimatization to hypoxia in animals (Aaron & Powell, 1993; Engwall & Bisgard, 1990; Ou et al., 1992; Tatsumi et al., 1992b; Ryan et al., 1993a; Vizek et al., 1987) and human subjects (Forster et al., 1974; Goldberg et al., 1992; Sato et al., 1992; Schoene et al., 1990; White et al., 1987; Serebrovska & Ivashkevich, 1992).

The study by Sato et al. (1992) in human subjects is particularly important as these workers minimized possible effects of hypoxic brain depression by establishing hyperoxic conditions before testing the hypoxic ventilatory response. They also controlled for changes at the central chemoreceptor by using a standardized hyperoxic end-tidal PCO_2 at the same level of ventilation for each subject. Under these conditions they showed a progressively rising ventilatory response to hypoxia during 6 days at high altitude which persisted for 4-7 days after return to sea level (Fig. 6). Such findings are compatible with increased response of the CB to hypoxia as an important, if not primary, mechanism of VAH.

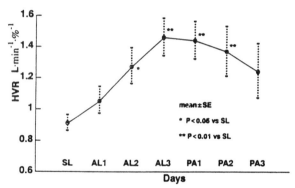

Figure 6. Hypoxic ventilatory response (HVR) in human subjects expressed as V_I/S_aO_2 at sea level (SL) and after approximately 1, 3, and 4-5 days at altitude (AL1, AL2, AL3, respectively) and after 1, 3, and 4-7 days post-altitude (PAL1, PAL2, PAL 3). Figure from Sato et al. (1992).

POSSIBLE MECHANISMS OF INCREASED CAROTID BODY RESPONSE TO HYPOXIA IN ACCLIMATIZATION

There have been few studies directed toward changes in CB hypoxic sensitivity during acclimatization. Those that have been carried out have focused on two areas, change in catecholaminergic modulation of the carotid body and efferent modulation of the CB via either the carotid sinus efferent or sympathetic efferents. Catecholaminergic modulation mechanisms could be mediated via efferents or could be intrinsic to the CB itself.

Olson et al. (1983) and Hanbauer et al. (1981) measured levels of catecholamines in the rat CB during prolonged hypoxia and found that dopamine (DA) was dramatically elevated in the CB and norepinephrine (NE) was also elevated, though to a less extent. Later Pequignot et al. (1987), showed that there was not only an increase in DA and NE levels, but their turnover rates were increased during chronic hypoxia. His group also found that CB DA turnover was at least partially under control of the sympathetic innervation to the CB (Pequignot et al., 1991). These studies strongly implicate some role for catecholaminergic mechanisms in mediating CB hypoxic sensitivity.

Carotid sinus nerve efferents are considered to be inhibitory to the CB and mediate their effects via DA release (O'Regan and Majcherczyk, 1983; Lahiri et al., 1984). After 3 to 7 weeks of hypoxia efferent activity in the carotid sinus nerve was found to be elevated (Lahiri, 1983, 1984). This finding would be incompatible with increased sensitivity to hypoxia. The effect of carotid sinus nerve efferents has been put in doubt by another study in acclimatized cats showing little effect of sinus nerve section on the increased hypoxic sensitivity of the acclimatized cat CB (Vizek et al., 1987). Carotid sinus nerve efferents are not required for increased CB afferent discharge during prolonged hypoxia in anesthetized goats (Nielsen et al., 1988). These findings do not support a major role for carotid sinus efferents in VAH, but do not rule out a role for intrinsic CB dopaminergic mechanisms.

Studies have been carried out to try to define the role of CB DA in VAH. Assuming an inhibitory role for DA on CB function, down-regulation of either DA release or receptor activity might be possible mechanisms involved in increasing hypoxic sensitivity of the CB. Two studies have failed to find a change in ventilatory response to infusions of DA suggesting no change in receptor activity during prolonged hypoxia in goats (Engwall & Bisgard, 1990; Ryan et al., 1993a). Carotid body DA blockade has provided equivocal results in goats suggesting that CB DA release might be involved in VAH (Bisgard et al.,1987). More convincing evidence for a similar mechanism was obtained by Tatsumi et al.(1992b), who found that increased maximal ventilatory response to hypoxia after CB DA blockade with domperidone was not further enhanced after VAH in cats. Thus, there is evidence for diminished dopaminergic inhibition having some role in increasing CB sensitivity to hypoxia during VAH. More research is needed to further elucidate this potential mechanism.

Noradrenergic mechanisms of VAH in the CB have also been examined recently. Inhibitory alpha-2 adrenergic receptors have been discovered in the cat CB (Kou et al., 1991). Cao et al. (1991) found that sensitivity to alpha-2 agonists was diminished in cats after 24 hours of hypoxia suggesting a down regulation of adrenergic inhibition in the cat CB could play a role in VAH. Goats have been found to have a similar CB alpha-adrenergic inhibitory response which can be shown by intracarotid infusions of NE (Pizarro et al., 1992). These findings served as the basis for studies of noradrenergic sensitivity to hypoxia and the role of sympathetic innervation of the CB in VAH in awake goats. Sensitivity to intracarotid NE infusion was found to be unchanged during and after VAH, and sympathetic denervation of the CB did not affect the time course of VAH, failing to support a role for noradrenergic mechanisms in VAH (Ryan et al., 1993a, 1993b).

In related studies beta-adrenergic blockade with propranolol had no effect on ventilatory acclimatization to 4,300 m in human subjects (Moore et al., 1987).

These studies suggest that intrinsic dopaminergic mechanisms may play a role in CB sensitivity to hypoxia during VAH, but do not provide support for neural efferents or noradrenergic CB mechanisms having a significant role in VAH. Other mechanisms intrinsic to the CB could play a role including increased activity of excitatory neuromodulators, inhibition of other inhibitory neuromodulators or a change in the expression of the transduction system itself.

VENTILATORY DEACCLIMATIZATION AFTER ALTITUDE SOJOURN

On return to normoxia, altitude sojourners maintain hyperventilation for at least 13 hours (Dempsey et al., 1979). It has been assumed that this continued hyperventilation (deacclimatization) was a manifestation of the same mechanism responsible for acclimatization. Studies in goats have shown that continued hyperventilation on return to normoxia only occurs if hypocapnic alkalosis has been allowed to develop during the hyperventilation of VAH. If arterial eucapnic conditions are maintained during hypoxia, then hyperventilation does not occur on return to normoxia (Bisgard et al., 1986b; Engwall & Bisgard, 1990; Ryan at al., 1993a). These studies suggest that it is likely there are separate mechanisms responsible for VAH and deacclimatization. VAH appears to be primarily initiated by CB mechanisms and perhaps other CNS stimuli while deacclimatization is secondary to the respiratory alkalosis that is caused by VAH, perhaps a resetting of the central chemoreceptors following compensation for the hypocapnic alkalosis.

SUMMARY

This brief review has attempted to provide an overview and update to readers on mechanisms of VAH. There now seems to be clear evidence for an important contribution from the CB in VAH. Indeed, in the goat and cat the CB seems to be the primary organ responsible for VAH. In humans it is difficult to be certain that the CB is as important as in the goat and cat because of inability to carry out invasive experiments. A few minutes after the onset of hypoxia humans experience hypoxic ventilatory decline possibly due to hypoxic brain depression, but later there is evidence for increased CNS facilitation during prolonged hypoxia. These phenomena likely affect the time course of VAH and may modulate the final level of ventilation. Nevertheless, recent available data showing evidence of increased ventilatory responses to acute hypoxia during and after VAH are compatible with a major role for the CB in VAH of humans.

The author wishes to thank the many colleagues who have contributed to the studies presented in this brief review. All of the studies quoted from the author's laboratory were supported by NIH grant HL15473.

REFERENCES

Aaron, E.A. & Powell, F.L. (1993). Effect of chronic hypoxia on hypoxic ventilatory response in awake rats. J. Appl. Physiol. 74:1635-1640.

Bascom, D.A., Clement, I.D., Cunningham, D.A., Painter, R., Robbins, P.A. (1990). Changes in peripheral chemoreflex sensitivity during sustained, isocapnic hypoxia. Respir. Physiol. 82:161-176.

Berkenbosch, A., Dahan, A., DeGoede, J., Olievier, I.C.W. (1992). The ventilatory response to CO_2 of the peripheral and central chemoreflex loop before and after sustained hypoxia in man. J. Physiol. (Lond.) 456:71-83.

Bisgard, G.E., Busch, M.A., Daristotle, L., Berssenbrugge, A., Forster, H.V. (1986a). Carotid body hypercapnia does not elicit ventilatory acclimatization in goats. Respir. Physiol. 65:113-125.

Bisgard, G.E., Busch, M.A., Forster, H.V. (1986b). Ventilatory acclimatization to hypoxia is not dependent on cerebral hypocapnic alkalosis. J. Appl. Physiol. 60:1011-1015.

Bisgard, G.E., Kressin, N.A., Nielsen, A.M., Daristotle, L., Smith, C.A., Forster, H.V. (1987). Dopamine blockade alters ventilatory acclimatization to hypoxia in goats. Respir. Physiol. 69:245-255.

Bouverot, P., & Bureau, M. (1975). Ventilatory acclimatization and CSF acid-base balance on carotid chemodenervated dogs at 3,550 m. Pflügers Arch. 361:17-23.

Busch, M.A., Bisgard, G.E., Forster, H.V. (1985). Ventilatory acclimatization to hypoxia is not dependent on arterial hypoxemia. J. Appl. Physiol. 58:1874-1880.

Busch, M.A., Mesina, J., Forster, H.V., Bisgard, G.E. (1983). The effects of unilateral carotid body excision on ventilatory control in goats. Respir. Physiol. 54:353-361.

Cao, H., Kou, Y.R., Prabhakar, N.R. (1991). Absence of chemoreceptor inhibition by alpha-2 adrenergic receptor agonist in cats exposed to low PO_2. FASEB J. 5:A1118.

Cao, K-Y., Zwillich, C.W., Berthon-Jones, M, Sullivan, C.E. (1992). Increased normoxic ventilation induced by repetitive hypoxia in conscious dogs. J. Appl. Physiol. 1992; 73:2083-2088.

Cruz, J.C., Reeves, J.T., Grover, R.F., Maher, J.T., McCullough, R.E., Denniston, J.C. (1980). Ventilatory acclimatization to high altitude is prevented by CO_2 breathing. Respir. 39:121-130.

Davies, D.G. (1978). Evidence for cerebral extracellular fluid [H+] as a stimulus during acclimatization to hypoxia. Respir. Physiol. 32:167-182.

Dempsey, J.A., & Forster, H.V. (1982). Mediation of ventilatory adaptations. Physiol. Rev. 62:262-346.

Dempsey, J.A., Forster, H.V., Bisgard, G.E., Chosy, L.W., Hanson, P.G., Kiorpes, A.L., Pelligrino, D.A. (1979). Role of cerebrospinal fluid [H+] in ventilatory deacclimatization from chronic hypoxia. J. Clin. Invest. 64:199-205.

Dempsey, J.A., Forster, H.V., Birnbaum, M.L., Reddan, W.G., Thoden, J., Grover, R.F., Rankin, J. (1972). Control of exercise hyperpnea under varying durations of exposure to moderate hypoxia. Respir. Physiol. 16:213-231.

Dempsey, J.A., Forster, H.V., DoPico, G.A. (1974). Ventilatory acclimatization to moderate hypoxemia in man. The role of spinal fluid [H+]. J. Clin. Invest. 53:1091-1100.

Dempsey, J.A., Forster, H.V., Gledhill, N., DoPico, G.A. (1975). Effects of moderate hypoxemia and hypocapnia on CSF [H+] and ventilation in man. J. Appl. Physiol. 38:665-674.

Easton, P.A., & Anthonisen, N.R. (1988). Ventilatory response to sustained hypoxia after pretreatment with aminophylline. J. Appl. Physiol. 64:1445-1450.

Easton, P.A., Slykerman, L.J., Anthonisen, N.R. (1986). Ventilatory response to sustained hypoxia in normal adults. J. Appl. Physiol. 61:906-911.

Easton, P.A., Slykerman, L.J., Anthonisen, N.R. (1988a). Recovery of the ventilatory response to hypoxia in normal adults. J. Appl. Physiol. 64:521-528.

Eger E.I.,II, Kellogg, R.H., Mines, A.H., Lima-Ostos, M., Morrill, C.G., Kent, D.W. (1968). Influence of CO_2 on ventilatory acclimatization to altitude. J. Appl. Physiol. 24:607-615.

Eldridge, F.L., Millhorn, D.E., Kiley, J.P. (1985). Antagonism by theophylline of respiratory inhibition induced by adenosine. J. Appl. Physiol. 59:1428-1433.

Engwall, M.J.A., & Bisgard, G.E. (1990). Ventilatory responses to chemoreceptor stimulation after hypoxic acclimatization in awake goats. J. Appl. Physiol. 69:1236-1243.

Engwall, M.J.A., Vidruk, E.H., Nielsen, A.M., Bisgard, G.E. (1988). Response of the goat carotid body to acute and prolonged hypercapnia. Respir. Physiol. 74:335-344.

Fencl, V., Gabel, R.A., Wolfe, D. (1979). Composition of cerebral fluids in goats adapted to high altitude. J. Appl. Physiol. 47:508-513.

Fordyce, W.E. & Tenney, S.M. (1984). Role of the carotid bodies in ventilatory acclimation to chronic hypoxia by the awake cat. Respir. Physiol. 58:207-221.

Forster, H.V., Bisgard, G.E., Klein, J.P. (1981). Effect of peripheral chemoreceptor denervation on acclimatization of goats during hypoxia. J. Appl. Physiol. 50:392-398.

Forster, H.V., Bisgard, G.E., Rasmussen, B., Orr, J.A., Buss, D.D., Manohar, M. (1976). Ventilatory control in peripheral chemoreceptor-denervated ponies during chronic hypoxemia. J. Appl. Physiol. 41:878-885.

Forster, H.V., Dempsey, .J.A. (1981). Ventilatory adaptations. In "Lung Biology in Health and Disease. Regulation of Breathing." T. Hornbein, ed. Dekker, New York.

Forster, H.V., Dempsey, J.A., Birnbaum, M.L., Reddan, W.G., Thoden, J., Grover, R.F., Rankin, J. (1971). Effect of chronic exposure to hypoxia on ventilatory response to CO_2 and hypoxia. J. Appl. Physiol. 31:586-592.

Forster, H.V., Dempsey, J.A., Chosy, L.W. (1975). Incomplete compensation of CSF [H+] in man during acclimatization to high altitude (4,300 m). J. Appl. Physiol. 38:1067-1072.

Forster, H.V., Dempsey, J.A., Vidruk,E., DoPico, G.A. (1974). Evidence of altered regulation of ventilation during exposure to hypoxia. Respir. Physiol. 20:379-392.

Forster, H.V., Soto, R.J., Dempsey, J.A., Hosko, M.J. (1975). Effect of sojourn at 4,300 m altitude on electroencephalogram and visual evoked response. J. Appl. Physiol. 39:109-113.

Gallman, E.A. & Millhorn, D.E. (1988). Two long-lasting central respiratory responses following acute hypoxia in glomectomized cats. J. Physiol. (Lond.) 395:333-347.

Goldberg, S.V., Schoene, R.B., Haynor, D., Trimble, B., Swenson, E.R., Morrison, J.B., Banister, E.J. (1992). Brain tissue pH and ventilatory acclimatization to high altitude. J. Appl. Physiol. 72:58-63.

Hanbauer, I., Karoum, F., Hellstrom, S., Lahiri, S. (1981). Effects of hypoxia lasting up to one month on the catecholamine content in rat carotid body. Neurosci. 6:81-86.

Huang, S.Y., Alexander, J.K., Grover, R., Maher, J.T., McCullough, R.E., McCullough, R.G., Moore, L.G., Sampson, J.B., Weil, J.V., Reeves, J.V. (1984). Hypocapnia and sustained hypoxia blunt ventilation on arrival at high altitude. J. Appl. Physiol. 56:602-606.

Kellogg, R.H. (1977). Oxygen and carbon dioxide in the regulation of respiration. Fed. Proc. 36:1658-1663.

Kou, Y.R., Ernsberger, P., Cragg, P.A., Cherniack, N.S., Prabhakar, N.R. (1991). Role of alpha-2 adrenergic receptors in the carotid body response to isocapnic hypoxia. Respir. Physiol. 83:353-364.

Lahiri, S., Smatresk, N., Pokorski, M., Barnard, P., Mokashi, A. (1983). Efferent inhibition of carotid body chemoreception in chronically hypoxic cats. Amer. J. Physiol. 245:R678-R683.

Lahiri, S., Smatresk, N., Pokorski, M., Barnard, P., Mokashi, A., McGregor, K.H. (1984). Dopaminergic efferent inhibition of carotid body chemoreceptors in chronically hypoxic cats. Amer. J. Physiol. 247:R24-R28.

Millhorn, D.E., Eldridge, F.L., Waldrop, T.G.(1980a). Prolonged stimulation of respiration by a new central neural mechanism. Respir. Physiol. 41:87-103.

Millhorn, D.E., Eldridge, F.L., Waldrop, T.G. (1980b). Prolonged stimulation of respiration by endogenous central serotonin. Respir. Physiol. 42:171-188.

Moore, L.G., Cymerman, A., Huang, S.Y., McCullough, R.E., McCullough, R.G., Rock, P.B., Young, A., Young, P., Weil, J.V., Reeves, J.T. (1987). Propranolol blocks metabolic rate increase but not ventilatory acclimatization to 4300 m. Respir. Physiol. 70:195-204.

Musch, T.I., Dempsey, J.A., Smith, C.A., Mitchell, G.S., Bateman, N.T. (1983). Metabolic acids and [H+] regulation in brain tissue during acclimatization to chronic hypoxia. J. Appl. Physiol. 55:1486-1495.

Nielsen, A.M., Bisgard, G.E., Vidruk, E.H. (1988). Carotid chemoreceptor activity during acute and sustained hypoxia in goats. J. Appl. Physiol. 65:1796-1802.

Olson, E.B.,Jr. (1987). Ventilatory adaptation to hypoxia occurs in serotonin-depleted rats. Respir. Physiol. 69:227-235.

Olson, E.B.,Jr. & Dempsey, J. (1978). Rat as a model for human-like ventilatory adaptation to chronic hypoxia. J. Appl. Physiol. 44:763-769.

Olson, E.B., Jr., Vidruk, E.H., Dempsey, J.A. (1988). Carotid body excision significantly changes ventilatory control in awake rats. J. Appl. Physiol. 64:666-671.

Olson, E.B.,Jr., Vidruk, E.H., McCrimmon, D.R., Dempsey, J.A. (1983). Monoamine neurotransmitter metabolism during acclimatization to hypoxia in rats. Respir. Physiol. 54:79-96.

O'Regan, R.G. & Majcherczyk, S. (1983) Control of peripheral chemoreceptors by efferent nerves. In "Physiology of the Peripheral Arterial Chemoreceptors"., H. Acker & R.G. O'Regan., eds., Elsevier, Amsterdam, pp 257-298.

Orr, J.A., Bisgard, G.E., Forster, H.V., Buss, D.D., Dempsey, J.A., Will, J.A. (1975). Cerebrospinal fluid alkalosis during high-altitude sojourn in unanesthetized ponies. Respir. Physiol. 25:23-37.

Ou, L.C., Chen, J., Fiore, E., Leiter, J.C., Brinck-Johnsen, T., Birchard, G.F., Clemons, G., Smith, R.P. (1992). Ventilatory and hematopoietic responses to chronic hypoxia in two rat strains. J. Appl. Physiol. 72:2354-2363.

Ou, L.C., St. John, W.M., Tenney, S.M. (1983). The contribution of central mechanisms rostral to the pons in high altitude ventilatory acclimatization. Respir. Physiol. 54:343-351.

Pequignot, J.M., Cottet-Emard, J.M., Dalmaz, Y., Peyrin, L. (1987). Dopamine and norepinephrine dynamics in rat carotid body during long-term hypoxia. J. Auton. Nerv. Sys. 21:9-14.

Pequignot, J.M., Dalmaz, Y., Claustre, J., Cottet-Emard, J.M., Borghini, N., Peyrin, L. (1991). Preganglionic sympathetic fibres modulate dopamine turnover in rat carotid body during long-term hypoxia. J. Auton. Nerv. Sys. 32:243-250.

Pizarro, J., Warner, M.M., Ryan, M.L., Mitchell, G.S., Bisgard, G.E. (1992). Intracarotid norepinephrine infusions inhibit ventilation in goats. Respir. Physiol. 90:299-310.

Ryan, M.L., Hedrick, M.S., Pizarro, J., Bisgard, G.E. (1993a). Carotid body noradrenergic sensitivity in ventilatory acclimatization to hypoxia. Respir. Physiol. 92:77-90.

Ryan, M.L., Hedrick, M.S., Pizarro, J., Li, Q., Bisgard, G.E. (1993b). Ventilatory acclimatization to hypoxia does not require sympathetic innervation to the carotid body in awake goats. FASEB J. 7:A396.

Sato, M., Severinghaus, J.W., Powell, F.L., Xu, F-D., Spellman, M.J.,Jr. (1992). Augmented hypoxic ventilatory response in men at altitude. J. Appl. Physiol. 73:101-107.

Schmeling, W.T., Forster, H.V., Hosko, M.J. (1977). Effect of sojourn at 3200 m altitude on spinal reflexes in young adult males. Aviat. Space. Environ. Med. 48:1039-1045.

Schoene, R.B., Lahiri, S., Hackett, P.H., Peters, R.M.,Jr., Milledge, J.S., Pizzo, C.J., Sarnquist, F.H., Boyer, S.J., Graber, D.J., Maret, K.H., West, J.B. (1984). Relationship of hypoxic ventilatory response to exercise performance on Mount Everest. J. Appl. Physiol. 56: 1478-1483.

Schoene, R.B., Roach, R.C., Hackett, P.H., Sutton, J.R., Cymerman, A., Houston, C.S. (1990). Operation everest II: ventilatory adaptation during gradual decompression to extreme altitude. Med. Sci. Sports. Exer. 22:804-810.

Serebrovskaya, T.V. & Ivashkevich, A.A. (1992). Effects of a 1-yr stay at altitude on ventilation, metabolism, and work capacity. J. Appl. Physiol. 73:1749-1755.

Severinghaus, J.W., Mitchell, R.A., Richardson, B.W., Singer, M.M. (1963). Respiratory control at high altitude suggesting active transport regulation of CSF pH. J. Appl. Physiol. 18:1155-1166.

Smith, C.A., Bisgard, G.E., Nielsen, A.M., Daristotle, L., Kressin, N.A., Forster, H.V., Dempsey, J.A. (1986). Carotid bodies are required for ventilatory acclimatization to chronic hypoxia. J. Appl. Physiol. 60:1003-1010.

Tatsumi, K., Pickett, C.K., Weil, J.V. (1992a). Effects of haloperidol and domperidone on ventilatory roll off during sustained hypoxia in cats. J. Appl. Physiol. 72:1945-1952.

Tatsumi, K., Pickett, C.K., Weil, J.V. (1992b). Possible role of dopamine in ventilatory acclimatization to high altitude. Am. Rev. Respir. Dis. 145:A677.

Vizek. M., Pickett, C.K., Weil, J.V. (1987). Increased carotid body hypoxic sensitivity during acclimatization to hypobaric hypoxia. J. Appl. Physiol. 63:2403-2410.

Weil, J.V. (1991). Control of ventilation in chronic hypoxia: role of peripheral chemoreceptors. In "Response and Adaptation to Hypoxia, Organ to Organelle". Lahiri, S., Cherniack, N.S., & Fitzgerald, R.S., eds.

Weiskopf, R.B., Gabel, R.A., Fencl, V. (1976). Alkaline shift in lumbar and intracranial CSF in man after 5 days at high altitude. J. Appl. Physiol. 41:93-97.

Weizhen, N., Engwall, M.J.A., Daristotle, L., Pizarro, J., Bisgard, G.E. (1992). Ventilatory effects of prolonged systemic (CNS) hypoxia in awake goats. Respir. Physiol. 87:37-48.

West, J.B. (1988). Rate of ventilatory acclimatization to extreme altitude. Respir. Physiol. 74: 323-333.

West, J.B. (1991). Acclimatizaton and Adaptation: Organ to Cell. In "Response and Adaptation to Hypoxia, Organ to Organelle". Lahiri, S., Cherniack, N.S., & Fitzgerald, R.S., eds.

West, J.B., Hackett, P.H., Maret, K.H., Milledge, J.S., Peters, R.M. Jr., Pizzo, C.J. Winslow, R.M. (1983). Pulmonary gas exchange on the summit of Mount Everest. J. Appl. Physiol. 55:678-687.

White, D.P., Gleeson, K., Pickett, C.K., Rannels, A.M., Cymerman, A., Weil, J.V. (1987). Altitude acclimatization: influence on periodic breathing and chemoresponsiveness during sleep. J. Appl. Physiol. 63:401-412.

Xu, F., Sato, M., Spellman, M.J.,Jr., Mitchell, R.A., Severinghaus, J.W. (1992). Topography of cat medullary ventral surface hypoxic acidification. J. Appl. Physiol. 73:2631-2637.

Xu, F.D., Spellman, M.J.,Jr., Sato, M., Baumgartner, J.E., Ciricillo, S.F., Severinghaus, J.W. (1991). Anomalous hypoxic acidification of medullary ventral surface. J. Appl. Physiol. 71:2211-2217.

CHEMOSENSITIVITY FROM THE LUNGS OF VERTEBRATES

Peter Scheid and Hashim Shams

Institut für Physiologie, Ruhr-Universität Bochum, 44780 Bochum, FRG

INTRODUCTION

It is well established today that arterial and central receptors sensitive to CO_2 and H^+ can affect breathing. However, it is likewise appreciated that these receptors alone cannot explain the adaptive changes of respiration in all experimental and natural conditions, particularly not during mild and moderate exercise, when both arterial (and probably central) PCO_2 and $[H^+]$ are decreased and thus ruled out as stimuli for exercise hyperpnea. The theory of Zuntz & Geppert (1886) of receptors sensitive to the PCO_2 in mixed venous blood has, therefore, long remained attractive (see Dejours, 1964) since mixed venous PCO_2 is certainly increased even during mild exercise. However, positive evidence for the existence of such receptors in mammals has never been provided.

A similar strategic placement for receptors would be in the lung itself, particularly if they were accessible to the inflowing blood. The observation of CO_2-sensitive receptors in the avian lung (Fedde & Peterson, 1970; see Scheid & Piiper, 1986) received, therefore, great interest even among mammalian physiologists. But although similar receptors have been observed in other non-mammalian air-breathing vertebrates (see Fedde & Kuhlmann, 1978), convincing evidence of their existence in mammalian lungs has, to our understanding, not been provided.

We will review the evidence of CO_2-sensitivity from the lungs of air-breathing vertebrates. We will, in particular, suggest that some apparent chemosensitivity originating from mammalian lungs is due to prostanoid mediators, particularly to thromboxane A_2.

PULMONARY CO_2-SENSITIVITY IN VERTEBRATE LUNGS

Birds

A number of early studies of the effects of altering intrapulmonary gas concentrations and of bilateral vagotomy have suggested that receptors which are involved in the control of breathing are present in the avian lung; and CO_2-sensitive afferents from the lung have indeed been recorded in the vagus nerve (see Fedde & Kuhlmann, 1978). It has, however, long been undecided whether these endings were specifically chemosensitive or were merely CO_2-sensitive mechanoreceptors. We have used the peculiar anatomy of the avian lung in an experimental model to investigate this question in the duck (Fedde et al., 1974a).

Arterial Chemoreceptors: Cell to System
Edited by R. O'Regan *et al*, Plenum Press, New York, 1994

The avian respiratory system consists of the gas exchanging parabronchial lung and a number of spacious air-sacs (Fig. 1; see Scheid, 1979). The parabronchi are long, narrow tubes, surrounded by the gas exchanging tissue and open at both ends to the secondary bronchi. The two sets of secondary bronchi connect to the primary bronchi, which depart from the trachea. There are two groups of airsacs: the cranial group (cervical, clavicular, cranial thoracic) is connected to the medioventral secondary bronchi; the caudal group (caudal thoracic, abdominal) connects directly to the main bronchus. All airsacs serve as bellows to ventilate the parabronchi during both inspiration and expiration. The advantage of this structural system for the study of pulmonary CO_2 receptors is that a mode of unidirectional ventilation of the parabronchial lung can be established by entering a constant flow of gas into the trachea which leaves a cannulated airsac of the caudal group, thus providing ventilation without motion. The CO_2 composition of this ventilating gas can rapidly be changed while vagal afferents are recorded (Fedde et al., 1974a). Vagal afferents

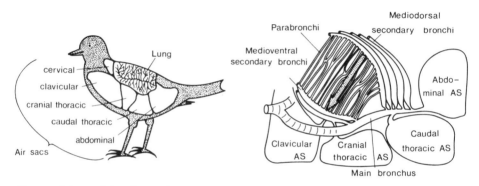

Figure 1. Schema of the avian respiratory system with lung and airsacs (left) and their connection to the bronchial system.

were found which reduced their firing rate in a predictable way when gas CO_2 fraction was increased or decreased in steps between 0 and about 0.10. If, on the other hand, the ventilatory outflow was obstructed so as to increase intrapulmonary pressure, these endings did not alter their firing rate (Fig. 2). We have, therefore, concluded that these receptors are true chemosensitive endings, and they have been termed *intrapulmonary chemoreceptors* (IPC). IPC respond to CO_2 even when the pulmonary circulation is occluded so that the stimulus cannot reach the arterial blood. There is conclusive evidence that IPC inhibit breathing (see Fedde and Kuhlmann, 1978). The mechanism by which CO_2 affects their firing rate remains unknown.

We found, like others (Molony, 1974), a second type of afferent vagal fibers which were mechanosensitive, but did not show CO_2 sensitivity (Fedde et al., 1974b). This lack in response to changes in pulmonary CO_2 concentration may be due to the location of these receptors outside the lung.

Reptiles

Reptiles respond with a first-breath increase in ventilation to elevation of inspired CO_2, suggesting CO_2 sensitivity in these animals as well. Single-unit recordings of vagal afferents have indeed shown that CO_2 sensitive receptors exist in lungs of the lizard (*Tupinambis nigropunctatus*; Fedde et al., 1977) and the turtle (Milsom & Jones, 1979). The lizard lung is sack-shaped, which allows for unidirectional ventilation like in birds. With this technique,

we found IPC in the tegu lung that resembled those in the avian lung: receptors that responded to CO_2 in the lung gas but did not respond to stretch. A second type of CO_2 sensitive endings was stretch receptors which displayed a mild CO_2 sensitivity (Fedde et al. 1977).

Amphibians

The respiratory response to CO_2 in the bullfrog appears to be due to CO_2-sensitive

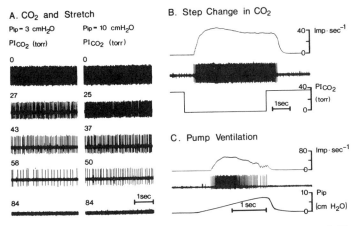

Figure 2. Intrapulmonary chemoreceptor in the duck lung. This vagal afferent responded in A to various steady levels of CO_2 (left) but not to stretch (right). It showed a rapid phasic response to a step change in PCO_2 and responded in C to cyclic pump ventilation of the animal with its cyclic variation in PCO_2.

mechanoreceptors in their lungs. IPC have, however, not been observed in these animals (Fedde & Kuhlmann, 1978).

Mammals

Unidirectional ventilation cannot be easily established in mammals. However, experiments in dogs with cardio-pulmonary bypass (Bradley et al., 1976) and pulmonary vascular occlusion suggested that changes in pulmonary gas CO_2 concentration affected respiration. The search for IPC in the cat remained unsuccessful (Kunz et al., 1976), and the CO_2 response was attributed to a CO_2 sensitivity of slowly adapting pulmonary stretch receptors (SAR), which are known to affect breathing. The firing rate of SAR has indeed been reported to be modulated by intrapulmonary CO_2 concentration (Mustafa and Purves, 1972; Schoener and Frankel, 1972; Sant-Ambrogio et al., 1974).

We have looked at this problem again using the dog with one vascularly isolated lung in which we could establish varied levels of CO_2 and record from vagal afferent fibers Mitchell et al., 1980). The other lung was vascularly intact, and served gas exchange, but was denervated. Hence, we could observe the reflex effect of changing intrapulmonary CO_2 concentration on breathing by recording the phrenic neurogram. Although both lung stretch and changes in arterial PCO_2 (via the gas exchanging lung) affected phrenic output in a predictable way, changing pulmonary PCO_2 in the vascularly isolated lung did neither affect breathing nor the activity of vagal afferents.

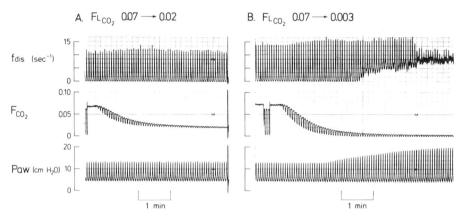

Figure 3. Response of a slowly adapting pulmonary stretch receptor in the dog to changing airway CO_2 concentration (FCO2) in the pump-ventilated vascularly isolated lung. In A, FCO2 was changed from 0.07 to 0.02, which did neither affect (integrated) discharge frequency of the fiber (fdis) nor airway pressure (Paw). When the change in FCO2 was, however, to near zero (0.003 in B), fdis became erratic, and Paw increased. (From Mitchell et al., 1980)

At first, this result was unexpected, particularly in the light of the literature evidence. However, we consistently found the amplitude of phrenic output and the phrenic burst frequency to diminish when the lung gas CO_2 fraction was reduced below about 0.01. And it was in this low CO_2 range that the vagal afferents responded with rather erratic frequency, and that the airway pressure increased (Fig. 3). We concluded that in this unphysiological condition with obstructed bronchial blood flow, the low airway PCO_2 will affect the bronchial smooth muscle and will thus stimulate the lung stretch afferents. This unphysiological reflex, which is typical for the isolated lung, may thus have no physiological significance. At that time we concluded that intrapulmonary CO_2 sensitivity did not exist in the lung of dogs, and probably not in other mammals (Mitchell et al., 1980).

New evidence for intrapulmonary CO_2 sensitivity of respiration in the dog came from experiments by Sheldon and Green (1982) in which pulmonary circulation was isolated from systemic circulation. Increases in either pulmonary blood flow or pulmonary arterial PCO_2 resulted in increases in breathing. This, and some notion that right ventricular CO_2 may have an effect on breathing, stimulated us to perform an investigation in the cat in which we loaded the venous blood with CO_2 (Orr et al., 1988). We used an oxygenator in a peripheral arterio-venous bypass to return CO_2-laden blood to the femoral vein, whereby the mixed venous PCO_2 was elevated by about 10 Torr. The anesthetized cat was pump-ventilated so as to maintain arterial PCO_2 constant, independent of CO_2 loading; the phrenic neurogram was recorded to investigate the respiratory effect of the venous loading procedure. Although the cats maintained their arterial CO_2 sensitivity, they did not display any response to the venous CO_2 loading. We concluded that there are no respiratory chemoreceptors in our experimental animals, neither in the larger veins, nor in the right heart, or the pulmonary circulation, up into the capillary bed. The apparent difference to the results of others, particularly those of Sheldon and Green (1982) could not be explained, although some differences in the experimental protocol were obvious: among them, the high CO_2 levels (up to 85 Torr) and the CO_2 elevation in the entire pulmonary circulation in the experiments of Sheldon and Green (1982). It should also be noted that their experiments necessitated quite extensive thoracic surgery (see below).

CARDIO-RESPIRATORY EFFECTS MEDIATED BY THROMBOXANE A_2

Acid infusion in the cat

During our CO_2 loading experiments (Orr et al., 1988) we used intravenous acid infusion to test for H^+ sensitivity of respiration (Orr et al., 1987). We observed that low-rate infusion of 0.25 molar HCl evoked unexpected cardio-respiratory effects, consisting of pulmonary hypertension and rapid shallow breathing, whereas increased tidal volume had been expected in response to the lowering of the venous and arterial blood pH. To investigate this reaction, we incorporated in the anesthetized cat an arterio-venous loop, from a femoral artery to a femoral vein, to infuse the acid; and we simultaneously infused, a few cm downstream from the acid infusion site, a stoichiometrically equal amount of NaOH, both at a rate of 0.2 mmol·min^{-1} (shunt flow, 20 ml·min^{-1}). Although the blood pH was normal before it re-entered the circulation, the cardio-respiratory effects remained the same: rapid-shallow breathing and pulmonary hypertension (Fig. 4). It was remarkable that these effects could only be observed upon the first acid infusion; the second, or any further, infusion showed a very attenuated response, if any.

Thromboxane A_2 mediates the effects of acid infusion

A possible candidate for these responses appeared to be thromboxane(Tx)A_2 which is synthesized in and released from various cells including blood cells and is known to be a potent vasoconstrictor. Our hypothesis was, thus, that the low pH created in blood at the very tip of the acid infusion catheter would stimulate, e.g., platelets to release TxA_2. The first acid infusion did indeed result in significantly elevated plasma levels of TxB_2 (the stable degradation product of TxA_2) which correlated with the cardio-respiratory effects. When the Tx synthase was blocked with Dazmegrel, both elevation of plasma TxB_2 and cardio-respiratory effects were eliminated. On the other hand, the TxA_2 mimetic, U46,619, evoked the same cardio-respiratory effects (without elevating Tx levels in blood). These experiments showed clearly the involvement of thromboxane A_2 in the effects that we had observed with acid infusion.

These results should also be considered when critically reading earlier reports on chemosensitivity of respiration. Intravenous infusion of strong acids has often been used as a tool to lower blood pH, and the respiratory effects, at least those in response to the first acid infusion, may be a mixture of the TxA_2 effects and the responses via arterial and central chemoreceptors.

The vagus nerve is involved in mediating the thromboxane effects

To test whether the cardio-respiratory effects of thromboxane are mediated by vagal afferents, we reversibly cold-blocked both vagus nerves in the cat before we applied the

TxA$_2$ mimetic U 46,619 (Shams & Scheid, 1990). After vagal blockade, U 46,619 did not evoke any effect on respiration, but the effects on pulmonary circulation remained unaffected (Fig. 5). We concluded that the respiratory effects of TxA$_2$ are mediated by vagal afferent fibers, whereas pulmonary hypertension is unrelated to vagal integrity. In a subsequent study, we recorded single-unit afferent activity and its response to injection of U 46,619 in fine strands of the vagus nerve in the cat and rabbit (Karla et al., 1992). In slowly adapting and rapidly adapting pulmonary stretch receptor endings, U 46,619 evoked only small activity changes, whereas C-fibers were invariably stimulated by this compound (Fig. 6). Since this response was unrelated to concomitant increases in airway pressure, we concluded that the effect of thromboxane was directly on the nerve ending and was not mediated through smooth muscle contraction.

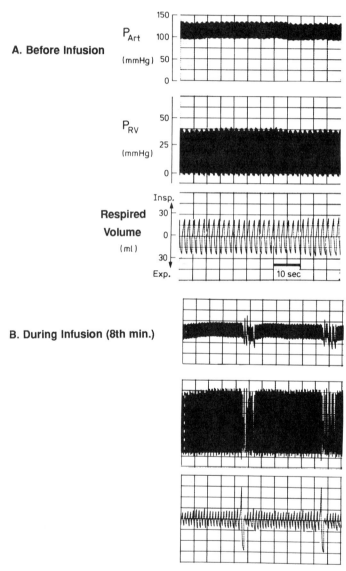

Figure 4. Response of the anesthetized cat to the first infusion of stoichiometrically equal amounts of HCl and NaOH into an arterio-venous loop. In A, systemic (PArt) and right ventricular blood pressure (PRV) were recorded together with respired volume in control conditions. The recording in B is during the 8th minute of acid-base infusion. (From Orr et al., 1987).

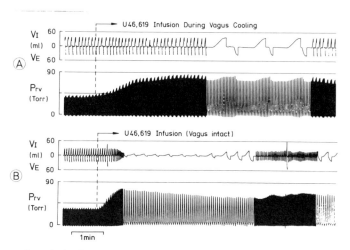

Figure 5. Response of respired volume (top trace) and right ventricular blood pressure (Prv; bottom panel) in the anesthetized cat to the thromboxane mimetic U 46,619. In A the vagus nerves are blocked by cooling to 1 °C. In B, the vagus nerves are re-warmed. (From Shams and Scheid, 1990).

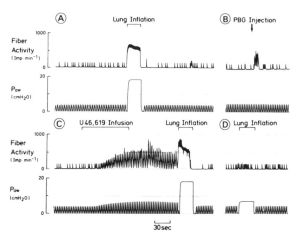

Figure 6. Response of a vagal C-fiber in the anesthetized cat to lung inflation (A), injection of phenyl-biguanide (PBG; B), and to infusion of U 46,619 (C). U 46,619 causes a strong increase in fiber activity and a small increase in airway pressure (Paw); however, elevation of Paw to a similar level in D does not evoke a comparable increase in fiber activity, suggesting that U 46,619 acts directly on the fiber, not via stretch. (From Karla et al., 1992).

Transient ventilatory responses to endotoxin

Release of TxA_2 has been reported during a variety of pathophysiological states including endotoxemia (Brigham, 1985; Kuhl et al., 1988; Winn et al., 1983), exposure to high altitude hypoxia (Richalet et al., 1991), monocrotoline-induced pneumotoxicity (Czer et al., 1986), pulmonary embolism (Garcia-Szabo et al., 1988; Schumacher et al., 1990), and airway reactions to ozone (Aizawa et al., 1985) or allergens (Beasley et al., 1989). Since it is well established that TxA_2 elicits bronchoconstriction and vasoconstriction in the lung, this eicosanoid has been implicated in mediating the alterations in airway resistance, compliance and pulmonary hypertension during these pathophysiological events. However, its implication in the concomitant respiratory alterations has not been studied. We have, therefore, used endotoxin infusion as a well established model for the adult respiratory distress syndrome (Brigham & Meyrick, 1986) to test the hypothesis that TxA_2 is released in this situation (Orr et al., 1993).

We have again used the cat and infused endotoxin (*E. coli*, strain B055) intravenously (1.6 mg·kg^{-1}, delivered over one minute). We found effects very similar to those with TxA_2 or U 46,619 infusion: rapid shallow breathing, pulmonary hypertension (and systemic hypotension); these effects were transient. Blocking prostanoid synthesis by indomethacin, or the TxA_2 receptor by Daltroban, eliminated any cardio-respiratory effect of endotoxin infusion. We concluded that TxA_2 is responsible for the early cardio-respiratory effects of endotoxin infusion. TxA_2 may similarly be involved in other pathophysiological situation.

CONCLUSION

This series of experiments shows clearly that TxA_2, which is released under a number of pathophysiological conditions, exerts effects on respiration which may interfere and override the normal chemosensitivity of respiration. Accepting that acid infusion has in this sense to be regarded as a pathophysiological condition, one is inclined to assume that some of the results reported on the pH sensitivity of respiration are contaminated by TxA_2 effects. It is remarkable, however, that acid (or endotoxin) infusion is effective only during the first infusion, and that this sensitivity does normally not recover in the run of an experimental day. In experiments necessitating acid infusion as an experimental tool, one should, therefore, repeat this infusion once or twice before collecting data to be used for analysis of respiratory chemosensitivity.

On the other hand, extensive thoracic surgery and mechanical irritation of the lung also lead to TxA_2 release. One wonders, therefore, whether some of the results obtained with cardio-pulmonary bypass and isolated pulmonary and systemic circulations might not be similarly contaminated by the release of TxA_2.

REFERENCES

Aizawa, H., K.F. Chung, G.D. Leikauf, I. Ueki, R.A. Bethel, P.M. O'Byrne, T. Hirose & J.A. Nadel (1985). Significance of thromboxane generation in ozone-induced airway hyperresponsiveness in dogs. J. Appl. Physiol. 59: 1918-1923.

Banzett, R.B., H.M. Coleridge & J.C.G. Coleridge (1978). I. Pulmonary CO_2 ventilatory reflex in dogs: effective range of CO_2 and results of vagal cooling. Respir. Physiol. 34: 121-134.

Beasley, R.C., R.L. Featherstone, M.K. Church, P. Rafferty, J.G. Varley, A. Harris, C. Robinson & S.T. Holgate (1989). Effect of a thromboxane receptor antagonist on PGD_2 and allergen-induced bronchoconstriction. J. Appl. Physiol. 66: 1685-1693.

Bradley, G.W., M.I.M. Noble & D. Trenchard (1976). The direct effect on pulmonary stretch receptor discharge produced by changing lung carbon dioxide concentration in dogs on cardio-pulmonary bypass and its action on breathing. J. Physiol. (London) 261: 359-373.

Brigham, K.L. & B. Meyrick (1986). Endotoxin and lung injury. Am. Rev. Respir. Dis. 133: 913-927.

Brigham, K. (1985). Metabolites of arachidonic acid in experimental lung vascular injury. Fed. Proc. 44: 43-45.

Czer, G.T., J. Marsh, R. Konopka & K.M. Moser (1986). Low-dose PGI_2 prevents monocrotoline-induced thromboxane production and lung injury. J. Appl. Physiol. 60: 464-471.

Dejours, P. (1964). Control of respiration in muscular exercise. In: Handbook of Physiology, Section 3: Respiration, edited by W.O. Fenn and H. Rahn, vol. 1. Washington, DC: American Physiological Society, pp. 631-648.

Fedde, M.R. & D.F. Peterson (1970). Intrapulmonary receptor response to changes in airway-gas composition in Gallus domesticus. J. Physiol. (London) 209: 609-625.

Fedde, M.R., R.N. Gatz, H. Slama & P. Scheid (1974a). Intrapulmonary CO_2 receptors in the duck: I. Stimulus specificity. Respir. Physiol. 22: 99-114.

Fedde, M.R., R.N. Gatz, H. Slama & P. Scheid (1974b). Intrapulmonary CO_2 receptors in the duck: II. Comparison with mechanoreceptors. Respir. Physiol. 22, 115-121.

Fedde, M.R., W.D. Kuhlmann & P. Scheid (1977). Intrapulmonary receptors in the tegu lizard: I. Sensitivity to CO_2. Respir. Physiol. 29: 35-48.

Fedde, M.R., W.D. Kuhlmann & P. Scheid (1977). Intrapulmonary receptors in the tegu lizard: II. Functional characteristics and localization. Respir. Physiol. 29: 49-62.

Fedde, M.R. & W.D. Kuhlmann (1978). Intrapulmonary carbon dioxide sensitive receptors: amphibians to mammals. In: Respiratory Function in Birds, Adult and Embryonic, edited by J. Piiper. Berlin, Heidelberg, New York: Springer, pp. 33-50.

Garcia-Szabo, R., A. Johnson & A.B. Malik (1988). Thromboxane increases pulmonary vascular resistance and transvascular fluid and protein exchange after pulmonary microembolism. Prostaglandins 35: 707-721.

Karla, W., H. Shams, J.A. Orr & P. Scheid (1992). Effects of the thromboxane A_2 mimetic, U 46,619, on pulmonary vagal afferents in the cat. Respir. Physiol. 87: 383-396.

Kuhl, P.G., J.M. Bolds, J.E. Loyd, J.R. Snapper & G.A. Fitzgerald (1988). Thromboxane receptor-mediated bronchial and hemodynamic responses in ovine endotoxemia. Am. J. Physiol. 254: R310-R319.

Kunz, A.L., T. Kawashiro & P. Scheid (1976). Study of CO_2 sensitive vagal afferents in the cat lung. Respir. Physiol. 27: 347-355.

Mitchell, G.S., B.A. Cross, T. Hiramoto & P. Scheid (1980). Effects of intrapulmonary CO_2 and airway pressure on phrenic activity and pulmonary stretch receptor discharge in dogs. Respir. Physiol. 40: 29-48.

Molony, V. (1974). Classification of vagal afferents firing in phase with breathing in Gallus domesticus. Respir. Physiol. 22: 57-76.

Mustafa, M.E.K.Y. & M.J. Purves (1972). The effect of CO_2 upon discharge from slowly adapting stretch receptors in lungs of rabbits. Respir. Physiol. 16: 197-212.

Orr, J.A., H. Shams, W. Karla, B.A. Peskar & P. Scheid (1993). Transient ventilatory responses to endotoxin infusion in the cat are mediated by thromboxane A_2. Respir. Physiol. 93: 189-201.

Orr, J.A., M.R. Fedde, H. Shams, H. Röskenbleck and P. Scheid (1988). Absence of CO_2-sensitive venous chemoreceptors in the cat. Respir. Physiol. 73: 211-224.

Orr, J.A., H. Shams, M.R. Fedde & P. Scheid (1987). Cardiorespiratory changes during HCl infusion unrelated to decreases in circulating blood pH. J. Appl. Physiol. 62: 2362-2370.

Richalet, J.-P., A. Hornych, C. Rathat, J. Aumont, P. Larmignat & P. Remy (1991). Plasma prostaglandins, leukotrienes, and thromboxane in acute high altitude hypoxia. Respir. Physiol. 85: 205-215.

Sant'Ambrogio, G., G. Miserocchi & J. Mortola (1974). Transient responses of pulmonary stretch receptors in the dog to inhalation of carbon dioxide. Respir. Physiol. 22: 191-197.

Scheid, P. & J. Piiper (1986). Control of breathing in birds. In: Handbook of Physiology, Section 3: The Respiratory System, Volume II: Control of Breathing, edited by A.P. Fishman, N.S. Cherniack & J.G. Widdicombe, Part 2. Bethesda, MD: American Physiological Society, pp. 815-832.

Scheid, P. (1979). Mechanisms of gas exchange in bird lungs. Rev. Physiol. Biochem. Pharmacol. 86: 137-186.

Schoener, E.P. & H.M. Frankel (1972). Effect of hyperthermia and $PaCO_2$ on the slowly adapting pulmonary stretch receptor. Am. J. Physiol. 222:68-72.

Schumacher, W.A., C.L. Heran & M.L. Ogletree (1990). Protamine-induced pulmonary hypertension in heparinized monkeys and pigs is inhibited by the thromboxane receptor antagonist, SQ 30,741. Eicosanoids 3: 87-93.

Shams, H., B.A. Peskar & P. Scheid (1988). Acid infusion elicits thromboxane A_2-mediated effects on respiration and pulmonary hemodynamics in the cat. Respir. Physiol. 71: 169-183.

Shams, H. & P. Scheid (1990). Effects of thromboxane on respiration and pulmonary circulation in the cat: role of vagus nerve. J. Appl. Physiol. 68: 2042-2046.

Sheldon, M.I. & J.F. Green (1982). Evidence for pulmonary CO_2 chemosensitivity: effects on ventilation. J. Appl. Physiol. 21: 1108-1116.

Winn, R., J. Harlan, B. Nadir, L. Harker & J. Hildebrandt (1983). Thromboxane A_2 mediates the lung vasoconstriction but not permeability after endotoxin. J. Clin. Invest. 72: 911-918.

Zuntz, N. & J. Geppert (1886). Über die Natur der normalen Atemreize und den Ort ihrer Wirkung. Arch. ges. Physiol. 38: 337-338.

HEYMANS' VISIT TO DUBLIN TO REVIEW "BUFFER" NERVE EXPERIMENTS

J.B. Moynihan and C.S. Breathnach

Department of Human Anatomy and Physiology, University College,
Earlsfort Terrace, Dublin 2, Ireland

On Wednesday, May 17th, 1939 Corneille Heymans delivered the ninth Purser Lecture in Dublin (Heymans, 1939). John Mallet Purser (1839-1929) was Professor of the Institute of Medicine (1879-1901) and sixteen years after retirement from the chair in which he established histology and physiology within the medical curriculum he was invited to take on the duties of Regius Professor of Physic (1917-1925) in the University of Dublin. After his death the admiration of his friends and pupils found expression in the foundation of the John Mallet Purser Memorial Lecture.

Although the discovery of the cardio-aortic depressor nerves had shown that the cardio-aortic vascular area, especially the aortic arch, was provided with pressoreceptive reflexogenic innervation which served to keep a balance between hypertension and hypotension and to maintain the normal blood pressure, the cardiovascular reactions to changes of the carotid-cephalic pressure were long attributed to the direct central influence of blood pressure acting on the activity of the cardiovascular centre in the brain stem. Contrary (incomplete) experimental evidence, although available from 1900, was ignored until Ewald Hering (1834-1918) in Prague established the existence of the carotid sinus mechanism by which the carotid blood pressure controls reflexly the activity of the cardiovascular centres and thus the systemic arterial blood pressure.

In 1939 it was necessary to define the term "carotid sinus" as a specially innervated area of the bifurcation of the common carotid artery. Within this area are the origins of the internal and external carotid and occipital arteries, the carotid bulb (which is a dilatation at the root of the internal carotid) and the carotid body or carotid ganglion which lies between the bifurcating arteries. This region is connected with the central nervous system by means of a distinct group of nerve fibres constituting the carotid sinus nerves.

The reflex regulation of blood pressure by means of the pressosensitivity of the carotid sinus was examined and established by techniques perfected in Heymans' laboratory. Although later experiments were carried out with a Dale Schuster pump, the isolated carotid sinuses, with their carefully preserved nerve supply, were perfused from another dog so that the pressure within the innervated sinus could be raised or lowered at will. Since the carotid sinus was connected to the animal only by intact nerves, it was possible to show that it is by reflexes due to changes in pressure originating within the carotid sinuses that the arterial blood pressure is regulated. The efferent limbs of the reflexes were the vagus and sympathetic nerves, the former providing the main control over heart rate. Sympathetic efferents controlled the vessels in the skin and muscles and especially in the splanchnic circulation.

Cross-circulation experiments might with fairness be termed the Belgian technique, for they were introduced by Leon Fredericq (1851-1933) into the study of respiratory control. Fredericq, like Heymans, was born and educated in Ghent, moving to Liege in 1879 to succeed Theodor Schwann as Professor of Physiology. By progressive cooling experiments he provided evidence in favour of location of the respiratory centre in the medulla oblongata, and in 1887 he began a series of confirmatory experiments by cross-circulation. In these experiments blood from the carotid artery of one dog (A) was directed into the head of a second dog (B), B's head receiving blood only from the first dog; ventilation of A with hypoxic gas mixtures produced dyspnoea in the second dog (B) (Fredericq, 1901).

The importance of arteriolar smooth muscle in regulating peripheral resistance has overshadowed venomotion. Heymans investigated the reflex regulation of venous tone by the carotid sinus reflexes using the technique of J.F. Donegan (1921). In Donegan's technique, all the tributaries to a vein were securely tied; a cannula introduced at the capillary end was used for access, and a cannula at the central end, after the blood was washed out, was attached to a water manometer, and changes in internal pressure were monitored. Alternatively, Ringer's solution from a reservoir kept in a water bath at $40^{\circ}C$ was allowed to flow continuously through the tied-off tube of vein, and the rate of flow of the fluid was recorded on a revolving drum by an electric drop recorder.

Mesenteric veins isolated from the general circulation, when perfused in situ, contract reflexly during lowered carotid sinus pressure and dilate if it is increased. Veins acting as capacitance vessels are subject to the carotid sinus reflexes. The humoral component of the sympathico-adrenal system, though "only an accessory regulating mechanism", was also fully explored. Other pressosensitive regions (atrial and pulmonary arterial), as described in the literature, were briefly reviewed. To examine the importance of the spleen in regulating the circulating blood volume, cross-circulation through carotid-jugular-splenic anastomoses was used to demonstrate the dependence of the action of the canine spleen as a blood-cell reservoir upon blood pressure and carotid sinus reflexes.

The lecturer then turned his attention to the role of the pressosensitive mechanisms of cardiovascular regulation in the adaptation of blood flow and blood supply to skeletal muscles during exercise, and to the cerebral and coronary circulations. Reduction in vasoconstrictive tone in exercising muscles is balanced by increased vasoconstriction elsewhere so that blood pressure is maintained at or near normal level. The pressoreactive mechanisms of blood pressure regulation protect the cerebral and coronary circulations against variations of arterial pressure; although blood flow measurements in these two circulatory systems were not recorded, with hindsight it is clear that Heymans was drifting towards the concept of autoregulation.

Experimental arterial hypertension produced in dogs by total excision of the buffer nerves or moderator fibres in the cardio-aortic and carotid sinus nerves was prevented by total sympathectomy, so that this particular canine variety could fairly be termed "essential neurogenic hypertension", quite distinct from the nephropathic variety which had recently been described by Goldblatt and his co-workers, and produced by "the liberation of a not very active vasopressor renal factor". But Heymans and his associates showed that the renal nerves also exerted an important influence by demonstrating an experimental neurogenic hypertension of renal origin, which he tentatively postulated might be more closely related to "the primary mechanism of essential hypertension in man". His diffidence was well-founded for, in spite of intensive investigation the interactions between the renin-angiotensin system, the sympathetic nervous system and the pressoreceptor reflexes in the regulation of arterial blood pressure have still to be elucidated (Reid, 1992).

Before finally surveying current knowledge of experimental arterial hypertension to convince his clinical auditors of "the bonds closely uniting physiology, pathology and experimental surgery in attempts to elucidate the mechanisms" of disease, he provided a schematic representation of the main functions of the pressosensitive vascular areas in the reflex regulation of blood pressure and blood supply.

Corneille Heymans was a worthy successor to the Nobel Laureates Hopkins, Adrian and Dale, and to Sharpey-Schafer, Almroth Wright, Ariens Kappers, Joseph Barcroft and Gordon Holmes as John Mallet Purser Lecturer for 1939.

REFERENCES

Donegan, J.F. (1921) The physiology of the veins. J. Physiol. (Lond.) 55:226-245.

Fredericq, L. (1901) Sur la cause de l'apnee. Archiv. Biol. (Paris)11:561-580.

Heymans, C. (1939) The regulation of blood pressure and vasomotor tone. Ir. J. Med. Sci. 166:717-728.

Reid, I.A. (1992) Interactions between ANG II, sympathetic nervous system, and baroreceptor reflexes in regulation of blood pressure. Am. J. Physiol. 262:E763-E778.

A BELATED CENTENNIAL TRIBUTE TO CORNEILLE HEYMANS

C. S. Breathnach

Department of Human Anatomy and Physiology,
University College Dublin, Earlsfort Terrace,
Dublin 2, Ireland

The importance of chemical stimuli in the regulation of pulmonary ventilation was well established by 1925, and the *direct* influence of carbon dioxide, oxygen and hydrogen ion concentration, alone or in combination, upon Flourens' *noeud vital* (1842) was the widely accepted interpretation of the cross-circulation experiments reported by Leon Fredericq in 1901, which showed that changes in activity of the respiratory centre were induced by varying the carbon dioxide concentration in the blood supplied to the perfused head.

However, Jean Francois Heymans and his son Corneille found that the medullary centre could be influenced *indirectly* (Heymans & Heymans, 1925; 1926). Perfusing the isolated head of a recipient dog by means of a donor dog, the perfused head being connected with the body of the recipient solely through the vagus nerves, Heymans *pere et fils* observed that asphyxia or anoxia of the *body* of the recipient induced a *reflex* stimulation of the respiratory centre in the perfused head, whereas hyperventilation was inhibitory. Nicotine injected into the recipient's body also provoked a reflex stimulation. By systematic experimentation, the origin of this chemoreflex stimulation was located in the region of the aortic arch, afferent fibres from which travelled in the vagus nerves. A decade elapsed before Comroe & Schmidt (1938) showed that the chemoreceptors involved reside in the aortic bodies.

While investigating the pressoreceptors of the carotid sinus Corneille Heymans and his colleagues (Heymans & Bouckaert, 1930; Heymans et al., 1930; Heymans et al., 1933) found that this area is also chemosensitive. Chemoreceptors here, they reported, act reflexly through the carotid sinus nerve (a branch of the glossopharyngeal nerve) mainly on the respiratory centre but also on the cardiovascular centre. Whereas the pressoreceptors proved to be located in the arterial wall of the sinus, the chemoreceptors are collected in the carotid body or *glomus caroticum*, the 'tasting' function of which was surmised independently by De Castro (1928) (whose speculative paper was not available to Heymans in Ghent).

Corneille Heymans (1963) recounted how "fortune favours the prepared mind". The primary observations on the aortic chemoreceptors were made during performance of experiments for other purposes, when the arrest of artificial ventilation of the *body* of the recipient dog induced a reflex stimulation of the respiratory centre in the perfused *head*. This wholly unexpected observation provided the impetus for a series of planned experiments which eventually led to the identification of the location and functions of the chemoreceptors in the aortic arch.

Arterial Chemoreceptors: Cell to System
Edited by R. O'Regan *et al*, Plenum Press, New York, 1994

Serendipity also helped in the identification of the carotid chemoreceptors (Heymans, 1963): at the end of a successful experiment designed to elucidate carotid sinus pressor sensitivity the animal was still in good shape, and the profitable son of a thrifty father decided not to waste an opportunity to carry out an unplanned experiment. One carotid sinus area of the dog was innervated, the other had been denervated. Potassium cyanide (a solution of which was nearby on the laboratory desk), when injected into the intact sinus, induced the expected forceful hyperpnoea. When similar amounts of cyanide were injected into the carotid artery on the denervated side, no hyperpnoea occurred. The alternate injections were repeated several times and the same respiratory responses were observed. A planned experiment the next morning confirmed the previous evening's observations (Heymans, 1963), and a series of experiments designed to establish the identity and functions of the chemoreceptors in the carotid body was undertaken (Heymans & Bouckaert, 1930; Heymans et al., 1930; Heymans et al., 1933).

These unexpected results contradicted firmly held opinions, and when Heymans recounted his experiments concerning the pressoreceptors regulating arterial blood pressure and the chemoreceptors acting on respiration to Carl Wiggers in New York in 1927, the revered physiologist challenged the young Belgian to demonstrate the truth of his assertions in an experimental animal, which he would be only too pleased to provide. The following day the visitor repeated his experiments, and Wiggers magnanimously agreed: "Heymans, the dog is right, textbooks are wrong!" (Heymans, 1963). Two years later, when Heymans joined European physiologists on the *Minnekahda* on their way to the Thirteenth International Congress of Physiological Sciences in Boston 'the respiratory physiologists of the old school were not prepared to accept his views' as they "talked shop" on board (Zotterman, 1968); they obviously believed in the motto of the Royal Society *Nullius in Verba*. In Zotterman's account (1968) of the voyage two important sidelights are worthy of mention: though 'the Spanish group was quite numerous' there is no hint of a priority claim for De Castro's extraordinarily perceptive functional interpretation of the innervation and microscopic structure of the *glomus caroticum* (De Castro, 1928); secondly, Heymans 'was always very entertaining, and had an enormous store of anecdotes, of which I remember only the following: "Mrs. Webster one morning found Mr. Webster (*The Webster Dictionary*) kissing her chambermaid, so she exclaimed 'Mr. Webster, I am surprised!' 'Mrs. Webster,' said Mr. Webster calmly, 'how many times have I to remind you about the proper use of these difficult words? *We* were surprised, *you* were astonished, my dear'". The unpredictable observation which surprised Heymans led to a discovery that astonished older physiologists.

At the Fourteenth Congress in Rome in 1932, there were still sceptics, and Klothilde Gollwitzer-Meier of Hamburg declared she would not accept his conclusions until she had seen the experiment performed (Neil, 1973). Although Heymans was understandably nervous that the demonstration would not go smoothly without a hitch, the cyanide worked equally well on one side and not at all on the other in the Italian laboratory before a distinguished audience, and Gollwitzer-Meier (1934) herself went on to provide the final proof in 1934 that carotid chemoreceptor reflexes are aroused only from the carotid body region of the bifurcation, whereas the pressoreceptor responses can be provoked only from the carotid sinus itself.

In remembering the pioneer experiments of Corneille Heymans, who died on 18 July 1968 in Ghent, the city where he had been born on 28 March 1892 and had lived all his life (Neil, 1973), it is right and fitting to recall that Walpole's *Three Princes of Serendip* made their discoveries, of things they were not in quest of, by accident and sagacity, *not* by accident alone but by accident and sagacity.

REFERENCES

Comroe, J.H. & Schmidt, C.F. (1938) The part played by reflexes from the carotid body in the chemical regulation of respiration in the dog. Am. J. Physiol. 121:75-97.

De Castro, F. (1928) Sur la structure et l'innervation du sinus carotidien de l'homme et des mammiferes. Nouveaux faits sur l'innervation et la fonction du glomus caroticum. Trab. Lab. Invest. Biol. Univ. Madrid 25:331-380.

Flourens, M.J.P. (1842)"Recherches experimentales sur les proprietes et les fonctions du systeme nerveux dans les animaux vertebres", 2nd.edn., Paris.

Fredericq, L. (1901) Sur la cause de l'apnee. Archiv. Biol. (Paris) 11:561-580.

Gollwitzer-Meier, K. (1934) Ueber die Erregung der Sinusnerven durch physiologische und pharmakologische Reize. Pflug. Arch. ges. Physiol. 234:342-361.

Heymans, C. (1963) A look at an old but still current problem. Annu. Rev. Physiol. 25:1-14.

Heymans, C. & Bouckaert, J.J. (1930) Sinus caroticus and respiratory reflexes.I.Cerebral blood flow and respiration. Adrenaline apnoea. J. Physiol. (Lond.) 69:254-266 and xiii-xiv.

Heymans, C., Bouckaert, J.J. & Dautrebande, L. (1930) Sinus carotidien et reflexes respiratoires.II. Archiv. Int. Pharmacodyn. 39:400-448.

Heymans, C.,Bouckaert, J.J. & Regniers, P. (1933)"Le sinus carotidien et la zone homologue cardio-aortique", Doin, Paris.

Heymans, J.-F. & Heymans, C. (1925) Sur le mechanisme de l'apnee reflexe ou pneumogastrique. C. R. Soc. Biol. 92:1335.

Heymans, J.-F. & Heymans, C. (1926) Recherches physiologiques et pharmacodynamiques sur la tete isolee du chien. Arch. Int. Pharmacodyn. 32:1-33.

Neil, E. (1973) An appraisal of the work of Corneille Heymans on baroreceptor and chemoreceptor reflexes. Arch. Int. Pharmacodyn. 202:suppl.:283-293.

Zotterman, Y. (1968) The Minnekahda Voyage, 1929. In "History of the International Congresses of Physiology, 1889-1968." W.O. Fenn, ed., Waverly Press, Bethesda, MD.

GLOMERA THAT ARE NOT CHEMOSENSITIVE?

Miriam Kennedy, John J. Smith, and Caoimhin S. Breathnach

Department of Human Anatomy and Physiology, University College,
Earlsfort Terrace, Dublin 2. Ireland

Arteriovenous shunts, or glomera, are a common feature in the vasculature of the skin, particularly in the corium of the fingertips, the nailbeds, around the limb joints, and over the scapula and coccyx.

The *painful subcutaneous tubercles* described by Wood in 1812 were shown by Masson in 1924 to be glomus tumours composed of prominent round- or spindle-shaped glomus cells surrounding vascular spaces lined by endothelium. Such a glomus tumour in an uncommon, encapsulated, benign neoplasm that reproduces in caricature the neuromyoarterial glomus of human skin. Though multiple glomus tumours have been described, the tumours are overwhelmingly solitary, and while they have been reported in trachea, mediastinum, stomach, kidney, female genital tract, muscle, joint capsule, bone, and in a presacral teratoma, they are most commonly described in the skin.

Glomus tumours appear as purple or red spots, several though rarely more than 10mm in diameter, which are typically painful. The characteristically lancinating pain is surprisingly severe in view of the small size of the tumour; it is remarkably incapacitating in tumours in the nailbed; in some cases the pattern of paroxysmal pain arises only after injury. While pain is not invariable, it is a fairly constant characteristic of diagnostic significance (Shugart et al., 1963). A paroxysm triggered by pressure or heat may be fleeting or day-long; it may last minutes or hours. Where multiple tumours are present, several may be painful (Moschella & Hurley, 1992). Total excision gives immediate relief from the paroxysm, but incomplete removal, a distinct hazard with subungual tumours, is invariably unsatisfactory.

Glomus tumours arise from a neuromyoarterial body, the Sucquet-Hoyer canal of anastomosis, containing contractile glomus cells. Under the light microscope the tumour is seen to be composed of blood vessels lined by normal endothelial cells and surrounded by sheets of uniform, round or oval glomus cells interspersed with many unmyelinated nerve fibres (Kohorn et al., 1986). Masson (1935) was the first to demonstrate the presence of myofibrils in glomus cells, and in the electron microscope they have been shown to resemble modified smooth muscle cells (Murad et al., 1968; Toker, 1969; Venkatachalam & Greally, 1969). The common features include numerous myofibrils, peripheral vesicles, fusiform condensations and prominent attachment bodies.

Ultrastructural studies of arterial chemosensory organs present a different picture. To overcome the conflicting ambiguities that have arisen, Eyzaguirre and Zapata (1984) avoid using Roman numerals; the typical and most prominent structure is the *glomus cell*. These ovoid cells have a large nucleus and abundant mitochondria; they are identifiable by two salient and concomitant features: formaldehyde induced fluorescence and an abundance of dense-core vesicles, characteristics which are common to catecholamine-containing cells. The sustentacular ('satellite' or 'capsule') cells are of glial lineage; these supporting cells usually enclose several glomus cells and the nerve terminals apposed to them by one or two fingerlike layers of cytoplasm.

The striking morphological differences between cutaneous glomus tumours and chemosensitive glomera is mirrored in the difference in pathological behaviour of the skin tumours and chemosensory tumours. Whereas cutaneous glomus tumours are benign, carotid body tumours are malignant; though in the majority of cases they are only locally invasive, late lymph node involvement does occur (McPherson et al., 1989). Moreover, carotid body tumours form only part of a complex pattern of paragangliomas, some of which may secrete catecholamines; while carotid body tumours are not actively secretory, other branchiomeric and aorticosympathetic paragangliomas may be clinically indistinguishable from phaeochromocytomas; resection, as in the case of cutaneous glomera, is the treatment of choice.

To conclude, the resemblance between cutaneous and chemosensitive glomera is superficial Glomus is "like a portmanteau - there are two meanings packed into one word" (Carroll, 1871)

REFERENCES

Carroll, L. (1871) Through the looking glass. Reprinted with Alice's adventures in wonderland. London, New York, Puffin Books, 1985. p274

Eyzaguirre, C., & Zapata, P. (1984) Perspectives in carotid body research. J. Appl. Physiol. 57:931-967.

Kohorn, E.I., Merino, M.J. & Goldenhersh, M. (1986) Vulval pain and dyspareunia due to glomus tumor. Obstet. Gynecol. 67:41S - 42S.

McPherson, G.A.D., Halliday, A.W. & Mansfield, A.O. (1989) Carotid body tumours and other cervical paragangliomas, diagnosis and management in 25 patients. Brit. J. Surg. 76:33-36.

Masson, P. (1924) Le glomus neuromyoarteriel des regions tactiles et ses tumeurs. Lyon. Chir. 21:257-280.

Masson, P. (1935) Le glomus cutanes de l'Homme. Bull. Soc. Franc. Derm. Syph. 42:1174-1245.

Moschella, S. L. & Hurley, H. J. (1992) "Dermatology." Philadelphia. Saunders. 3rd edition. pp. 1783-1784.

Murad, T.M., von Haam, E. & Murthy, M.S.N. (1968) Ultrastructure of a hemangiopericytoma and a glomus tumor. Cancer 22:1239-1249.

Shugart, R.R., Soule, E.H. & Johnson, E.W., Jr. (1963) Glomus tumor. Surg. Gyn. Obst. 117:334-340.

Toker, C. (1969) Glomangioma, an ultrastructural study. Cancer 23:487-492.

Venkatachalam, M.A. & Greally, J.G. (1969) Fine structure of glomus tumor: similarity of glomus cells to smooth muscle. Cancer 23:1176-1184.

Wood, W. (1812) On painful subcutaneous tubercle. Edinburgh Med. J. 8:883.

ELECTROTONIC COUPLING BETWEEN CAROTID BODY GLOMUS CELLS

L. Monti-Bloch,[1,2] Veronica Abudara,[1,2] and C. Eyzaguirre[1]

[1]Department of Physiology, University of Utah School of Medicine, Salt Lake City, Utah, USA and [2]Department of Physiology, Facultad de Medicina, Universidad de la Republica, Montevideo, Uruguay

INTRODUCTION

The carotid body detects chemical changes in the blood such as PO_2, PCO_2 and pH, and generates afferent discharges in the carotid nerve. During stimulation, the glomus cells release endogenous substances (ACh, catecholamines, and neuropeptides) toward the carotid nerve terminals. To understand how secretion occurs, we have studied the electric connections between glomus cells at rest and during activity elicited by 'natural' stimuli, or the transmitters (Monti-Bloch et al., 1990, 1993). In other secretory organs, adjoining cells are electrically coupled and they uncouple (fully or partially) during secretion (for refs. see Bennett & Spray, 1985; Hertzberg & Johnson, 1988; Bennett et al., 1991).

METHODS

Carotid bodies, removed from anesthetized rats, were transferred to a Lucite chamber mounted on an inverted Nomarski microscope. The preparation was superfused with physiological saline equilibrated with oxygen (about 300 torr in the chamber) at 30-32°C. Pairs of adjacent cells were impaled for simultaneous intracellular recordings. Electric pulses of either polarity were alternatively delivered to each cell through the recording electrodes. Lactic acid, dopamine (DA), ACh, bethanechol and nicotine were applied upstream. Hypoxia was induced by applying sodium dithionite ($Na_2S_2O_4$), or superfusing with 100% N_2. For acidic-hypercapnic stimulation, the solution was equilibrated with 100% CO_2

RESULTS

The resting parameters of Cell 1 were statistically similar to those of Cell 2. Their E_Ms were 10 to -64 mV and R_Os varied from 24.1-3,500 MΩ. The coupling coefficients (K_Cs) ranged from 0.003 to 1.0. K_C was calculated as the ratio between the voltage transferred to Cell 2 (E_2) and the voltage applied to Cell 1 (V_1) or E_2/V_1 (Bennett, 1966). This report deals only with K_C.

Current-voltage (I-V) curves were linear for the 'on' and transferred currents suggesting that the coupling junctions are symmetric or ohmic. Most cells in the pairs reacted similarly to different stimuli (e.g. both uncoupled), but a minority behaved differently (e.g. one cell uncoupled and the other became better coupled).

Hypoxia

Boluses (100 μl) of $Na_2S_2O_4$ 1-10 mM lowered the saline PO_2 to 91-124 torr. Superfusion with 100% N_2 lowered it to 25-81 torr. Dithionite and N_2 reduced coupling in about 70% of the cells, N_2 being more effective. Uncoupling appeared dependent on the bath PO_2 since N_2 was more effective than dithionite and decreased PO_2 more than $Na_2S_2O_4$.

Acidification

We applied boluses of lactic acid 0.2 to 1.0 mM or superfused with 100% CO_2. Lactic acid reduced pH_o by 0.01 to 0.1 units. CO_2 drastically lowered pH_o to 5.5. Both lactic acid and CO_2, weak organic acids, lower the intracellular pH of glomus cells and their effects on the E_M and the R_O are similar (Eyzaguirre et al., 1989; He et al., 1990, 1991a, b). Lactic acid and CO_2 were equally effective uncouplers in about 80% of the pairs. The uncoupling effect of organic acids has been repeatedly reported in other systems.

Transmitters (ACh and DA)

DA (40-320 μg) and ACh (50-100 μg) were applied upstream in 100 μl boluses. Both agents reduced coupling in 58% of the cells and were either ineffective or increased it in the rest. There were no differences between the effects of both substances. To test if the effects of ACh were nicotinic or muscarinic, we applied nicotine (5-10 μg) and the muscarinic agonist bethanechol (50-100 μg). Both drugs uncoupled 90% of the pairs, bethanechol being more effective, although it increased coupling in two cells. Nicotine was weaker but consistent as uncoupler.

In summary, cell uncoupling occurred in about 70% of the cases, the maximum being a reduction of 83%. Fewer cells (about 25%) developed stronger coupling. The maximum increase was 69%. Significant uncoupling occurred during hypoxia, acidity, nicotine and bethanechol. The effects of DA were marginally significant whereas ACh had variable effects. The mean decrease in coupling for all cells (-0.13 ± 0.003) was highly significant (p < 0.001).

DISCUSSION

There is agreement that intercellular communication occurs through active channels forming the gap junctions connecting adjoining cells (Bennett & Spray, 1985; Hertzberg & Johnson, 1988; Sperelakis & Cole, 1989). Gap junctions between glomus cells (McDonald, 1981) may be responsible for intercellular coupling. Uncoupling may have been produced by closing of the connecting channels, which would explain the decrease in intercellular conductance.

Two mechanisms may be responsible for uncoupling: (1) A decrease in intracellular pH (pH_i) and (2) Increases in intracellular calcium ($[Ca^{2+}]_i$). Both mechanisms play important roles in intercellular coupling (Bennett & Spray, 1985; Hertzberg & Johnson, 1988; Sperelakis & Cole, 1989). Of the stimuli employed, acid and CO_2 reduce intracellular pH, and they effectively uncoupled glomus cells. Hypoxia was also an uncoupler, but its effect on the pH_i of glomus cells is less consistent (Biscoe et al., 1989; Buckler et al., 1991; He et al., 1990, 1991a, b; Iturriaga et al., 1992). We do not know if the other agents employed in this study affect pH_i.

Usually an increase in $[Ca^{2+}]_i$ is important in uncoupling neighbouring cells (Bennett & Spray, 1985; Hertzberg & Johnson, 1988; Sperelakis & Cole, 1989). In the carotid body, Biscoe et al., (1989) and Sato et al., (1991) have shown an increase in $[Ca^{2+}]_i$ during applications of NaCN and Na-dithionite. However, Donnelly and Kholwadwala (1992) have shown a decrease in $[Ca^{2+}]_i$ during hypoxia. Our own studies have shown a dual effect of hypoxia (induced by Na-dithionite) on $[Ca^{2+}]_i$. We found an initial decrease followed by a marked increase (Zhang et al., 1992). Therefore, if hypoxia does not induce clear changes in pH_i, hypoxia uncoupling may have been due to increased $[Ca^{2+}]_i$. We do not have information on the effects of other stimuli on $[Ca^{2+}]_i$. However, Biscoe, et. al., (1989) reported some effects of carbachol (an ACh analogue) on $[Ca^{2+}]_i$, but they were inconsistent, which may partly explain the variable uncoupling effects of ACh in our experiments.

Another coupling factor is cAMP. An increase in $[cAMP]_i$ uncouples cell pairs (Hax et al., 1974; Flagg-Newton et al., 1981). This has been shown in retinal horizontal cells as a result of cAMP microinjections, application of forskolin (adelynate cyclase activator) or by inhibiting the inactivating enzyme phosphodiesterase with isobutylmethylxanthine (Lasater & Dowling, 1985, Neyton et al., 1985). In glomus cells, cAMP may be important. Its cellular levels are increased during hypoxia (Wang et al., 1991) and this may contribute to cell uncoupling as in other tissues.

However, fully understanding intercellular coupling in glomus cells is bound to be difficult. Virtually any stimulus acts via complex pathways. For instance, ACh releases dopamine from the cells, thus acting by more than one mechanism. Hypoxia releases multiple transmitters (see Fidone & Gonzalez, 1986) that in turn can affect the cells via autoreceptors (Eyzaguirre et al., 1990). Therefore, a single agent, influencing cell coupling, may act by different pathways, some of which are still unknown.

This communication, supported by grant NS 07938 from NIH, is based on work recently published (Monti-Bloch et al., 1993).

REFERENCES

Bennett, M.V.L.(1966). Physiology of electronic junctions. Ann. N. Y. Acad. Sci. 137:509-539

Bennett, M.V.L., Barrio, L. C., Bargiello, T. A., Spray, D. C., Hertzberg, E. & Saez, J. C. (1991). Gap junctions : New tools, new answers, new questions. Neuron 6:305-320.

Bennett, M.V.L. & Spray, D. C. (1985). "Gap Junctions", Cold Spring Harbor Laboratory.

Biscoe, T. J., Duchen, M. R., Eisner, D. A., O'Neill, S. C. & Valdeolmillos, M. (1989). Measurements of intracellular Ca^{2+} in dissociated type I cells of the rabbit carotid body. J. Physiol. (Lond.) 416:421-434.

Buckler, K. J., Vaughan-Jones, R. D., Peers, C. & Nye, P. C. G. (1991). Intracellular pH and its regulation in isolated type I carotid body cells of the neonatal rat. J. Physiol. (Lond.) 436:107-129.

Donnelly, D. F. & Kholwadwala, D. (1992). Hypoxia decreases intracellular calcium in adult rat carotid body glomus cells. J. Neurophysiol. 67:1543-1551.

Eyzaguirre, C., Monti-Bloch, L., Baron, M., Hayashida, Y. & Woodbury, J. L., (1989). Changes in glomus cell membrane properties in response to stimulants and depressants of carotid nerve discharge. Brain Res. 477:265-279.

Eyzaguirre, C., Monti-Bloch, L. & Woodbury, J. W. (1990). Effects of putative neurotransmitters of the carotid body on its own glomus cells. Eur. J. Neurosci. 2:77-88.

Fidone, S. J. & Gonzalez, C. (1986). Initiation and control of chemoreceptor activity in the carotid body, In: Handbook of Physiology, The Respiratory System, Vol. II, sect 3, Am Physiol. Soc., Bethesda, MD.

Flagg-Newton, J. L., Dahl, G & Loewenstein, W. R. (1981). Cell junction and cyclic AMP. I. Upregulation of junctional membrane permeability and junctional membrane particles by cyclic nucleotide treatments. J. Membr. Biol. 63:105-121.

Hax, W. M. A., Van Venrooji, G. E. & Vossenberg, J. B. (1974). Cell communication: A cyclic AMP-mediated phenomenon. J. Membr. Biol. 19:253-266.

He, S.-F., Wei, J.-Y. & Eyzaguirre, C. (1990). Intracellular pH of cultured carotid body cells. In "Arterial Chemoreception", C. Eyzaguirre, S. J. Fidone, R. S. Fitzgerald, S. Lahiri and D. M. McDonald, eds., SpringerVerlag, New York.

He, S.-F., Wei, J.-Y. & Eyzaguirre, C. (1991a). Intracellular pH and some membrane characteristics of cultured carotid body cells. Brain Res. 547:258-286.

He, S.-F., Wei, J.-Y. & Eyzaguirre, C. (1991b). Effects of relative hypoxia and hypercapnia on intracellular pH and membrane potential of cultured carotid body cells. Brain Res. 556:333-338.

Hertzberg, E. L. & Johnson, R. G. (1988). Gap Junctions. In "Modern Cell Biology", vol. 7, Alan R. Liss, New York.

Iturriaga, R., Rumsey, W. L., Lahiri, S., Spergel, D. & Wilson, D. F. (1992). Intracellular pH and oxygen chemoreception in the cat carotid body in vitro. J. Appl. Physiol. 72:2259-2262.

Kessler, J. A., Spray, D. C., Saenz, J. C. & Bennett, M. V. L. (1985). Development and regulation of electrotonic coupling between cultured sympathetic neurons. In "Gap Junctions", M. V. L. Bennett and D. C. Spray, eds Cold Spring Harbour Laboratory.

Lasater, E. M. & Dowling, J. E. (1985). Electric coupling between pairs of isolated fish horizontal cells is modulated by dopamine and cAMP. In "Gap Junctions", M. V. L. Bennett and D. C. Spray, eds., Cold Spring Harbour Laboratory.

McDonald, D. M. (1991. Peripheral chemoreceptors: structure-function relationships of the carotid body. In "Regulation ofBreathing", T. F. Hornbein, ed., vol. 17 of "Lung Biology in Health and Disease". C. Lenfant, exec. ed., Marcel Decker, New York.

Monti-Bloch, L. & Eyzaguirre, C. (1990). Effects of natural stimuli, chemical agents and transmitters on glomus cell membranes and intracellular communications. In "Arterial Chemoreception", C. Eyzaguirre, S. J. Fidone, R. S. Fitzgerald, S. Lahiri and D. M. McDonald, eds., Springer-Verlag, New York.

Monti-Bloch, L., Abudara, V. & Eyzaguirre, C. (1993). Electrical communication between glomus cells of the rat carotid body. Brain Res. in press.

Neyton, J., Piccolino, M. & Gerschenfeld, H. M. (1985). Neurotransmitter-induced modulation of gap junction permeability in retinal horizontal cells. In "Gap Junctions", M. V. L. Bennett and D. C. Spray, eds., Cold Spring Harbour Laboratory.

Sato, M., Ikeda, K., Yoshizaki, K. & Koyano, H. (1991). Response of cytosolic calcium to anoxia and cyanide in cultured glomus cells of newborn rabbit carotid body. Brain Res. 551:327-330.

Sperelakis, N. & Cole, W. C. (1989). "Cell Interations and Gap Junctions", CRC Press.

Spray, D. C. & Bennett, M. V. L. (1985). Physiology and pharmacology of gap junctions. Ann. Rev. Physiol. 47:281-303.

Wang, W. J., Cheng, G. F., Yoshizaki, K., Dinger, B. & Fidone, S. (1991). The role of cyclic AMP in chemoreception in the rabbit carotid body. Brain Res. 540:96-104.

Wilding, T. J., Cheng, B. & Roos, A. (1992). pH regulation in adult rat carotid body glomus cells. J. Gen. Physiol. 100:593-608.

Zhang, X.-Q., Pang. L. & Eyzaguirre, C. (1992). Effects of hypoxia induced by $Na_2S_2O_4$ on K^+ and Ca^{2+} activities of cultured carotid body glomus cells. Soc. Neurosci. Abstr. 18:1198.

CO-BINDING CHROMOPHORES IN OXYGEN CHEMORECEPTION IN THE CAROTID BODY

S. Lahiri, D. K. Ray, D. Chugh, R. Iturriaga, and A. Mokashi

Department of Physiology, University of Pennsylvania School of Medicine, Philadelphia, PA 19104-6085, USA

INTRODUCTION

The mechanism of O_2 chemoreception in the carotid body (CB) is not clear. Previously, we provided evidence (Mulligan et al., 1981; Mulligan & Lahiri, 1982; Shirahata et al., 1987) that inhibitors of mitochondrial oxidative phosphorylation specifically blocked the excitatory response to hypoxia. We further demonstrated that it is the energy production rather than O_2 consumption alone that is critical. More recently, Duchen and Biscoe (1992) showed similar responses of glomus cell $[Ca^{2+}]_i$ to hypoxia. With the discovery of O_2 sensitive K^+ channels in glomus cells (e.g., Lopez-Barneo et al., 1988; Delpiano and Heschler, 1989), Gonzalez et al. (1992) discounted the metabolic hypothesis of O_2 chemoreception. A distinction between the two hypotheses can be made by applying appropriate ratios of CO/O_2 to the carotid body and measuring chemosensory and/or glomus cell responses. CO specifically prevents reaction of cytochrome oxidase (Keilin, 1970) with O_2 and should manifest a hypoxia-like effect on the one hand, as shown by Joels and Neil (1962), and binding with hemoglobin-like pigment, would behave like O_2 and reverse the stimulatory effect of hypoxia, as proposed by Lloyd et al. (1968). We tested these predictions using the cat carotid body perfused and superfused in vitro with cell-free physiological solution and recording the chemosensory responses.

METHODS

Carotid bodies were vascularly isolated, and dissected out with the carotid sinus nerves, perfused and superfused in a small chamber in vitro, and chemosensory discharges were recorded (see Iturriaga et al., 1990). All Tyrode's solutions containing $NaHCO_3$ were equilibrated with appropriate gases (O_2, CO_2, CO and N_2). Only the perfusate contained CO. Two protocols were conducted: (a) Without light exposure, the CB was tested with hypoxia first, and then maintaining the same level of hypoxia, Tyrode containing CO was administered. The results provided the time-course of effects of CO. Intermittently, the carotid body was exposed to strong white light to test the effect of photodissociation of CO-complex. (b) the CB was perfused with PCO of about 100 Torr and at a PO_2 of about 100 Torr which did not stimulate chemosensory discharge. After interruption of perfusate flow, the preparation was alternately exposed to light.

Arterial Chemoreceptors: Cell to System
Edited by R. O'Regan *et al*, Plenum Press, New York, 1994

149

RESULTS AND DISCUSSION

Figure 1 shows the effects of transition from hypoxia to the same level of hypoxia plus high PCO of 300 Torr. Hypoxia (PO_2 = 50 Torr) stimulated the chemosensory discharge, an effect which was not light sensitive. The effect of high CO consisted of two parts: an immediate suppression of the chemosensory discharge followed by an excitation which was suppressed by white light. Also note that the excitation by CO was less than that due to moderate hypoxia.

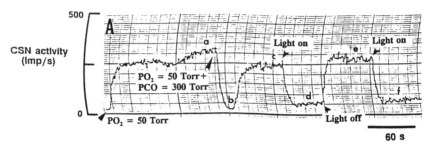

Figure 1. Metabolic effects on O_2 chemoreception, as mediated by CO. Effect of perfusate PCO of 300 Torr on the hypoxia effect on the chemosensory discharge. Sequence of events: (a) PO_2 = 50 Torr without light; (b) PO_2 = 50 Torr + PCO = 300 Torr without light; c) without light; (d) with light; (e) without light; and (f) with light. Light inhibited chemosensory excitation by PCO 300/PO_2 50; but the effect of hypoxia per se appeared to be inhibited throughout by CO.

Photodissociation of CO-complex prevented the chemosensory excitation caused by CO acting through respiratory pigments like cytochrome oxidase. However, CO continued to inhibit the chemosensory response to hypoxia per se. That CO, even when dissociated from cytochrome oxidase, prevented hypoxic excitation, suggests that CO was still bound to another pigment(s) and blocked O_2 chemoreception. Similar studies with lower PCO of 50-60 Torr suppressed the pre-existing hypoxic excitation but did not induce a similar photodissociable effect of light of CO-complex in the carotid body.

One lesson from these results is that high PCO/PO_2 ratio elicited chemosensory discharge of moderate intensity, blockable by visible light, consistent with the expected metabolic effects of CO on cytochrome oxidase (Keilin, 1970). These effects per se, however, do not preclude possible contribution of other pigments to chemosensory excitation. In further studies, using various wavelengths of light, we found that the photodissociation action spectra corresponded to the well-known characteristic absorption spectra of cytochrome oxidase (Keilin, 1970). We take this as incontrovertible evidence for the metabolic hypothesis of O_2 chemoreception. (Lahiri et al., 1993a)

Taken together, we believe that interference with the oxidative metabolism of the chemoreceptor cell contributes to O_2 chemoreception, contrary to the view expressed by Gonzalez et al. (1992). Once the phosphate-potential in the cell is disturbed, there are ways, involving ATPases and ion-pumps by which cellular excitability, cell $[Ca^{2+}]$ and neurotransmitter release can be controlled.

Another lesson from the CO effects relates to suppression of hypoxic chemosensory excitation as seen in the transition from hypoxia to carbonylation with hypoxia and in the steady-state effects of CO on hypoxia. A part of the effect could be due to the binding of CO with a hypothetical heme-pigment in the chemoreceptor cell membrane and behaving like O_2, reversing hypoxic chemoreception, as originally postulated by Lloyd et al. (1968). More recently, the glomus cell membrane has been found to contain a special K^+ channel whose conductance is diminished during "hypoxia" (Lopez-Barneo et al., 1988; Ganfornina et al., 1992; Delpiano and Heschler, 1989; Peers, 1990), leading to cell depolarization.

Lopez-Lopez et al. (1992) also reported that the "hypoxic" effect is partially reversed by PCO of about 70 Torr. This "hypoxic" PO_2 range (150 Torr to 80 Torr) in the extracellular medium is admittedly far above the arterial hypoxic PO_2 range (60 Torr to 30 Torr) and, therefore, above cellular PO_2 (Lahiri et al., 1993b). There may be other factors like cyclic AMP which may lower O_2-affinity for the K^+O_2 channel, but this hypothesis has not been tested. The question then arises as to how low PO_2 raises cellular cyclic AMP and where this O_2 sensor lies. Since ATP has not been found to have any effect on K^+O_2 conductance and metabolic inhibitors including high PCO stimulate chemosensory discharge, a gap in the knowledge is obvious. A direct relationship between K^+O_2 channel and chemosensory discharge remains to be established.

Another explanation for the inhibitory effect of CO is that it would be expected to bind with the cytosolic guanylate cyclase containing heme, stimulate cyclic GMP production which, in turn, could augment the specific protein kinase and protein phosphorylation and, ultimately, the physiological response. This particular pathway has been well worked out for NO which is endogenously produced in the carotid body. NO is inhibitory to hypoxic chemosensory excitation (Fidone et al., 1993; Katayama et al., 1993; Prabhakar et al., 1993). The complexes of guanylate cyclase with CO and NO are likely to be photodissociable corresponding to the absorbance spectrum of the complex, which should manifest itself in the action spectrum. Accordingly, photodissociation should reverse inhibition, and result in excitation of the chemosensory discharge. This was not seen in most of our experiments except in one trial which is illustrated in Figure 2. The idea in this experiment was to create certain range of concentrations of bound CO which, when photodissociated, would provide sufficient signal in the chemosensory discharge. Another interpretation of this result is that photodissociation of CO-complex made O_2 available, and the chemoreceptor came "alive" and was able to respond.

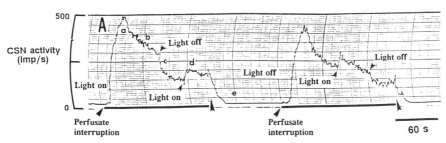

Figure 2. Light exposure excited chemosensory discharge during interruption of perfusate flow with CO. Superfusate, free of CO, washed away CO and created an appropriate PCO/PO_2 to show the excitatory photodissociation effect. That is, absence of light decreased and presence of light increased of excitation, which is incompatible with the metabolic hypothesis.

PERSPECTIVES

The fact that high PCO/PO_2 ratio stimulates carotid chemoreceptor discharge with action spectrum corresponding to cytochrome oxidase provides strong evidence in favor of the metabolic hypothesis of O_2 chemoreception. Excitation by CO cannot be explained by any other mechanism than by intracellular release of Ca^{2+} because the CO-complex with the putative membrane heme would rverse the K^+ conductance decrease and cell depolarization during hypoxia, diminishing the Ca^{2+} entry and neurotransmitter release and ultimately the neural discharge.

We thank Suzanne Hyndman and Mary Pili for preparing the manuscript. The work was supported by the grant HL-43413-05. D. K. Ray and D. Chugh were recipients of fellowship from T32 HL-07027-18.

REFERENCES

Delpiano, M.A. & J. Hescheler. (1989) Evidence for a PO_2-sensitive K^+ channel in the type I cell of the rabbit carotid body. FEBS Lett. 249: 195-198.

Duchen, M.R. & T.J. Biscoe. (1992) Mitochondrial function in type I cells isolated from rabbit arterial chemoreceptors. J. Physiol. (London) 450: 13-31.

Fidone, S., Z.-Z. Wang, B. Dinger & S. Stenaas. (1993) The role of nitric oxide (NO) in carotid chemoreceptor efferent inhibition. This volume.

Ganfornina, M.D. & J. Lopez-Barneo. (1991) Single K^+ channels in membrane patches of arterial chemoreceptor cells are modulated by O_2 tension. Proc. Natl. Acad. Sci. 88: 2927-2930.

Gonzalez, C., L., Almaraz, A. Obeso & R. Rigual. (1992) Oxygen and acid chemoreception in the carotid body chemoreceptors. Trends in Neurosci. 15: 146-153.

Iturriaga, R., W.L. Rumsey, A. Mokashi, D. Spergel, D.F. Wilson & S. Lahiri. (1991) In vitro perfused-superfused cat carotid body for physiological and pharmacological studies. J. Appl Physiol. 70: 1393-400.

Joels, N. & E. Neil. (1962) The action of high tensions of carbon monoxide on the carotid chemoreceptors. Arch. Int. Pharmacodyn. 130: 528-534.

Katayama, M., D. Chugh, A. Mokashi, D. Ray, D. Bebout & S. Lahiri. (1993) NO mimics O_2 in the carotid body chemoreception. This volume.

Keilin, D. (1970) The history of cell respiration and cytochrome. London: Cambridge University Press, pp. 221-327.

Lahiri, S. (1981) Chemical modification of carotid body chemoreception by sulfhydryls. Science 212: 1065-1066.

Lahiri, S., R. Iturriaga, A. Mokashi., D.K. Ray & D. Chugh (1993a) CO reveals dual mechanisms of O_2 chemoreception in the cat carotid body. Respir. Physiol. 94: 227-240

Lahiri, S., W.L. Rumsey, D.F. Wilson & R. Iturriaga. (1993b) Contribution of in vivo microvascular PO_2 in the cat carotid body chemotransduction. J. Appl. Physiol. (in press).

Lloyd, B.B., D.J.C. Cunningham & R.C. Goode. (1968) Depression of hypoxic hyperventilation in man by sudden inspiration of carbon monoxide. In: Arterial Chemoreceptors, edited by R.W. Torrance. Oxford: Blackwell Scientific Publications. pp. 145-148.

Lopez-Barneo, J., J. R.Lopez-Lopez, J. Urena & C. Gonzalez. (1988) Chemotransduction in the carotid body: K^+ current modulated by PO_2 in type I chemoreceptor cells. Science 241: 580-582.

Lopez-Lopez, J.R. & C. Gonzalez. (1992) Time course of K^+ current initiation by low oxygen in the chemoreceptor cells of adult rabbit carotid body. FEBS Lett. 299: 251-254.

Mulligan, E., S. Lahiri & B.T. Storey. (1981) Carotid body O_2 chemoreception and mitochondrial oxidative phosphorylation. J. Appl. Physiol. 51: 438-446.

Mulligan, E. & S. Lahiri. (1982) The separation of carotid chemoreceptor responses to O_2 and CO_2 by oligomycin and antimycin A. Am. J. Physiol. 240: C200-C206.

Peers, C. (1990) Effect of D600 on hypoxic suppression of K^+ current in isolated type I carotid body cells of the neonatal rat. FEBS Lett. 271: 37-40.

Prabhakar, N.R. (1993) "Neurotransmitters in the carotid body" This volume.

Shirahata, M., S. Andronikou & S. Lahiri. (1987). Differential effects of oligomycin on carotid chemoreceptor responses to O_2 and CO_2 in the cat. J. Appl. Physiol. 63: 2084-2092.

Snyder, S.H. (1992) Nitric oxide: first in a new class of neurotransmitters? Science 257: 494-496.

ACTIONS OF NICOTINIC AGONISTS ON ISOLATED TYPE I CELLS OF THE NEONATAL RAT CAROTID BODY

Chris Peers[1], Christopher N. Wyatt[1] and Keith J. Buckler[2]

[1]Department of Pharmacology, Leeds University, Leeds, UK and
[2]University Laboratory of Physiology, Parks Road, Oxford, UK

INTRODUCTION

Although catecholamines are believed to be the primary chemosensory transmitters, acetylcholine (ACh) is also present in type I cells, and is released during stimulation of the carotid body (Eyzaguirre & Zapata, 1968; Fidone & Gonzalez, 1986). Effects of exogenous ACh vary with species (Fidone et al., 1990), but in the rat and cat, excitatory effects such as increased carotid sinus nerve activity or the stimulation of catecholamine release are observed (Shaw et al., 1989; Kholwadwala & Donnelly, 1992). These effects are mediated by nicotinic ACh receptors (nAChRs). Here, we have examined the actions of nicotinic agonists on isolated type I cells to determine whether nAChRs are present on these cells, and how their activation might lead to the reported excitation of the intact carotid body.

METHODS

Type I cells were enzymatically isolated as previously described (e.g. Wyatt & Peers, 1993). Whole-cell patch-clamp recordings were made at room temperature (21-24°C) from cells perfused with HEPES-buffered solutions as reported elsewhere (Peers, 1991). In another series of experiments intracellular free Ca^{2+} concentration ($[Ca^{2+}]_i$) was measured using the fluorescent indicator Indo-1. These studies were performed at 37°C in HCO_3^-/CO_2 buffered solutions (see Buckler & Vaughan-Jones, 1993, for further details).

RESULTS

In voltage-clamp studies, bath-applied nicotine or dimethylphenylpiperazinium (DMPP) evoked transient inward currents in type I cells (e.g. Fig. 1A). These currents were abolished by 3μM mecamylamine, showed strong rectification and were also observed when extracellular Ca^{2+} replaced Na^+ (see Wyatt & Peers, 1993). These features indicate that type I cells possess functional, neuronal-type nAChRs (c.f. Vernino et al., 1992). In current-clamp, when the membrane potential is not held constant, nicotine caused reversible depolarization of type I cells (Fig. 1B), to approximately -20mV. When applied to Indo-1-containing cells, DMPP evoked a rapid rise of $[Ca^{2+}]_i$ which could be inhibited by mecamylamine (Fig. 1C).

Arterial Chemoreceptors: Cell to System
Edited by R. O'Regan *et al*, Plenum Press, New York, 1994

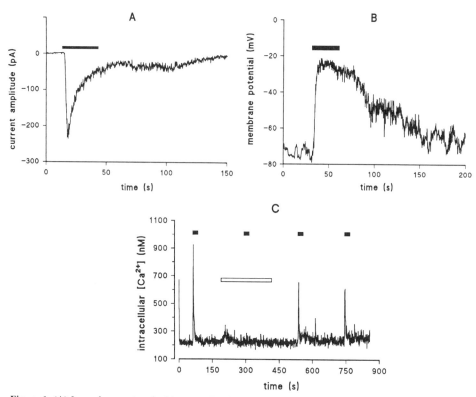

Figure 1. (A) Inward current evoked in a type I cell by bath-applied nicotine (300μM). (B) Membrane depolarization caused by bath-applied nicotine (100μM). (C) Rapid rises of intracellular [Ca^{2+}] caused by bath application of 100μM DMPP. In each trace, period of application of agonist is indicated by the solid horizontal bars. In (C) open bar indicates period of exposure to 1μM mecamylamine.

DISCUSSION

These studies demonstrate that nAChRs are present on isolated type I cells of the neonatal rat carotid body, consistent with the earlier identification of α-bungarotoxin sites localised on rat type I cells (Chen & Yates, 1984). Our findings are also consistent with the excitatory action (elevation of carotid sinus nerve discharge and release of catecholamines) of cholinergic agonists on the intact rat carotid body (Shaw et al., 1989; Kholwadwala & Donnelly, 1992). The rise of [Ca^{2+}]$_i$ seen following application of DMPP may arise in part from Ca^{2+} influx through the nAChR pore itself (Wyatt & Peers, 1993), but it is also likely that Ca^{2+} influx occurs through L-type Ca^{2+} channels opened by the depolarization following nAChR activation, since the release of catecholamines evoked by carbachol (a non-selective AChR agonist) can be partially inhibited by the L-type Ca^{2+} channel antagonist nitrendipine (Shaw et al., 1989). The location of nAChRs on 'presynaptic' type I cells provides a means by which ACh may have an enhancing influence on carotid body chemotransduction.

This work was supported by The Wellcome Trust

REFERENCES

Buckler, K. J. & Vaughan-Jones, R. D. (1993). Effects of acidic stimuli on intracellular calcium in isolated type-I cells of the neonatal rat carotid body. Pflugers Archiv. (in press).

Chen, I. L. & Yates, R. D. (1984). Two types of glomus cell in the rat carotid body as revealed by alpha-bungarotoxin binding. J. Neurocytol. 13:281-302.

Eyzaguirre, C. & Zapata, P. (1968). The release of acetylcholine from carotid body tissues. Further study on the effects of acetylcholine and cholinergic blocking agents on the chemosensory discharge. J. Physiol. 195:589-607.

Fidone, S. & Gonzalez, C. (1986). Initiation and control of chemoreceptor activity in the carotid body. In The Respiratory System, Handbook of Physiology, Cherniack, N. S. & Widdicombe, J. G., eds, Sect. 3, vol. II, pp 247-312. American Physiological Society, Bethesda, MD.

Fidone, S., Gonzalez, C., Obeso, A., Gomez-Nino, A. & Dinger, B. (1990). Biogenic amine and neuropeptide transmitters in carotid body chemotransmission: experimental findings and perspectives. In Hypoxia: The Adaptations (eds Sutton, J. R., Coattes, G. & Remmers, J. E.) pp 116-126. Marcel-Decker, London.

Kholwadwala, D. & Donnelly, D. F. (1992). Maturation of carotid body chemoreceptor sensitivity to hypoxia: in vitro studies in the newborn rat. J. Physiol. 453:461-474.

Peers, C. (1991). Hypoxic suppression of K^+ currents in type I carotid body cells: selective effect on the Ca^{2+}-activated K^+ current. Neurosci. Lett. 119:253-256.

Shaw, K., Montague, W. & Pallot, D. J. (1989). Biochemical studies on the release of catecholamines from the rat carotid body in vitro. Biochim. Biophys. Acta 1013:42-46.

Vernino, S., Amador, M., Luetje, C. W., Patrick, J. & Dani, J. A. (1992). Calcium modulation and high calcium permeability of neuronal nicotinic acetylcholine receptors. Neuron 8:127-134.

Wyatt, C. N. & Peers, C. (1993). Nicotinic acetylcholine receptors in isolated type I cells of the neonatal rat carotid body. Neurosci. 54:275-281.

Ca^{2+}-ACTIVATED K^+-CHANNELS FROM ISOLATED TYPE I CAROTID BODY CELLS OF THE NEONATAL RAT

Christopher N. Wyatt and Chris Peers

Department of Pharmacology, Leeds University, Leeds, U.K.

INTRODUCTION

Over the past five years, the patch-clamp technique has been applied to type I cells isolated from carotid bodies of rats and rabbits (e.g. Duchen et al., 1988; Lopez-Barneo et al., 1988; Delpiano & Hescheler, 1989; Peers, 1990a; Stea & Nurse, 1991). Our previous studies, using type I cells from rats (approximately 10 days old) have shown that whole-cell K^+ currents can be subdivided into two types; a Ca^{2+}-activated, charybdotoxin-sensitive current, IK_{Ca}, and a Ca^{2+}-independent, voltage-gated current, IK_V (Peers, 1990a,b). Of these, IK_{Ca} can be inhibited by chemostimuli such as hypoxia (Peers, 1990b), acidity (Peers, 1990a; Peers and Green, 1991) or the respiratory stimulant doxapram (Peers, 1991). Here, we describe the properties of the single Ca^{2+}-activated K^+ channels which underlie the macroscopic IK_{Ca}, and show that doxapram can inhibit this channel without the involvement of a second messenger system.

METHODS

Type I cells were enzymatically isolated and maintained in culture as previously described (Peers, 1990a). Single channel activity was recorded in outside-out membrane patches (Hamill et al., 1981), filtered at 1 or 2KHz and stored on tape for subsequent analysis using PAT software (J. Dempster, Strathclyde University, Scotland). Solutions exposed to the cytosolic face of patches always contained, inter alia, 120mM K^+, 2mM ATP and 0.1-1.0µM Ca^{2+}. Extracellular solutions were usually of standard composition (Peers, 1990a) but for some experiments K^+ was raised from 5mM to 120mM (Na^+ replacement). Channel amplitudes and activity were determined from all-point histograms of the digitised data. Since patches always contained multiple channels, activity is expressed as NP_0 (number of channels multiplied by open probability) rather than just P_0 since we could not always accurately determine the number of channels in a given patch.

RESULTS

Channels were identified in outside-out patches which had a slope conductance of 180-190pS and reversed at 0mV in symmetrical 120mM K^+. When external K^+ was reduced to

Arterial Chemoreceptors: Cell to System
Edited by R. O'Regan *et al*, Plenum Press, New York, 1994

5mM, the extrapolated reversal potential was close to E_K, indicating the presence of a K^+ channel. At any given Ca^{2+} concentration, channel activity increased with depolarization, and at any given membrane potential channel activity was highest when intracellular Ca^{2+} was high. For example, NP_0 at 0mV (5mM external K^+) was 0.0010 ±0.0002 at pCa 7 (n=7 patches) and at pCa 6, NP_0 was 0.627 ± 0.110 (n=19; p<0.005, unpaired t-test). In 5 patches, bath application of charybdotoxin (100nM) to the extracellular face of channels reduced activity by approximately 80%. These data indicate that this channel is a high-conductance Ca^{2+}-activated K^+ channel which underlies the macroscopic IK_{Ca} described previously (Peers, 1990a).

Bath application of doxapram (30-300μM) inhibited channel activity in outside-out patches in a concentration-dependent manner. In the presence of doxapram, openings were interrupted by brief closures (or blocking events), and at the highest concentration, the apparent single channel amplitude appeared to be substantially reduced (Fig. 1). This effect of apparently reduced amplitude arose presumably because of the bandwidth limitations of our recording system (low-pass filter, 1 or 2KHz cut-off) and is consistent with doxapram producing a flickery block of Ca^{2+}-activated K^+ channels in type I cells.

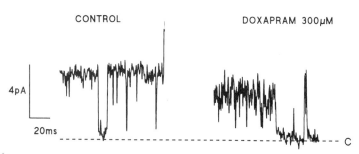

CONTROL   DOXAPRAM 300μM

4pA

20ms

Figure 1. Ca^{2+}-activated K^+ channel activity recorded from an outside-out membrane patch (pCa 6, 0mV membrane potential, external K^+ 5mM) before and during bath application of 300μM doxapram. Dashed line marks current level when channel is closed.

DISCUSSION

Our present studies have identified a Ca^{2+}-dependent, voltage- and charybdotoxin-sensitive, high conductance K^+ channel which underlies the previously reported macroscopic IK_{Ca} (Peers, 1990a). IK_{Ca} can be selectively inhibited by chemostimuli (Peers, 1990a,b), and we have also shown here that these channels can be directly inhibited by doxapram, which causes a 'flickery' channel blockade (c.f. Davies et al., 1991). Although NP_0 values were low, it is noteworthy that we never isolated a single channel in any given patch: instead we always noted multiple channel activity, suggesting that these channels are present at high density in the type I cell plasma membrane.

Although these studies are in agreement with our previous whole-cell recordings, they contrast with those of Ganfornina and Lopez-Barneo (1991) who have shown, using type I cells from adult rabbits, that hypoxia selectively inhibits a lower-conductance K^+ channel which is insensitive to intracellular Ca^{2+}. In rabbit type I cells, this effect is suggested to alter the firing frequency of spontaneously active cells, thereby regulating Ca^{2+} influx and transmitter release (Lopez-Barneo et al., 1988). In rat type I cells, where spontaneous action potentials have not been reported, blockade of the Ca^{2+}-activated K^+ channels described here could lead to cell depolarization, activation of voltage-gated Ca^{2+} channels and hence an influx of Ca^{2+} which is required for stimulation of transmitter release.

These studies were supported by The Wellcome Trust

REFERENCES

Davies, N. W., Pettit, A. I., Agarwal, R. & Standen, N. B. (1991). The flickery block of ATP-dependent potassium channels of skeletal muscle by internal 4-aminopyridine. Pflugers Archiv. 419:25-31.

Delpiano, M. A. & Hescheler, J. (1989). Evidence for a pO_2-sensitive K^+ channel in the type-I cell of the rabbit carotid body. FEBS Lett. 249:195-198.

Duchen, M.R., Caddy, K. W. T., Kirby, G. C., Patterson, D. L., Ponte, J. & Biscoe, T. J. (1988). Biophysical studies of the cellular elements of the rabbit carotid body. Neurosci. 26:291-311.

Ganfornina, M. D. & Lopez-Barneo, J. (1991). Single K^+ channels in membrane patches of arterial chemoreceptor cells are modulated by O_2 tension. Proc. Natl. Acad. Sci. USA 88:2927-2930.

Hamill, O. P., Marty, A., Neher, E., Sakmann, B. & Sigworth, F.J. (1981). Improved patch-clamp techniques for high-resolution current recordings from cells and cell-free membrane patches. Pflugers Archiv. 391:85-100.

Lopez-Barneo, J., Lopez-Lopez, J. R., Urena, J. & Gonzalez, C. (1988). Chemotransduction in the carotid body: K^+ current modulated by pO_2 in type I chemoreceptor cells. Science 241:580-582.

Peers, C. (1990a). Selective effect of lowered extracellular pH on Ca^{2+}-dependent K^+ currents in type I cells isolated from the neonatal rat carotid body. J. Physiol. 422:381-395.

Peers, C. (1990b). Hypoxic suppression of K^+ currents in type I carotid body cells: selective effect on the Ca^{2+}-activated K^+ current. Neurosci. Lett. 119:253-256.

Peers, C. (1991). Effects of doxapram on ionic currents recorded in isolated type I cells of the neonatal rat carotid body. Brain Res. 568:116-122.

Peers, C. & Green, F.K. (1991). Intracellular acidosis inhibits Ca^{2+}-activated K^+ currents in isolated type I cells of the neonatal rat carotid body. J. Physiol. 437:589-602.

Stea, A. & Nurse, C. A. (1991). Whole-cell and perforated-patch recordings from O_2-sensitive rat carotid body cells grown in short- and long-term culture. Pflugers Archiv. 418:93-101.

CULTURING CAROTID BODY CELLS OF ADULT CATS

Machiko Shirahata[1,2], Brian Schofield[1], Beek Y. Chin[1], and Thomas R. Guilarte[1]

Departments of [1]Environmental Health Sciences and [2]Anesthesiology/Critical Care Medicine, The Johns Hopkins University, Baltimore, MD 21205, USA

INTRODUCTION

Recently patch clamp techniques or optical fluorometric techniques have been applied to freshly dissociated or cultured carotid body glomus cells to understand chemosensory mechanisms of the carotid body. Results were not consistent. The inconsistency of the available data may result from various reasons. Firstly, the studied cells might have been heterogeneous due to the difficulty of differentiating between dissociated glomus cells and sheath cells. Secondly, culture conditions may alter characteristics of the glomus cells. Thirdly, differences in the age and species used to generate the available data make the interpretation more difficult. The purpose of this study is to standardise our culture techniques to overcome these difficulties.

METHODS

Adults cats of either sex (1.8-3 kg) were anesthetized with pentobarbital (30-40 mg/kg). Both carotid bodies were excised and cleaned under a dissecting microscope. The tissues were incubated in Ham's F12 medium containing 0.1-0.2 % collagenase in the CO_2 incubator (5 % CO_2 in air) at 37 °C for 1 hour. The tissues were gently triturated, and the cell suspension was centrifuged (100-200 g, 5 min). The pellet was resuspended in the defined culture medium (Bottenstein and Sato's N_2: Bottenstein et al.,1979) and divided into 8 to 10 small wells, some of which contained glass-coverslips. The wells and coverslips had been previously treated with poly-D-lysine and then coated with diluted Matrigel^{TM} (1/10). The cells were usually kept up to 1 month, and culture medium was changed two times a week.

To assess function of the cultured glomus cells, secretion of dopamine and expression of tyrosine hydroxylase were monitored. For the measurement of dopamine culture medium was changed to 50 µl of Krebs solution. The cells were exposed to either 5% CO_2/95% air or 5% CO_2/95% N_2 at 37°C. After 1 hour 40 µl of Krebs solution was collected for dopamine measurement. Culture medium was added to the wells, and cells were given a one hour rest period in the CO_2 incubator. The cells then received a second gas exposure, and the same procedure was employed to collect the second sample. The samples were stored at -80°C until dopamine was measured using HPLC with electro-chemical detection. To examine the expression of tyrosine hydroxylase the cultured cells were fixed with 4% paraformaldehyde, and the cell membrane was permeabilized with 80% acetone/20% water. Standard immunohistological techniques with avidin-biotin-peroxidase were applied using monoclonal antibody to tyrosine hydroxylase raised in mouse hybridoma cells (dilution: 1/600).

To identify living glomus cells in culture we used two surface markers which are specific for neurons and for Schwann cells: fluorochrome conjugated tetanus toxin fragment (Neurotag^{TM}) and anti-galactocerebroside. The specificity of anti-galactocerebroside to sheath cells was studied in both fixed cultured cells and fixed tissue section. Cells or tissues were double stained for tyrosine hydroxylase and for anti-galactocerebroside by immunohistological techniques. Localisation of the staining was carefully examined with a light microscope. To label live cells Neurotag Red^{TM} was added in the culture medium (20 μg/ml). Then anti-galactocerebroside was applied (2 μg/ml), and new medium containing fluorescein-conjugated anti-mouse IgG (50 μg/ml) followed. The coverslips with cells were transferred to the chamber used for patch clamp study and the cells were examined with a fluorescent microscope.

RESULTS

Carotid body cells from adults cats were successfully cultured for up to 37 days. In this culture condition extension of processes was usually seen within 24 hours. Clusters tended to be spherical throughout the culture period. Cultured glomus cells synthesized dopamine. In cells cultured for 2-3 days dopamine secretion was 47 ± 21 and 279 ± 45 fmole/well/hour during normoxia and hypoxia (mean $\pm$ SEM, n=6), respectively. An increase in dopamine secretion during hypoxia was observed after 1 week and 1 month. As expected from dopamine secretion glomus cells expressed tyrosine hydroxylase at all times during culture period. The shape of the glomus cells and processes were well observed with this staining. Isolated glomus cells had rather well developed processes, and they retained their neuron-like morphology up to 30 days. Glomus cells in clusters also showed processes within the cluster or extending out from the cluster.

Double stained tissue and cells were carefully examined, and we found that no cells which expressed tyrosine hydroxylase had galactocerebroside on their surface. In culture application of Neurotag Red^{TM} and anti-galactocerebroside combined with fluorescein-conjugated anti-mouse IgG clearly distinguished between glomus cells and sheath cells. With phase contrast image only it was extremely hard to differentiate between glomus cells and sheath cells.

DISCUSSION

This is the first report of culturing glomus cells of adult cats. Although glomus cells from other species have been cultured, proper culture conditions for neural cells differ not only from one tissue to another, but the species and age of the animals influence the survival and growth of the cells as well (Banker et al., 1991). We introduced the usage of serum-free media (Bottenstein's N_2) which is known to support growth of nerve cells. Since the components of serum vary from batch to batch, elimination of serum assures a constant culture environment. Matrigel^{TM} is known to support cell growth and differentiation in many cell types. Although we diluted it to 1/10, clusters tended to keep spherical form for 1 month. When Matrigel^{TM} was used, cells attached to the glass very well and they were not rinsed away by the flow of superfusion. This is advantageous to expose cells to different environment by superfusion during patch clamp studies or fluorometric measurement of ions. Glomus cells cultured in the condition described above produced dopamine, and dopamine release increased in response to hypoxia. Tyrosine hydroxylase was expressed in glomus cells at all times during the culture period. The results indicate that these glomus cells were healthy and functioning in a manner similar to glomus cells *in situ* in terms of dopamine synthesis and secretion. In addition, the immunofluorescent studies described above showed that glomus cells can be easily identified by applying Neurotag™ and anti-galactocerebroside combined with fluorescein-conjugated anti-mouse IgG.

One of the problems of using primary culture for physiological studies is the heterogeneous population of the cell types. Differentiation between dissociated glomus cells and sheath cells is quite difficult, because their shapes and sizes are alike. We found that anti-galactocerebroside selectively bound to sheath cells, but not glomus cells. In culture, rhodamine conjugated tetanus toxin fragment labelled both glomus and sheath cells. With a combination of these labelling agents we could effectively differentiate the two type of cells.

Investigation of glomus cell function is essential to clarify the mechanisms of carotid body chemoreception. At the same time results obtained from cells have to be explained in the context of the responses of the carotid body *in vivo*. Since abundant *in vivo* physiological data using adult cats are available, the culture and identification methods of glomus cells from adult cats described here will be extremely useful for conducting further *in vitro* physiological studies.

This work was supported by HL 47044 and HL 10342.

REFERENCES

Banker, G. & Goslin, K. (1991). Culturing nerve cells. Cambridge, MA: The MIT press

Bottenstein, J.E. & Sato, G.H. (1979). Growth of a rat neuroblastoma cell line in serum-free supplemented medium. Proc. Natl. Acad. Sci. U.S.A. 76:514-517.

PLASTICITY IN CULTURED ARTERIAL CHEMORECEPTORS: EFFECTS OF CHRONIC HYPOXIA AND CYCLIC AMP ANALOGS

Colin A. Nurse, Adele Jackson, and Anthony Stea

Department of Biology, McMaster University, Hamilton, Ontario, Canada, L8S 4K1

INTRODUCTION

Exposure of humans and animals to chronic hypoxia causes hypertrophy of the chemosensory carotid body (McGregor et al., 1988), and sensitization of the ventilatory reflex (Barnard et al., 1987; Nielsen et al., 1987). The underlying mechanisms are unclear but are likely to involve the glomus or type 1 cells, which are now generally considered to be the oxygen sensors (Gonzalez et al., 1992). These structural and functional changes may be triggered by the direct, chronic stimulation of glomus cells by low PO_2, perhaps acting via the intracellular second messenger cAMP (see Wang et al. 1991). To address this we investigated whether chronic exposure of carotid body cultures to hypoxia (6% O_2) or cAMP analogs leads to modification in glomus cells properties that may explain carotid body plasticity during ventilatory acclimatization.

METHODS

The procedures for long-term culture of glomus cells from the carotid bodies of 5-12 day old rats have been previously described (Nurse, 1990; Stea et al., 1992). For the first 2 days all cultures were grown in a normoxic (20% O_2) environment; thereafter, some of them were either transferred to a hypoxic environment (6% O_2) or treated with 1 mM dibutyryl cAMP during normoxia. At the end of the treatment period cultures were fixed and prepared for immunocytochemistry (Nurse, 1990), or mounted for patch clamp/whole-cell recording (Stea et al., 1992). Glomus cells were identified using antibodies against tyrosine hydroxylase (TH), and visualized with a fluorescein-conjugated secondary antibody (Nurse, 1990). Neurofilament proteins (NF 68kd and NF 160kd) were labelled with mouse monoclonal antibodies (Boehringer Mannheim, Montreal) at a concentration of 5-10 µg/ml and visualized with a Texas red-conjugated goat anti-mouse IgG (Cappel, Malvern, PA). For detection of GAP-43, a monoclonal antibody (9-1E12; a gift from Dr. D.J. Schreyer) was used at a final concentration of 1:20000, and visualized with a Texas red-conjugated secondary antibody.

RESULTS

During whole cell recordings, the most obvious modification in glomus cells grown under chronic hypoxia was the increased magnitude of the inward Na^+ current (Stea et al., 1992). This current is normally small (< 50pA) or absent in rat glomus cells, but reached values of ca. 500 pA after 1 week in chronic hypoxia. Blockade of the outward K^+ current, with Cs^+ and tetraethylammonium (TEA) in the pipette, revealed Ca^{2+} currents that were also enlarged following chronic hypoxia. However, only the Na^+ (but not Ca^{2+} nor K^+) current density was significantly increased when the peak currents were normalized to account for the increased glomus cell size during chronic hypoxia (Stea et al., 1992; Mills & Nurse, 1993). These effects could be mimicked qualitatively by growing normoxic cultures in the continuous presence of the membrane-permeable cAMP analog, dibutyryl cAMP (dbcAMP; 1 mM).

The above cellular adaptations to chronic hypoxia resemble the plasticity that occurs when related chromaffin cells differentiate into neurons following exposure to Nerve Growth Factor (see Stea et al., 1992). It was therefore of interest to investigate whether hypoxia (and/or dbcAMP) could regulate expression of the plasticity-associated protein GAP-43 (Skene, 1990), and other markers of neuronal differentiation. Figure 1a,b illustrate that following chronic hypoxia some TH+ glomus cells (Fig. 1a) express GAP-43 immunoreactivity (Fig. 1b), which is virtually undetectable in control, normoxic cultures (not shown). Treatment of normoxic cultures with 1 mM dbcAMP (Figs. 1 c,d,e,f), enhanced not only GAP-43 expression (Fig. 1d), but also neurite processes (Fig. 1c) and neurofilament (NF) expression (Fig. 1f).

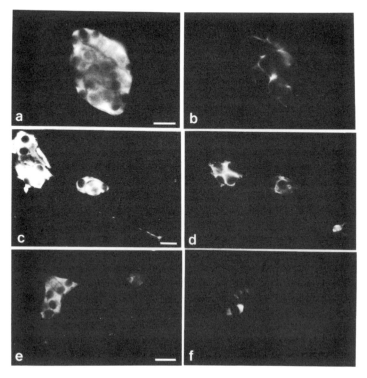

Figure 1. Expression of GAP-43 and neurofilament (NF 68 kd) in glomus cells grown under certain conditions. Figs. a,c,e represent fields containing glomus cells stained for TH-immunoreactivity and visualized with a fluorescein filter set; a, chronic hypoxia for 8 days; c,e, 1 mM dbcAMP present. Figs. b,d,f are the same fields as in a,c, and e respectively, but stained for GAP-43 (b,d) and NF 68 kd (f), and visualized with Texas red. Bar represents 20 μm.

DISCUSSION

These studies indicate that chronic hypoxia induces a variety of physiological and morphological changes (summarized in Fig. 2) in carotid body chemoreceptors, that could be mediated in part by elevation of intracellular cAMP. The fact that these changes occurred *in vitro* indicates that influences from the rest of the cardiovascular and nervous systems were not involved. We obtained evidence for glomus cell hypertrophy and a selective increase in Na^+ (but not Ca^{2+} nor K^+) channel density (see also, Stea et al., 1992; Mills & Nurse, 1993). Doubtless, these cellular modifications contribute to the increased size and chemosensitivity of the carotid body during ventilatory acclimatization to hypoxia (Barnard et al., 1987; McGregor et al., 1988).

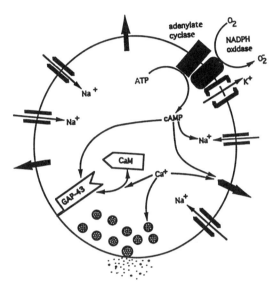

Figure 2. Schematic diagram summarizing the effects of chronic hypoxia on glomus cells. During hypoxia, interactions with the membrane-bound O_2-sensor protein (NADPH oxidase) are thought to close a subset of K^+ channels and activate adenylate cyclase. The production of cAMP (from ATP) probably leads to a cascade of events including, upregulation of Na^+ channel density and GAP-43, a calmodulin (CaM) binding protein which facilitates neurotransmitter release. Elevation of intracellular Ca^{2+} may complement cAMP and cause cellular hypertrophy.

Interestingly, chronic hypoxia appeared to upregulate the plasticity-associated protein GAP-43 in glomus cells. Though GAP-43, which is known to bind calmodulin, has frequently been associated with axonal regeneration and synaptic remodelling (Skene, 1990), there is evidence for its involvement in neurotransmitter release (e.g. Dekker et al., 1989). Thus, increased GAP-43 expression during chronic hypoxia may also contribute to enhanced neurotransmitter release from glomus cells, and increased respiratory drive during acclimatization to hypoxia.

Finally, we provide evidence that during treatment with cAMP analogs postnatal glomus cells have the capacity for neuronal differentiation (i.e., express NF and elaborate neurites), though this potential may not be fully expressed during exposure to chronic hypoxia.

We acknowledge the assistance of Cathy Vollmer and Lynn Macintyre, and thank Dr. D. Schreyer for the gift of GAP-43 antibody. This work was supported by grants from Heart and Stroke Foundation of Ontario, NSERC, NIH, and Dysautonomia Foundation.

REFERENCES

Barnard, P., Andronikou, S., Pokorski, M., Smatresk, N. & Lahiri, S. (1987). Time-dependent effect of hypoxia on carotid body chemosensory function. J. Appl. Physiol. 63: 685-691.

Dekker, L., DeGraan, P., Oestreicher, A., Versteeg, D. & Gispen, W. (1989). Inhibition of noradrenaline release by antibodies to B-50 (GAP-43). Nature 342: 74-76.

Doupe, A., Landis, S. & Patterson, P. (1985). Environmental influences in the development of neural crest derivatives: Glucocorticoids, growth factors, and chromaffin cell plasticity. J. Neurosci.5: 2119-2142.

Gonsalez, C., Almaraz. L., Obeso, A. & Rigual, R. (1992). Oxygen and acid chemoreception in the carotid body chemoreceptors. TINS 15: 146-153.

McGregor, K., Gil, J. & Lahiri, S. (1984). A morphometric study of the carotid body in chronically hypoxic rats. J. Appl. Physiol. 57: 1430-1438.

Mills, L. & Nurse, C. (1993). Chronic hypoxia in vitro increases volume of carotid body chemoreceptors. NeuroReport 4: 619-622.

Neilsen, A., Bisgard, G. & Vidruk E. (1988). Carotid chemoreceptor activity during acute and sustained hypoxia in goats. J. Appl. Physiol. 65: 1796-1802.

Nurse, C. (1990). Carbonic anhydrase and neuronal enzymes in cultured glomus cells of the carotid body of the rat. Cell Tissue Res. 261: 65-71.

Stea, A., Jackson, A. & Nurse, C. (1992). Hypoxia and dbcAMP but not nerve growth factor induce Na^+ channels and hypertrophy in chromaffin-like arterial chemoreceptors. Proc. Natl. Acad. Sci. USA 89: 9469-9473.

Skene, J. (1990). GAP-43 as a 'calmodulin' sponge and some implications for calcium signalling in axon terminals. Neurosci. Res., Suppl. 13: S112-S125.

Wang, Z.-Z., Stensaas, L.J., deVente, J., Dinger, B. & Fidone, S.J. (1991). Immunocytochemical localization of cAMP and cGMP in cells of the rat carotid body following natural and pharmacological stimulation. Histochem. 96: 523-530.

CAROTID BODY CHEMORECEPTION: ROLE OF EXTRACELLULAR Ca^{2+}

Rodrigo Iturriaga and Sukhamay Lahiri

Department of Physiology, University of Pennsylvania, Philadelphia, USA, and Laboratory of Neurobiology, Catholic University of Chile, Santiago, Chile

INTRODUCTION

In stimulus secretion-coupling, the excitable cells may depolarize first, opening voltage-gated calcium channels and allowing Ca^{2+} to enter the cells, activating exocytosis of vesicles and secretion of transmitters, which then act on the target cells. Applying the same model to the carotid body (CB), the role of the $[Ca^{2+}]_o$ has been investigated in the raising of $[Ca^{2+}]$ in the glomus cell (GC) and chemosensory excitation. But the results have been controversial (Buckler & Vaughan-Jones, 1993; Duchen & Biscoe, 1992; Donnelly & Kholwadwala, 1992; Gonzalez et al., 1992; Shirahata & Fitzgerald, 1991). Two different mechanisms have been proposed for the GC $[Ca^{2+}]_i$ rise observed during hypoxia: release of Ca^{2+} from mitochondria (Duchen and Biscoe, 1992) and Ca^{2+} entry from the extracellular space through voltage-gated channels (Shirahata & Fitzgerald 1991; Gonzalez et al., 1992).

We tested the above hypotheses using our in vitro cat CB preparation. We compared the effects of Tyrode perfusate containing Ca^{2+} 2mM, Tyrode nominally free of Ca^{2+} and Tyrode nominally free of Ca^{2+} plus EGTA (1mM) on the CB chemosensory response to hypoxia. For comparison, we also tested the effects of hypercapnia and nicotine.

METHODS

The carotid bifurcations with the CBs were perfused and superfused in vitro as previously described (Iturriaga et al., 1991). The CBs were perfused with Tyrode solution equilibrated at PO_2 of 120 Torr, PCO_2 of 30 Torr and pH 7.40. The chemosensory discharge was recorded from the whole carotid sinus nerve. The responses to hypoxia (PO_2 of 50 Torr), hypercapnia (PCO_2 of 60 Torr at pH 7.15) and to nicotine (bolus of 1 μg in 0.2 ml) were assessed during perfusion with Tyrode with $[Ca^{2+}]$ 2mM, during perfusion with Tyrode nominally free of Ca^{2+} (replaced by Mg^{2+} 2mM) or during perfusion with Tyrode nominally free of Ca^{2+} plus EGTA 1mM.

Arterial Chemoreceptors: Cell to System
Edited by R. O'Regan *et al*, Plenum Press, New York, 1994

RESULTS

Figure 1 shows the effects of nominally Ca^{2+} free medium on the CB chemosensory responses to hypoxia, hypercapnia and nicotine. During perfusion with Tyrode with $[Ca^{2+}]$ 2mM, hypoxia and hypercapnia rapidly increased the discharge after a short latency to maximal levels which showed a slight adaptation to hypoxia and a large one to hypercapnia (Fig. 1A). Nicotine caused a sharp increase in the chemosensory discharge. Nominally Ca^{2+} free medium greatly reduced the responses to hypercapnia and to nicotine, but only moderately reduced the hypoxic response (Fig. 1B). Following perfusion with Tyrode with Ca^{2+}, the hypoxic response was exaggerated, but the hypercapnic response was partially recovered. The response to nicotine was almost completely restored (Fig. 1C).

Perfusion with Tyrode nominally free of Ca^{2+} plus EGTA (1 mM) promptly reduced the chemosensory baseline activity. The responses to hypoxia, hypercapnia and nicotine were almost abolished. The hypoxic response was completely restored when EGTA was removed from the perfusate, but the hypercapnic response remained reduced.

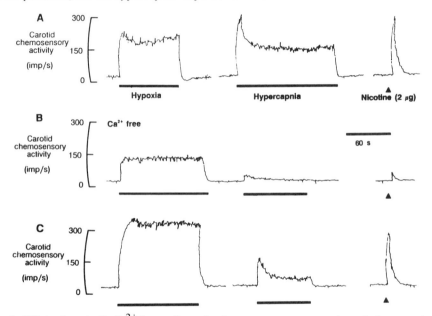

Figure 1. Effects of nominally Ca^{2+} free media on the chemosensory responses to hypoxia, hypercapnia and nicotine. A. Control perfusion with $[Ca^{2+}]$ 2mM. B. After 30 min of perfusion with nominal free Ca^{2+} medium (Ca^{2+} was replaced by Mg^{2+}). C. Recovery during perfusion with $[Ca^{2+}]$ 2mM (10 min).

DISCUSSION

The role of Ca^{2+} in the GC response to hypoxia is not well established. Duchen & Biscoe (1992) found that hypoxia increased $[Ca^{2+}]_i$, whereas Donnelly & Kholwadwala (1992) reported that hypoxia reduced $[Ca^{2+}]_i$. Shirahata & Fitzgerald (1991) and Gonzalez et al. (1992) concluded from their experiments on the whole CB that the entry of Ca^{2+} through voltage-gated channels is critical for the hypoxic response. In their model, hypoxia should depolarize the GC first, opening voltage-gated Ca^{2+} channels and allowing Ca^{2+} to enter the cell. However, Duchen and Biscoe (1992) presented data showing that hypoxia releases Ca^{2+} from an intracellular store, presumably from the mitochondria.

Our results show that a very low $[Ca^{2+}]_i$ (nominally Ca^{2+} free media) was enough to maintain the O_2 chemoreception. However, in the absence of $[Ca^{2+}]_o$ (nominally Ca^{2+} free media plus EGTA) the hypoxic response was greatly reduced. We are aware of the possibility that $[Ca^{2+}]_o$ could influence the cells and the nerve terminals differently in the whole CB than in the isolated cells. In spite of that possibility we concluded that at the same low $[Ca^{2+}]_o$ the hypoxic response seems to be less vulnerable than the hypercapnic and nicotinic responses, suggesting that hypoxia may release Ca^{2+} from an intracellular store in addition to Ca^{2+} entry.

The participation of Ca^{2+} in the CB chemoreception of CO_2-H^+ is also unclear. Gonzalez et al. (1992) proposed that acid hypercapnia reduces the GC pH_i which activates Na^+-H^+ exchange, leading to a rise in $[Na^+]_i$ and influx of Ca^{2+} via a Ca^{2+}-Na^+ exchanger working in reverse mode. However, Buckler & Vaughan-Jones (1993) measuring $[Ca^{2+}]_i$ in neonatal rat GC reported that acid hypercapnia depolarizes the cells, probably by decreasing the K^+ conductance, and leading Ca^{2+} entry through voltage-gated channels. Our results suggest that a common mechanism for raising $[Ca^{2+}]_i$ does not account for our observed temporal separation of the chemosensory responses to O_2 and CO_2 in the presence of low $[Ca^{2+}]_i$.

Supported in part by NHI grant HL 43413-04.

REFERENCES

Buckler, K.J. & Vaughan-Jones, R.D. (1993). Increasing PCO_2 raises $[Ca^{2+}]_i$ through voltage-gated Ca^{2+} entry in isolated carotid body glomus cells of the neonatal rat. J. Physiol. (Lond.) 459: 272P.

Donnelly, D.F. & Kholwadwala, D. (1992). Hypoxia decreased intracellular calcium in adult rat carotid body glomus cells. J. Neurophysiol. 67:1543-1551.

Duchen, M.R. & Biscoe, T.J. (1992). Relative mitochondrial membrane potential and $[Ca^{2+}]_i$ in type I cells isolated from the rabbit carotid body. J. Physiol. (Lond.) 450:33-61.

Gonzalez, C., Almaraz, L., Obeso, A. & Rigual, R. (1992). Oxygen and acid chemoreception in the carotid body chemoreceptors. Trends in Neurosci. 15:146-153.

Iturriaga, R., Rumsey, W.L., Mokashi, A., Spergel, D., Wilson, D.F. & Lahiri, S. (1991). In vitro perfused-superfused cat carotid body for physiological and pharmacological studies. J. Appl. Physiol. 70:1393-1400.

Shirahata, M. & Fitzgerald, R.S. (1991). Dependency of hypoxic chemotransduction in cat carotid body on voltage-gated calcium channels. J. Appl. Physiol. 71:1062-1069

CYTOSOLIC CALCIUM IN ISOLATED TYPE I CELLS OF THE ADULT RABBIT CAROTID BODY: EFFECTS OF HYPOXIA, CYANIDE AND CHANGES IN INTRACELLULAR pH.

M. Roumy.

URA CNRS 649, Laboratoire de Physiologie, Faculte de Medecine, 133, Route de Narbonne, F-31062 - Toulouse - Cedex, France.

INTRODUCTION

It has been suggested (Bernon et al., 1983; Biscoe et al., 1989; Roumy & Leitner, 1977) that cytosolic calcium concentration ($[Ca^{2+}]_i$) in type I cells controls the rate of release of a sensory transmitter and thus spike frequency in chemoafferent units. As the neurotransmitter has not yet been identified the question of its excitatory or inhibitory nature remains unsettled. Nevertheless, there must exist a unique relationship between changes in type I cells $[Ca^{2+}]_i$ and variations of chemoafferent activity during stimulation if cytosolic calcium is to play such a critical role. I therefore measured $[Ca^{2+}]_i$ of isolated type I cell clusters during hypoxia (PO_2 down to 10 torr). However, as carotid body cells consume oxygen, there is, *in vivo*, a gradient of PO_2 between blood an tissue, which magnitude is still a subject of debate, that might significantly differ from that between medium and isolated cells. Consequently, I also used cyanide which behaves as an inert gas at physiological pH, and thus equilibrates between blood and carotid body tissue or medium and cell clusters within a few tenths of a second with no concentration gradient (Forster, 1968). It should be remembered that cyanide already excites the chemoafferent units at $10\mu M$ concentration (Krilov & Anichkov, 1968 ; Leitner & Roumy, unpublished results). Finally the effects of changes in intracellular pH (pH_i) thought to be involved in the chemoafferent response to CO_2, were also studied.

METHODS

The left carotid body was excised from anaesthetized adult rabbits (2 - 3 kg) and incubated for 1 h at 38.5° C with a mixture of collagenase, hyaluronidase and deoxyribonuclease. It was then rinsed 4 times in 1 ml of medium at room temperature and mechanically dispersed. The cells were resuspended in 0.1 ml of medium containing 1-2μM of the permeant acetoxymethylester of the fluorescent calcium probe Fluo-3 (Minta et al., 1989). The cell suspension was deposited on a microscope coverslip for simultaneous cell attachment and Fluo-3 loading (30 min at room temperature). The coverslip formed part of the lid of the experimental chamber which was mounted on the stage of an upright epifluorescence microscope. Cells were viewed with a 100 : 1.32 oil-immersion objective.

Arterial Chemoreceptors: Cell to System
Edited by R. O'Regan *et al*, Plenum Press, New York, 1994

Fluo-3 fluorescence was excited at 488 nm and emitted light measured above 515 nm. Quenching of Fluo-3 fluorescence with $MnCl_2$ (5 mM) served to estimate $[Ca^{2+}]_i$. The cells were superfused at 35° C with a medium containing (in mM) : NaCl: 140; KCl: 4.5; $MgCl_2$: 0.75; $CaCl_2$: 2; glucose: 5; HEPES: 10; pH was 7.40 and bovine serum albumin was added at 0.1% final concentration. Hypoxia was obtained by equilibrating the medium to a known absolute pressure under vigorous agitation. The relationship between PO_2 and pressure was determined polarographically in preliminary experiments. Changes in pH_i were achieved by adding weak bases (NH_4Cl or benzylamine, 10mM) or acids (acetic or propionic, 10mM) to the medium while maintaining its pH to 7.40.

RESULTS

Fourteen cell clusters were superfused with an hypoxic medium (PO_2 = 10 torr) for 7 to 16 min. In 12 clusters fluorescence did not change. In 3 of these clusters temperature was raised to 37.5° C but hypoxia had still no effect (Figure 1).In the 2 remaining clusters hypoxia (10 torr) caused a brisk, 30 % increase in fluorescence after more than 5 min and 40 s latency, respectively.

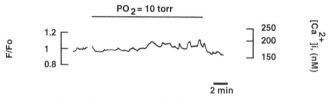

Figure 1. Effect of hypoxia on $[Ca^{2+}]_i$ in a cell cluster at 37.5° C.

In six cell clusters NaCN 10 µM was superfused for 4 to 12 min, with no effects upon $[Ca^{2+}]_i$. At 0.1 and 1 mM, NaCN always raised $[Ca^{2+}]_i$, the increase being larger at 1 mM. In 4 clusters NaCN 50 µM was tested : it caused a small increase in fluorescence after 2 to 3 min latency in 3 clusters and an 8 min superfusion was without effect in the fourth.

In the carotid body type I cells, NH_4Cl raises pH_i with partial recovery when the perfusion was maintained and reduces pHi below control when the cells are returned to normal medium (Buckler et al., 1991). In 13 cell clusters, fluorescence rose during NH_4Cl superfusion. In 4 clusters in which fluorescence was calibrated, the increase in $[Ca^{2+}]_i$ was 50 to 100 nM. When the cells were returned to normal medium, $[Ca^{2+}]_i$ decreased towards its control value so that no effect of the decrease in pH_i could be identified. Indeed, acetic and propionic acids did not affect $[Ca^{2+}]_i$.. Benzylamine, which did not caused acidification after its withdrawal produced an identical change in $[Ca^{2+}]_i$. In the absence of extracellular calcium, NH_4Cl had no effect upon $[Ca^{2+}]_i$.

DISCUSSION

In the present experiments I find that :
(i) hypoxia (10 torr) and cyanide (10 µM) which both excite chemoafferent units had no effect upon $[Ca^{2+}]_i$
(ii) cyanide (0.1, 1 mM) and alkaline pH_i which have opposite effects upon chemoafferent activity raised $[Ca^{2+}]_i$
(iii) acid and alkaline pH_i increases and decreases, respectively, chemoafferent activity (Rumsey et al., 1991) but acid pH_i had no effect upon type I cells $[Ca^{2+}]_i$.

These results do not support the idea that $[Ca^{2+}]_i$ in type I cells is a major determinant of chemoafferent discharge frequency through its action on the rate of release of a sensory neurotransmitter.

In addition, the lack of effect of hypoxia and cyanide (10 μM) upon $[Ca^{2+}]_i$ together with the absence of a reduction in ATP content during hypoxia (Verna et al., 1990) suggest that a depression of oxidative metabolism may not be involved in the chemoafferent response to hypoxia.

This work has been supported by the Centre National de la Recherche Scientifique. I thank Ms C. Fortun for editing the manuscript.

REFERENCES

Bernon, R., Leitner, L.M., Roumy, M., Verna, A. (1983). Effects of ion-containting liposomes upon the chemoafferent activity of the rabbit carotid body superfused in vitro. Neurosci. Lett. 35 : 289-295.

Biscoe, T.J., Duchen M.R., Eisner, D.A., O'Neill, S.C., Valdeolmillos, M. (1989). Measurement of intracellular Ca^{2+} in dissociated type I cells of the rabbit carotid body. J. Physiol. (Lond.) 416 : 421-434.

Buckler, K.J., Vaughan-Jones, R.D., Peers, C., Nye, P.G.C. (1991). Intracellular pH and its regulation in isolated type I carotid body cells of the neonatal rat. J. Physiol. (Lond.) 436: 107-129.

Forster, R.E. (1968). The diffusion of gases in the carotid body. In "Arterial chemoreceptors." R.W. Torrance, ed., Blackwell, London.

Krylov, S.S. & Anichkov, S.V. (1968). The effects of metabolic inhibition on carotid chemoreceptors. In "Arterial chemoreceptors." R.W. Torrance, ed., Blackwell, London.

Roumy, M. & Leitner, L.M., (1977). Role of calcium ions in the mechanism of arterial chemoreceptor excitation. In "Chemoreception in the carotid body." H. Acker et al, ed.., Springer, Berlin.

Rumsey, W.L., Iturriaga, R., Spergel, D., Lahiri, S., Wilson, D.F. (1991). Intracellular pH and chemoreception in the isolated perfused and superfused cat carotid body. In "Neurobiology and Cell Physiology of Chemoreception," P.G. Data, S. Lahiri & H. Acker, eds., Plenum Press, New York.

Verna A., Talib, N., Roumy, M., Pradet, A. (1990). Effects of metabolic inhibitors and hypoxia on the ATP, ADP and AMP content of the rabbit carotid body in vitro : the metabolic hypothesis in question. Neurosci. Lett. 116 : 156-161.

CHARACTERIZATION OF MEMBRANE CURRENTS IN PULMONARY NEUROEPITHELIAL BODIES: HYPOXIA-SENSITIVE AIRWAY CHEMORECEPTORS

Charlotte Youngson[1], Colin Nurse[2], Herman Yeger[1] and Ernest Cutz[1]

[1]Department of Pathology, The Research Institute, Hospital for Sick Children and the University of Toronto, 555 University Ave, Toronto, Ontario, M5G 1X8; [2]Department of Biology, McMaster University, 1280 Main St.W, Hamilton, Ontario L8S 4K1

INTRODUCTION

Neuroepithelial bodies (NEB) are composed of clusters of innervated amine and peptide containing cells located within the airway epithelium of human and animal lungs (Fig. 1A). Because of their location, direct studies on NEB are difficult, and their precise function has remained a mystery. NEB are most numerous during the perinatal period and they may play an important role in the transition from intrauterine to post-natal life. Based on alterations of NEB amine content both in vivo (Lauweryns & Cokelaere, 1973, Lauweryns et al 1977) and in vitro (Cutz et al, 1993), it has been postulated that NEB function as hypoxia-sensitive airway chemoreceptors responding to hypoxic stimuli by releasing their amine content. We recently obtained direct support for this transducer function following the demonstration that the outward K^+ current in cultured NEB was suppressed by acute exposure to hypoxia (Youngson et al, 1993). Presented here is a description of the membrane properties of NEB cells and a consideration of the similarities they share with arterial chemoreceptors, that is the carotid body (CB) glomus cells.

METHODS

Rabbit NEB cultures were prepared from the lungs of late gestational fetal rabbit. The cell dissociation procedure for culturing NEB cells, whole-cell recording and data analysis were as described previously (Youngson et al, 1993). The composition of the standard extracellular bathing solution was (mM): 140 NaCl, 3 KCl, 1.5 $CaCl_2$, 1 $MgCl_2$, 5 glucose, 10 HEPES. The composition of the intracellular pipette solution was (mM): 140 KCl, 1 $CaCl_2$, 10 EGTA, 10 HEPES, 4 ATP. To block the inward Ca^{2+} current, the Ca^{2+} in the external bathing solution was replaced by Co^{2+}. For application of hypoxic stimulus, N_2 was bubbled continuously for 20-40 minutes into a closed reservoir containing extracellular solution which was then used to perfuse the cultures (PO_2: 25-30 mmHg).

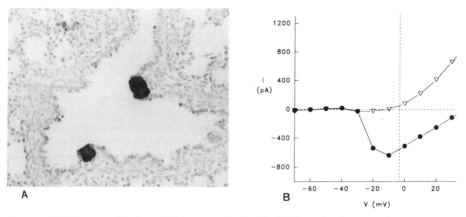

Figure 1. (A) Low magnification of 26 day gestational fetal rabbit lung showing several NEB positively immunostained with an antibody against 5-HT (x300). (B) I-V relation for a cultured NEB cell. Voltage clamp currents were measured from a holding potential of -60 mV to various test potentials. The outward (triangles) and inward (circles) currents were activated between -20 and -30 mV.

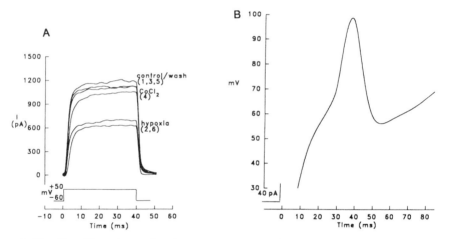

Figure 2. The effect of hypoxia on cultured NEB cell and the contribution the calcium-activated K+ current makes to the hypoxic response. (A) K+ currents were recorded by voltage steps to +50 mV from a holding potential of -60 mV. The same cell was cycled between normoxic (PO_2: 150 mmHg), hypoxic (PO_2: 25-30 mmHg) and normoxic stimuli (1,2,3) followed by Co^{2+} replacing Ca^{2+} in the extracellular bathing medium (4), and finally an additional normoxic and hypoxic stimulus (5,6). (B) Current clamp recording from NEB cell. Action potentials (approximately 100 mV) were elicited when a 5 ms depolarizing current was applied to cell.

RESULTS

Under voltage clamp, depolarizing voltage steps from a holding potential of -60 mV activated both fast transient inward and prolonged outward current in NEB cells. The I-V relation (Fig.1B) shows that both inward (solid circles) and outward (open triangles) currents were activated around -30 mV. We showed previously, using conventional channel blockers, that the inward current in NEB consists largely of a transient Na^+ and a prolonged Ca^{2+} components whereas the outward current is carried by K^+ ions (Youngson et al, 1993). To test whether NEB cells were sensitive to hypoxia, we first recorded whole cell currents using a normoxic perfusate and then switched to a hypoxic one. Hypoxia reversibly suppressed the outward K^+ current by 25-30% (n=12): an example is illustrated in Fig 2A. where the same cell was cycled through normoxic and hypoxic stimuli.

The possible contribution of the Ca^{2+}-activated K^+ current to the hypoxia-sensitive component of the K^+ current (Peers, 1990) was investigated with the use of extracellular Co^{2+} to block the Ca^{2+}-activated K^+ current. Substitution of extracellular Ca^{2+} by Co^{2+} resulted in a less than 10% suppression in total K^+ current, suggesting a relatively small contribution of Ca^{2+}-activated K^+ current to the overall K^+ current in these cells. Yet, following a subsequent hypoxic stimulus, a large (30%) reversible suppression of K^+ current occurred. Taken together these data do not support the view that the effect of hypoxia is mediated solely by the Ca^{2+}-activated K^+ current. The effect of hypoxia on the K^+ current was unique as neither the Na^+ current nor the Ca^{2+} current were effected.

Under current clamp mode, action potentials were elicited when a depolarizing stimulus was applied to NEB cells. The mean amplitude of action potentials was 132.3 $\pm$ 10 mV (mean $\pm$ SEM; n=8) (Fig. 2B). We have previously shown that the action potential frequency and the slope of the pacemaker potential in NEB cells were increased by hypoxia (Youngson et al, 1993) as previously reported in rabbit glomus cells (Lopez-Lopez et al, 1989).

DISCUSSION

The purpose of the study was to define further the membrane properties of pulmonary NEB and their membrane response to hypoxia. These studies show that NEB cells have excitable properties and display voltage-activated currents typical of neuroendocrine cells. In addition, they contain an O_2-sensitive K^+ current similar to that described in glomus cells of the CB (Lopez-Barneo, 1989). Thus, this membrane property may well be a basic property of O_2-chemoreceptors regardless of their location (pulmonary airway or arterial blood).

The function of NEB as hypoxia-sensitive airway chemoreceptors may be to act as an auxiliary chemoreceptor during the perinatal when arterial chemoreceptors are resetting. In support of this is the relative abundance of NEB during this developmental period. In addition, many fetal rabbit NEB are able to elicit all-or-nothing action potentials in contrast to fetal rabbit glomus cells which appear to lack inward Na^+ current electrical excitability (Hescheler et al, 1989). Thus it is conceivable that in the late fetal period, the airway chemoreceptors (NEB cells) display a broader sensitivity for PO_2 than arterial chemoreceptors.

REFERENCES

Cutz, E., Spiers, V., Yeger, H., Newman, C., Wang, D. & Perrin, D.G. (1993). Cell biology of pulmonary neuroepithelial bodies - validation of an in vitro model. Anat. Rec. 236:4-52.

Hescheler, J., Delpiano, M.A., Acker, H. & Pietruschka, F. (1989). Ionic currents on type-1 cells of the rabbit carotid body measured by voltage-clamp experiments and the effect of hypoxia. Brain Res. 486:79-88.

Lauweryns, J.M., Cokelaere, M., Deleersynder, M. & Liebens, (1977). Intrapulmonary neuroepithelial bodies in newborn rabbits: influence of hypoxia, hyperoxia, hypercapnia, nicotine, reserpine, L-DOPA and 5-HTP. Cell Tiss. Res. 182:425-440.

Lauweryns, J.M. & Cokelaere, M. (1973). Intrapulmonary neuro-epithelial bodies: hypoxia-sensitive neuro (chemo-) receptors. Experientia 29:1384-1386.

Lopez-Barneo, J., Lopez-Lopez, J.R., Urea, J. & Gonzalez, C. (1988). Chemotransduction in the carotid body: K^+ current modulated by PO_2 in type I chemoreceptor cells. Science 241:580-582.

Lopez-Lopez, J., Gonzalez, C., Urena, J. & Lopez-Barneo, J. (1989). Low PO_2 selectively inhibits K^+ channel activity in chemoreceptor cells of the mammalian carotid body. J. Gen. Physiol. 93:1011-1015.

Peers, C. (1990). Hypoxic supression of K^+ current in type 1 carotid body cells: selective effect on the Ca^{2+}-activated K^+ current. Neurosci. Lett. 119:253-256.

Youngson, C., Nurse, C., Yeger, H., & Cutz, E. (1993). Oxygen sensing in airway chemoreceptors: demonstration of hypoxia-sensitive K^+ current and O_2 sensor protein. Nature (Lond) 365:153-155.

IONIC CURRENTS ON ENDOTHELIAL CELLS OF RAT BRAIN CAPILLARIES

Marco. A. Delpiano

Max-Planck-Institut für molekulare Physiologie, Rheinlanddamm 201,
44139 Dortmund, Germany

INTRODUCTION

It is generally accepted that endothelial cells lining the inner surface of the vascular tree release vasoactive substances in response to low critical values of the arterial oxygen partial pressure. Although much is known about the electrical membrane properties of endothelial cells (Revest & Abbott, 1992) less is known about the intimate transduction mechanism which initiates O_2-chemoreception. Ionic currents of endothelial cells from rat brain capillaries were studied in voltage-clamp experiments to find out whether the response to hypoxia could be also related to changes in the membrane conductance as known on carotid body type-I cells (Lopez-Barneo et al., 1988; Hescheler et al., 1989). Here, it is shown that endothelial cells from rat brain capillaries contain PO_2-modulated K^+ channels.

MATERIALS AND METHODS

Transmembrane currents were characterized by patch-clamp experiments on endothelial cells isolated from rat brain capillaries and cloned by Pietruschka et al. (1990). Cells were superfused in a small chamber (400 µl) with an extracellular solution (E1) consisting of (in mM): NaCl 135, KCl 5.6, $CaCl_2$ 2.5, $MgCl_2$ 1.2, glucose 5.5, HEPES 10, adjusted with NaOH and sucrose to pH=7.4 and 300 mOsm respectively. Borosilicate pipettes were used with a resistance of 2-5 MΩ when filled with an intracellular solution (P1) consisting of (in mM): K^+-aspartate 80, KCl 50, EGTA 10, $MgCl_2$ 1.2, N_2ATP 1.5, HEPES 10, adjusted to pH=7.2 and 290 mOsm respectively. Voltage stimulation and current control were performed as previously reported (Hescheler et al., 1989).

RESULTS AND DISCUSSION

Outward and Inward Currents

Membrane currents elicited by 10 mV test pulses from a holding potential of -60 mV to various membrane potentials are shown in Fig. 1A. The superimposed currents show large outward and small inward components. The outward traces exhibit delayed activation while inward traces activate and inactivate much faster. Plotting outward and inward currents

Arterial Chemoreceptors: Cell to System
Edited by R. O'Regan *et al*, Plenum Press, New York, 1994

versus test pulses revealed their current-voltage (I-V) properties (Fig. 1B). The I-V curve for outward currents shows positive to -30 mV (filled triangle) a clear outward rectification. These currents were blocked by external TEA (5 mM) or internal Cs^+ (5 mM) and their equilibrium potential showed dependence on $[K^+]_o$. Therefore, they are mediated by voltage-gated K^+ channels. They seem to be modulated also by internal Ca^{2+} and ATP as their conductance is depressed by Ca^{2+} blockers and sulphonylurea derivatives (Fig. 2A). The inward currents (filled circle) exhibit a clear U-shaped I-V relationship with a maximum of 80 pA at about -12 mV. They are carried by Ca^{2+} ions through low and high voltage-gated channels (Delpiano & Cavalis, 1993). These cells did not express Na^+ currents as assumed previously (Delpiano, 1992). Low voltage-gated Ca^{2+} currents have a peak maximum of about -40 pA at -25 mV and were neither affected by antagonists nor agonists of the dihydropyridine derivatives but blocked by amiloride (50 μM) and Ni^{2+} (40 μM) (Delpiano & Cavalis, 1993).

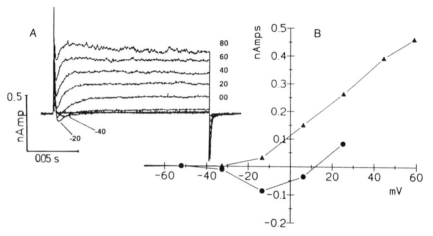

Figure 1. Current traces and I-V curve obtained from voltage-clamp experiments on endothelial cells. In (A) outward currents from 0 to 80 mV and inward currents at -20 and -40 mV test potentials are shown. In (B) the respective I-V relationship for outward (triangle) and inward (circle) currents can be seen.
Effect of hypoxia and NaCN

To examine the effect of hypoxia, cells clamped at -60 mV were continuously stimulated with a ramp pulse from -120 to 90 mV at a rate of 0.25 Hz. When the PO_2 was decreased from 300 to 20 Torr the amplitude of the outward K^+ current increased reversibly in 60 % of all experiments (Fig. 2A). The input resistance was also affected as shown in the slope increase of the ohmic components (Fig. 2A, left to 0.5 s). Probably this decrease in membrane resistance could be related to volume changes of the cell as suggested in cardiac cells (Tareen et al., 1991). In 30% of the cells hypoxia reduced K^+ conductance as reported in type-I cell (Lopez-Barneo, 1988; Hescheler et al., 1989) and recently in other PO_2-sensing cells (Post et al., 1993, Youngson et al., 1993). Cells exposed to NaCN (1 mM) show similar changes in K^+ conductance as hypoxia (Fig. 2B). In type-I cells cyanide enhances the K^+ conductance, reduces Ca^{2+} currents and hyperpolarizes cells (Biscoe & Duchen, 1989;

Hescheler et al., 1989). These changes have been ascribed to cyanide-induced intracellular Ca^{2+} release. This release has been proposed to be the initial sensing step in O_2-chemotransduction (Biscoe & Duchen, 1990). Albeit both hypoxia and cyanide may act upon same metabolic processes the resulting response may not necessarily be achieved through same pathways. In type-I cells hypoxia decreases K^+ currents while cyanide increases it. In endothelial cells more probably changes in intracellular ATP could involved rather than release in Ca^{2+}, since hypoxia in presence of Ca^{2+} blockers still changed K^+ conductance but not when of tolbutamide or glibenclamide were present.

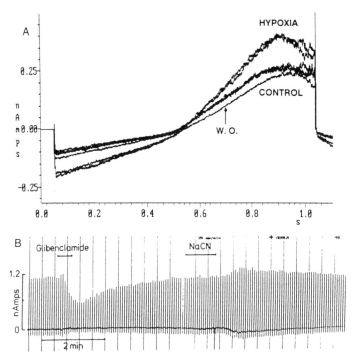

Figure 2. Effect of hypoxia, cyanide and glibenclamide on outward currents produced with repetitive ramp pulses at a holding potential of -60 mV. In (A) stationary currents starting at -120 mV (0.025 s) and ending at 90 mV (1.15 s) show the reversible effect of hypoxia. Note washing out (w.o.) after restoring control PO_2. In (B) the chart recording illustrates the effect of 0.2 mM glibenclamide and 1 mM NaCN on outward currents.

CONCLUSION

1. Endothelial cells of rat brain capillaries possess outward currents sensitive to hypoxia and cyanide.
2. Three different K^+ channels seem to be present: voltage-gated, Ca^{2+}-dependent and ATP-dependent.
3. Cells contain low and high voltage-gated Ca^{2+} channels but do not express Na^+ channels.

REFERENCES

Acker, H., Pietruschka, F. & Deutscher, J. (1990). Endothelial cell mitogen released from HT29 tumour cells grown in monolayer or multicellular spheroid culture. Br. J. Cancer 62:376-377.

Biscoe, T.J. & Duchen, M.R. (1989). Electrophysiological responses of dissociated type-I cells of the rabbit carotid body to cyanide. J. Physiol. (Lond.) 413:447-468.

Biscoe, J.T. & Duchen, M.R. (1990). Cellular basis of transduction in carotid chemoreceptors. Am. J. Physiol. 258:L271-L278.

Delpiano, M.A. (1992). Do endothelial cells contain similar PO_2-regulated channels as found in carotid body type-I cells?. Eur. J. Neurosci. (Suppl.) 5:64.

Delpiano, M.A. & Cavalis, A. (1993). Evidence for low voltage-activated calcium channels on endothelial cells from rat brain capillaries. Eur. J. Neurosci. (Suppl.) 6:85.

Hescheler, J., Delpiano, M.A., Acker, H. & Pietruschka, F. (1989). Ionic currents on type-I cells of the rabbit carotid body measured by voltage-clamp experiments and the effect of hypoxia. Brain. Res. 486:79-88.

Lopez-Barneo, J., Lopez-Lopez, J.R., Urena, J. & Gonzalez, C. (1988). Chemotransduction in the carotid body: K^+ current modulated by Po_2 in type I chemoreceptor cells. Science 241:580-582.

Post, J.M., Hume, J.R., Archer, S.L. & Weir, E.K. (1992). Direct role for potassium channel inhibition in hypoxic pulmonary vasoconstriction. Am. J. Physiol. 262:C882-C890.

Revest, P.A. & Abott, N.J. (1992) Membrane ion channels of endothelial cells. TIPS 13:404-407.

Tareen, F.M., Ono, K., Noma, A. & Ehara, T. (1991). α-adrenergic and muscarinic regulation of the chloride current in guinea-pig ventricular cells. J.Physiol. (Lond.) 440:225-241.

Youngson, C., Nurse, C., Yeger,H. & Cutz, E. (1993). Characterization of membrane currents in pulmonary neuroepithelial bodies-hypoxia-sensitive airway chemoreceptors. Nature 365: 153-155.

UROKINASE AND ITS RECEPTOR: MARKERS OF MALIGNANCY?

Patrick J Gaffney[1], David A Cooke[2] and Kevin G Burnand[2]

[1]Division of Haematology, National Institute for Biological Standards and Control, Potters Bar, Hertfordshire, EN6 3QG, UK.
[2]Department of Surgery, St Thomas' Hospital, London, SW1, UK

INTRODUCTION

For many years it has been known that abnormal coagulation and fibrinolytic activity existed in the environs of malignant tumours. Whether these activities affected the invasiveness and metastatic activity of tumours has been in question for some time. The advent of precise assays for individual components of both coagulation and fibrinolysis has allowed a more precise analysis of the individual components of those systems which seem relevant to malignancy. While this report may not seem to fit ideally into an international meeting on Arterial Chemoreception it is felt that a wider perspective on receptors in disease may not go amiss. Thus we present herein a brief overview on the role of one component of the human fibrinolytic system, urinary-type plasminogen activator, uPA (also known as urokinase in the UK) and its receptor, called uPA receptor (e.g. u-PAR) in human malignancy. A brief comment is also given on a role for tissue plasminogen activator (tPA) in malignancy.

FIBRINOLYSIS AND BREAST TUMOURS

While ovarian tumours were first demonstrated to specifically release uPA (Astedt & Holmberg, 1976) the finding (Gelister et al., 1986) that malignant colorectal tumours preferentially contain uPA rather than its companion plasminogen activator called, tissue plasminogen activator (tPA), stimulated work on breast tumours by a number of groups. These workers demonstrated a preponderance of uPA rather than tPA in malignant breast tumours (Layer et al., 1987; Evers et al., 1982; inter alia). Disease free interval following surgery for breast cancer was shown to be inversely related to urokinase level in the primary tumour (Janieke et al., 1989). Fig 1 shows in a step graph manner that mortality in a group (n = 50) of women following mastectomy/lumpectomy correlated directly with urokinase and inversely with tPA levels in the primary tumour. It is evident, in agreement with the data of Janieke and colleagues (1989), that high levels of uPA in the primary tumour yielded poor disease free interval and high mortality while levels of tPA suggested the reverse. These and other data in a variety of malignant tissues (for review see Duffy, 1993) has led to a consensus that high levels of uPA in the primary tumour indicated a poor prognosis for the patient.

The identification (Vassalli et al., 1985) of a receptor for uPA, denoted urokinase receptor (u-PAR) having a high density in malignant cells and capable of binding both single and two chain urokinase (Cubellis et al., 1986) has led to considerable interest in the interaction of the urokinase with its receptor and the development of fibrinolytic activity on the surface of malignant cells. The u-PAR has been purified and cloned (Behrendt et al., 1990; Rolden et al., 1990). While it seems that uPA itself may be a valuable prognostic marker for the outcome of breast cancer (Duffy, 1983) it seems also to be an indication of patient prognosis in lung (Oka et al., 1991), bladder (Hasui et al., 1992) and colonic (Ganesh et al., 1992) cancers. Thus uPA may be a prognostic marker for solid cancers in general.

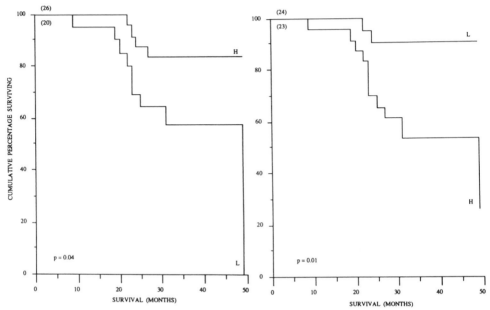

Figure 1 Left side: survival step graphs of patients grouped by high (H) and low (L) tPA activity (above and below 1.0 iu/mg tissue respectively) in homogenates of malignant human breast tissue. Right side: survival step graphs of the same patient group according to high (H) and low (L) uPA activity (above and below 0.25 iu/mg tissue respectively).

UROKINASE ITS RECEPTOR AND MALIGNANCY. A HYPOTHESIS

The question arises concerning the role which urokinase and its receptors may be playing in tumour invasion and metastasis. The major biological activity of urokinase is its ability to activate plasminogen to plasmin, which is a broad-spectrum hydrolytic enzyme capable of degrading a number of basement membrane proteins. Plow et al. (1986) have demonstrated that many cells bind plasminogen and insinuate a receptor for plasminogen on a number of the transformed and malignant cells examined. While urokinase is secreted from cells as its single chain inactive precursor called single chain urinary-type plasminogen activator (SCuPA) it has been shown that SCuPA when bound to the cell surface via its receptor (u-PAR) can directly activate plasminogen (Ellis et al., 1989). Thus, as shown in the speculative diagram in Fig 2, cells rich in bound SCuPA and plasminogen can generate plasmin which should degrade various components of basement membrane (lamirin, fibronectin etc.) and also activate metalloproteases (Tryggvason et al., 1987) which are known to be involved in tumour invasiveness. Whether urokinase is related to metastasis is a matter of controversy. The clinical data shown in Fig 1 suggests that disease-free interval depends inversely on urokinase in the primary tumours while there is also evidence that tumours which secrete high levels of tissue plasminogen activator (tPA) are directly related to a lack of metastasis leading to a good patient prognosis. However most workers believe (see review by Duffy, 1993) that high uPA enhances metastasis, this data depending on work with uPA specific antibodies and transfecting poorly metastatic cells with the uPA gene. In part of Fig 2 we suggest that high tPA secreting cells may digest the fibrin-platelet network which surround cells during the metastatic journey from one organ to another via the blood stream. Gorelik (1992) has demonstrated that this fibrin network enhances metastasis. Thus high levels of uPA in the primary tumour may be a major influence on tissue invasion while tPA levels secreted by the malignant cell may inhibit the metastatic phenomenon. A number of the very elegant experiments conducted on uPA gene transfection of cells ignored the effect on tPA secretion of the same cell lines (Yu & Schultz, 1990). Thus the complete plasminogen activator profile of the primary tumour cell may be necessary to fully understand the combined invasive and metastatic phenomena. It is interesting to note that a poor prognosis in breast cancer is not alone related to high uPA levels but also to low tPA levels (Fig 1). It is suggested here that future transfection experiments of low metastatic cells should include not only the uPA gene but also the tPA gene.

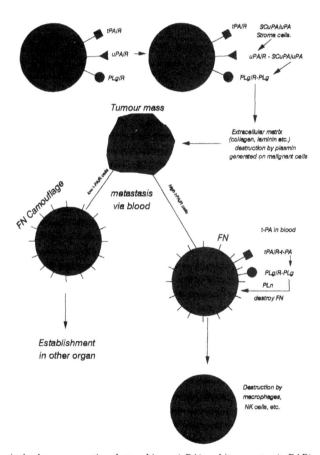

Figure 2 Hypothetical scheme suggesting that urokinase (uPA) and its receptor (u-PAR) play a part in tumour invasiveness and growth by generating plasmin from cell bound plasminogen. It also shows that tPA/plasminogen and their respective receptors (tPA/R and Plg/R) may inhibit metastasis via the fibrin-dependent fibrinolytic pathway which destroys the fibrin/platelet protective layer on malignant cells ensuring their destruction in the circulation.

Regardless of the outcome of such experiments it is clear that uPA is a valuable prospective marker in breast cancer and indeed in a variety of other solid tumours. Assay of this protease may become routine in order to select patients who would maximally benefit from further adjuvant chemotherapy. The suggestion in Fig 2 relating tPA-induced fibrinolysis to metastasis requires further validation and clarification. However the notion that relevant plasmin activity is located at invasive foci of malignant tumours conjures up therapeutic notions which relate to plasmin quenching with targeted plasmin inhibitors. Such experiments in a suitable animal model may yield valuable therapeutic interventions in human malignancy, especially in the case of inoperable tumours.

REFERENCES

Astedt, B. & Holmberg, L. (1976). Immunological identity of urokinase and ovarian carcinoma plasminogen activator released in tissue culture. Nature 261: 595-597.

Behrendt, N., Ronne, E., Ploug, M. et al. (1990). The human receptor for urokinase plasminogen activator. NH_2 terminal amino acid sequence and glycosylation variants. J. Biol. Chem. 265: 6453-6460.

Cubellis, M. V., Nolli, M. L., Cassani, G. & Blasi, F. (1986). Binding of single chain prourokinase to the urokinase receptor of human U937 cells. J. Biol. Chem. 261: 15819-15822.

Duffy, M. J. (1993). Urokinase-type plasminogen activator and malignancy - Review. Fibrinolysis 7: 295-302.

Ellis, V., Scully, M. F. & Kakkar, V. V. (1989). Plasminogen activator initiated by single-chain urokinase-type plasminogen activator. Potentiation by U937 monocytes. J. Biol. Chem. 264: 2185-2188.

Evers, J. L., Patel, J., Madeja, J. et al. (1982). Plasminogen activator activity composition in human breast cancer. Cancer Res. 42: 219-226.

Ganesh, S., Verspaget, H., Sier, C. et al. (1992). Prognostic relevance of mucosal plasminogen activator levels in colorectal cancer. Fibrinolysis 6: (Suppl. 2), 103.

Gelister, J., Mahmoud, M., Lewin, M. R., Gaffney, P. J. & Boulos, P. B. (1986). Plasminogen activators in human colorectal neoplasms. Br. Med. J. 293: 728-731.

Gorelik, E. (1992). Protective effect of fibrin on tumour metastasis. Fibrinolysis 6: (Suppl. 1), 35-38.

Hasui, Y., Marutsuka, K., Suzumiya, J. et al. (1992). The content of urokinase-type plasminogen activator as a prognostic factor in urinary bladder cancer. Int. J. Cancer 50: 871-873.

Janicke, F., Schmitt, M., Ulm, K., Gossner, W. & Graeff, H. (1989). Urokinase-type plasminogen activator antigen and early relapse in breast cancer. Lancet ii: 1049.

Layer, G. T., Cederholm-Williams, S. A., Gaffney, P. J. et al. (1987). Urokinase - the enzyme responsible for invasion and metastasis in human breast carcinoma. Fibrinolysis 1: 237-240.

Oka, T., Ishida, T., Nishino, T. & Sugimachi, K. (1991). Immunohistochemical evidence of urokinase-type plasminogen activator in primary and metastatic tumours of pulmonary adenocarcinoma. Cancer Res. 51: 3522-3525.

Plow, E. F., Freaney, D. E., Plescia, J. & Miles, L. A. (1986). The plasminogen system and cell surfaces: evidence for plasminogen and urokinase receptors on the same cell type. J. Cell Biol. 103: 2411-2420.

Roldan, A. L., Cubellis, M. V., Masucci, M. T. et al. (1990). Cloning and expression of the receptor for human urokinase plasminogen activator, a central molecule in cell surface, plasmin-dependent proteolysis. EMBO J. 9: 467-474.

Tryggvason, K., Hoyhtya, M. & Salo, T. (1987). Proteolytic degradation of extracellular matrix in tumour invasion. Biochim. Biophys. Acta 907: 191-217.

Vassali, J.-D., Baccino, D. & Berlin, D. (1985). A cellular binding site for the Mr 55,000 form of the human plasminogen activator, urokinase. J. Cell Biol. 100: 86-92.

Yu, H. & Schultz, R. M. (1990). Relationship between secreted urokinase plasminogen activator activity and metastatic potential in murine B16 cells transfected with human urokinase sense and artisense genes. Cancer Res. 50: 7623-7633.

ELECTROCHEMICAL MEASUREMENT OF RAPID DOPAMINE RELEASE IN PERFUSED CAT CAROTID BODY DURING ONSET OF HYPOXIA

Donald G. Buerk[1] and Sukhamay Lahiri[2]

[1]Department of Ophthalmology, [2]Department of Physiology and the Institute for Environmental Medicine , University of Pennsylvania School of Medicine, Philadelphia, PA 19104, USA

INTRODUCTION

Evidence that dopamine (DA) may play a role in carotid body (CB) chemotransduction has been reviewed by Eyzaguirre and Zapata (1984). Gonzalez et al. (1992) recently reviewed current theories for O_2 and acid chemotransduction mechanisms. Using CBs incubated with radiolabelled tyrosine, it has been shown that hypoxia releases DA from a newly synthesized pool, and that its release is dependent on Ca^{2+} (Fidone et al., 1982; Gonzalez & Fidone, 1977; Rigual et al., 1991). Acidic conditions or elevated K^+ also cause DA release in superfused cat and rabbit CBs.

Radiolabelling techniques have been useful for characterizing DA release from the CB. However, they are too slow to follow the time course of rapid DA release kinetics with different stimuli. Recent advances in electrochemical methods for measuring DA and other catecholamines have been made, which can provide more spatially detailed and more rapid time resolved measurements. For example, Donnelly (1993) recently reported measurements of catecholamine release from a superfused rat CB preparation using a carbon fiber microelectrode. In the present study, DA was measured in perfused cat CBs with shallowly recessed gold microsensors coated with a thin film of electroconductive Nafion polymer. Dopamine currents increased immediately with the onset of hypoxia and were correlated with increases in chemosensory nerve discharge.

METHODS

Metal-filled glass microelectrodes were constructed with shallow recesses (< 5 μm) and small tips (< 5 μm), modifying the PO_2 microelectrode design of Whalen et al. (1967). Gold cathodes were plated, then coated with a thin (< 1 μm) Nafion membrane by dipping in a solution of Nafion dissolved in propyl alcohol. DA was detected electrochemically by amperometry at $+150$ mV, similar to the DA oxidation potential found with a carbon fiber microelectrode by Donnelly (1993). Calibrations were performed in deoxygenated isotonic saline by sequentially adding DA to a recirculating system. Linear calibration curves were obtained. Sensitivities ranged between 0.2 to 0.65 picoampere per μM of DA for microsensors with tips between 5 to 8 μm.

Cat CBs were perfused in Tyrode (21% O_2, PCO_2 38 Torr, HCO_3^- 21.4 mM, pH 7.4 at 37 °C) using experimental methods described by Iturriaga et al. (1991). Neural discharge (ND) was measured from the carotid sinus nerve with bipolar platinum electrodes, using electronics for counting impulses each second. After inserting the DA microsensor approximately 200 μm deep into the CB, a hypoxic stimulus was produced either by interrupting perfusate flow (stop flow technique) or by switching to a low PO_2 (< 40 Torr) equilibrated Tyrode solution. Dopamine currents and ND were tape recorded, then digitized and analyzed by computer.

RESULTS

Examples for a flow interruption and a hypoxic perfusion experiment are shown in Fig.

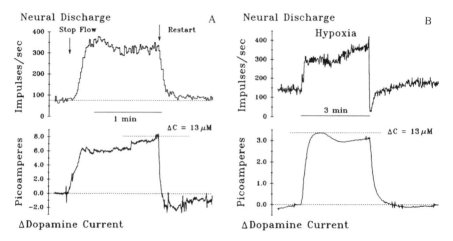

Figure. 1. A: Increases in neural discharge (top) and dopamine current (bottom) during flow interruption. B: Increases in neural discharge (top) and change in dopamine current (bottom) during hypoxic perfusion.

1. As shown in Fig. 1A, there was a rapid component of DA release observed within the first 10 to 20 sec after flow interruption. The mean rate was 0.71 ± 0.11 (SE) μM/sec (19 measurements, 8 cat CBs). This rapid component of DA release either preceded or occurred along with increases in ND. After the initial rapid release, DA increased more slowly, with a mean of 0.16 ± 0.02 μM/sec, reaching a maximum of 20.1 ± 2.5 μM after 90 sec. We did not see any appreciable decline in the rate or magnitude of DA release responses to repeated flow interruption measurements over a time course of 1 to 2 hours.

As shown in Fig. 1B, rapid DA release was also observed during hypoxic perfusion. The DA release was sustained during the hypoxic stimulus. Some variation in the maximum DA level was seen, probably due to changes in flow with prolonged hypoxia. Usually, the maximum DA levels were smaller than measured during flow interruption. Chemostimulation by nicotine did not cause any measurable DA release.

DISCUSSION

Changes in DA could be detected in CB tissue using recessed, thin-film Nafion coated DA microsensors with excellent temporal resolution and with accuracy in nM ranges. We found that the magnitude of DA release in the cat CB was over 10 times greater than reported for rat CB by Donnelly (1993). The time course of DA release measured in our cat CB experiments was much faster than in rat CB, where peak DA release with hypoxia was reported to occur 30 seconds or more after the maximum ND response (Donnelly, 1993). In our cat CB experiments, the very rapid kinetics of DA release which preceded or closely paralleled rapid increases in neural discharge are more consistent with the suspected neurotransmitter role for DA. Since we found that nicotine excited the cat CB without DA release, other neurotransmitters are also involved. Our electrochemical detection technique can be used to quantify the coupling between CB tissue hypoxia and DA release, or to study whether DA release occurs with other chemostimulants.

Supported by NSF award BCS 91-96021 and HL-43413-04 from NIH.

REFERENCES

Donnelly, D.F. (1993) Electrochemical detection of catecholamine release from rat carotid body in vitro. J. Appl. Physiol. 74:2330-2337.

Eyzaguirre, C., & P. Zapata.(1984) Perspectives in carotid body research. J. Appl. Physiol. 57:931-957.

Fidone, S., C. Gonzalez, & K. Yoshizaki. (1982) Effects of low oxygen on the release of dopamine from the rabbit carotid body in vitro. J. Physiol. (London) 333:93-110.

Gonzalez, C. & S. Fidone. (1977) Increased release of ^{3}H-dopamine during low O_2 stimulation of rabbit carotid body in vitro. Neurosci. Lett. 6:95-99.

Gonzalez, C., L. Almaraz, A. Obeso, and R. Rigual. (1992) Oxygen and acid chemoreception in the carotid body chemoreceptors. Trends in Neurosci. 15:146-153.

Iturriaga, R., W.L. Rumsey, A. Mokashi, D. Spergel, D.F. Wilson, & S. Lahiri. (1991) In vitro perfused-superfused cat carotid body for physiological and pharmacological studies. J. Appl. Physiol. 70:1393-1400.

Rigual, R., J.R. López-López, & C. Gonzalez. (1991) Release of dopamine and chemoreceptor discharge induced by low pH and high PCO_2 stimulation of the cat carotid body. J. Physiol. (London) 433:519-531.

Whalen, W.J., J. Riley, & P. Nair. (1967) A microelectrode for measuring intracellular PO_2. J. Appl. Physiol. 23:798-801.

HYPOXIA-INDUCED CATECHOLAMINE RELEASE FROM RAT CAROTID BODY, IN VITRO, DURING MATURATION AND FOLLOWING CHRONIC HYPOXIA

David F. Donnelly[1] and Thomas P. Doyle[2]

Department of Pediatrics, [1]Section of Respiratory Medicine and [2]Section of Cardiology, Yale University School of Medicine, New Haven, CT, 06510, USA

INTRODUCTION

Although it is well established that peripheral chemosensitivity is reduced in the newborn period compared to the adult, the reason for the reduced sensitivity is unclear. Two speculations are that low sensitivity is due to: 1) high tonic catecholamine secretion (Hertzberg et al., 1990), and 2) low secretory response to hypoxia (Donnelly 1993). To begin to address these speculations we measured free tissue catecholamine levels at different ages and, in adults, following chronic hypoxia in rat carotid bodies, *in vitro*, using Nafion-coated, carbon fiber microelectrodes.

METHODS

Carotid bodies and a portion of the sinus nerves were harvested from anesthetized rats of 4 age groups: 1d (n=6), 2d (n=6), 6d (n=5), and 20-30d (n=11). The tissue was placed in a dilute collagenase solution for removal of connective tissue and then superfused in a perfusion chamber (HEPES-buffered saline, 33-34°C, 2.5ml/min). PO_2 was monitored by a membrane-covered, platinum wire electrode. Single unit, sinus nerve recordings were obtained using a suction electrode applied to the cut peripheral end of the sinus nerve (Kholwadwala & Donnelly, 1992). Catecholamine electrodes were fabricated from single 10µ carbon fibers insulated in glass pipettes and polarized to +160 mV. At the start of each run the electrode was advanced into the tissue and allowed to stabilize. The tissue catecholamine levels were measured during control, hypoxia (1min, $PO_2 \approx 0$ Torr, at nadir) and recovery. After each experimental run the electrode was calibrated in saline containing 0 and 2µM dopamine.

RESULTS

In 20-30d animals, advancement of the carbon fiber electrode into the tissue caused a large increase in electrode current, which settled to a steady-state in 2-3 min (2.59±0.35 µM, mean±SEM). During hypoxia catecholamine increased 14.8±1.6 µM, and single fiber nerve activity increased from 1.8±0.5 Hz to 14.5±1.2 Hz (Fig. 1a).

In young animals, both the nerve activities and catecholamine responses were significantly less than the adult (Fig. 1b). Resting catecholamine tissue levels were 0.58±0.09, 0.53±0.14 and 0.54±0.12 µM for 1, 2 and 6d rats, respectively. The hypoxia-induced increase peaked at 1.47±0.42, 2.60±0.51 and 4.46±0.88 µM (p<0.05 vs adult, t-test). Baseline nerve activity was 0.6±0.2, 0.5±0.2 and 0.8±0.3 Hz and increased to 4.5±0.6, 5.2±0.9 and 10.5±1.6 Hz for 1, 2 and 6d rats during hypoxia.

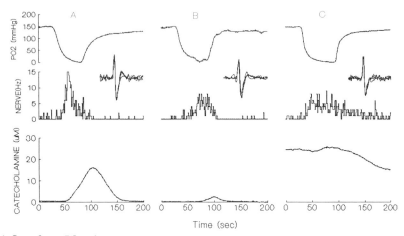

Figure 1. Superfusate PO_2, chemoreceptor nerve activity and tissue catecholamine levels as a function of time for 3 carotid bodies. (A) Response from a normal 21d rat. (B) Response from a normal 2d rat. (C) Response from a chronically hypoxic 22d rat. Inset: superimposed oscillographic sweeps.

For rats raised in a low oxygen environment (F_IO_2=0.09, n=9, 20-28d), chemoreceptor nerve activity and catecholamine levels were different than both normal adult and newborn rats (Fig. 1c). Baseline catecholamine levels were greatly elevated in chronically hypoxic rats (14.4±1.3 µM) and only increased slightly during hypoxia (15.6±2.2 µM)(Fig. 1c). Single fiber baseline nerve activity was not significantly different than that of adult rats raised in normoxia (2.7±1.2 Hz). During hypoxia, peak nerve activity increased by approximately 60% of normal to 8.2±4.3 Hz.

DISCUSSION

These results demonstrate that developmental changes occur in the regulation of carotid body free tissue catecholamine concentration. They complement previous results which argued for a close association between catecholamine release and changes in nerve activity (Donnelly 1993; Gonzalez & Fidone, 1977). The present work further extends this argument by showing an enhanced hypoxia-induced catecholamine release over the same time period during which nerve responsiveness is increasing due to maturation.

This conclusion is not consistent, however, with that reached by Hertzberg et al. (1990) who demonstrated that dopamine turnover rates were high after birth but decreased to adult levels by 6 hours of age. They suggested that the low hypoxia sensitivity at birth may be caused by a tonic, dopamine-induced inhibition. Although our data do not support this conclusion we have no datum to directly address the early developmental period (0-6 hours after birth). Nevertheless, developmental changes in hypoxia sensitivity occur well beyond 6 hours after birth (Eden & Hanson, 1987a; Kholwadwala & Donnelly, 1992) and it is this increase in activity which we find correlated to changes in catecholamine secretion.

In an attempt to better resolve this issue, experiments were conducted on carotid bodies of rats raised in a hypoxic environment. Chronic hypoxia impairs the maturation of chemosensitivity (Eden and Hanson, 1987b) and cause dopamine turnover to be enhanced well beyond 6 hours of age (Hertzberg et al., 1992). We found that basal catecholamine levels were greatly elevated in these carotid bodies and that the secretory response to hypoxia was less. The nerve response to hypoxia was diminished compared to controls, however not to the same degree observed in newborn rats. Despite the elevated baseline catecholamine levels, baseline nerve activity was unchanged, and this suggests that under some conditions nerve activity and catecholamine levels may be dissociated. The reason for this dissociation is obscure and its resolution awaits further study.

REFERENCES

Donnelly, D.F. (1993) Electrochemical detection of catecholamine release from rat carotid body, in vitro. J. Appl. Physiol. 74: 2330-2337.

Eden, G.J., & Hanson, M.A. (1987a) Maturation of the respiratory response to acute hypoxia in the newborn rat. J. Physiol. (London) 392: 1-9.

Eden, G.J., & Hanson, M.A. (1987b) Effects of chronic hypoxia from birth on the ventilatory response to acute hypoxia in the newborn rat. J. Physiol. (London) 392: 11-19.

Gonzalez, C., & Fidone, S. (1977) Increased release of ^{3}H-dopamine during low O_2 stimulation of rabbit carotid body in vitro. Neurosci. Lett. 6: 95-99.

Hertzberg, T., Hellstrom, S., Lagercrantz, H., & Pequignot, J.M. (1990) Development of the arterial chemoreflex and turnover of carotid body catecholamines in the newborn rat. J. Physiol. (London) 425: 211-225.

Hertzberg, T., Hellstrom, S., Holgert H., Lagercrantz, H., & Pequignot, J.M. (1992) Ventilatory response to hyperoxia in newborn rats born in hypoxia- possible relationship to carotid body dopamine. J. Physiol. (London) 456: 645-654.

Kholwadwala, D., & Donnelly, D.F. (1992) Maturation of carotid chemoreceptor sensitivity to hypoxia: in vitro studies in the newborn rat. J. Physiol. (London) 453: 461-473.

ASSESSMENT OF Na+ CHANNEL INVOLVEMENT IN THE RELEASE OF CATECHOLAMINES FROM CHEMORECEPTOR CELLS OF THE CAROTID BODY

A. Rocher, A. Obeso, B. Herreros and C. González.

Departamento de Bioquímica y Biología Molecular y Fisiología, Facultad de Medicina, Universidad de Valladolid, 47005 Valladolid, Spain

INTRODUCTION

Carotid body (CB) chemoreceptors are sensory receptors which are activated by decreases in P_aO_2 and pH (or increases in P_aCO_2) and thereby they initiate reflexes directed to maintain adequate O_2 levels and contribute to pH homeostasis. Type I cells of the CB are the primary chemoreceptor elements which release neurotransmitters (e.g. catecholamine; CA) upon stimulation. In this stimulus coupling process (i.e. chemotransduction) there are many aspects unsolved. Even when the presence of voltage-dependent ionic channels in chemoreceptor cells is well documented (Lopez-Barneo et al., 1988; Duchen et al., 1988) some models for the chemotransduction (Biscoe and Duchen 1990) do not incorporate a functional significance for tetrodotoxin (TTX)-sensitive Na^+ channels (but see Gonzalez et al., 1992). On the other hand, although dialysed cells generate Na^+-dependent action potentials (Lopez-Lopez et al., 1989), the appearance of spikes has never been reported in conventional intracellular recordings (see Gonzalez et al., 1992). To obviate the difficulties of the electrophysiological experiments, in the present work we have expanded our preliminary neurochemical study with veratridine (Rocher et al., 1988) and we have explored the effects of Na^+ channels blockage with TTX on the release of CA induced by hypoxia.

METHODS

Carotid bodies were isolated from adult rabbits (New Zealand white; 1.5-2.5 Kg) and incubated with [3,5-^{3}H]tyrosine (20 μM, 30 Ci/mmol) to label the CA stores. The CBs were transferred to precursor-free solution to wash out the precursor for 2 h. Thereafter, the solutions were renewed every 10 min and collected for analysis in [^{3}H]CA content. Test solution were intercalated as shown in RESULTS. The standard solution was a HEPES buffered Tyrode equilibrated with 100% O_2. In Na^+-free solutions NaCl was replaced by equimolar amounts of choline chloride. Results are expressed as cpm present in the samples, or as the evoked release by a test solution in relation to that obtained in basal conditions (see Obeso et al., 1992 for details).

RESULTS

The time course of the effect of veratridine (an alkaloid known to increase Na[+] permeability of excitable membranes) on the release of [³H]CA from the CB is shown in Fig. 1A. Incubation of CB with medium containing veratridine (50 µM) produced an increase in the [³H]CA output which reached a maximum after 10 to 15 min and then declined to a new level about three times basal release. The dose-response curve for veratridine has the appearance shown in Fig. 1B, which is similar to the reported effect of this drug in the adrenal medulla (Kirpekar & Prat, 1979).

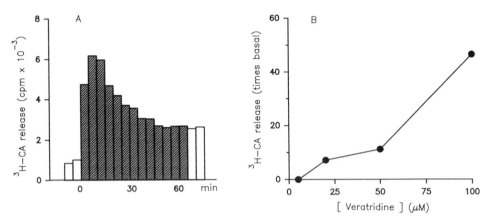

Figure 1. Effect of veratridine on the [³H]CA release from CB. (A) Time course of action of 50µM veratridine (hatched bars). (B) Dose-dependence of veratridine effect. Each point represent [³H]CA in a 10 min collection period.

The selectivity of the action of veratridine on Na[+] channels was assessed by testing for its Na[+] and Ca²[+] dependence and its sensitivity to TTX (Table I). The release of [³H]CA was inhibited by TTX by more than 98%, was absent in Na[+]-free solution and Ca²[+]-dependent by about 93%. The observed dependence on extracellular Na[+] and the inhibition by TTX demonstrates that the effect of veratridine on the CB is mediated by activation of voltage-dependent Na[+] channels in type I cells.

Table I. Na[+] and Ca²[+]-dependence of veratridine effect and inhibition by TTX of [³H]CA release induced by veratridine and hypoxia.

Incubating conditions	[³H]CA evoked release	% reduction
Veratridine	17.0 ± 0.9 [a]	--- ---
Veratridine + 1 µM TTX	0.3 ± 0.1 [a]	98
Veratridine, Na[+]-free	0.0[a]	100
Veratridine, Ca²[+]-free	1.4 ± 0.3 [a]	92
Hypoxia (10% O₂)	2.8 ± 0.5 [b]	----
Hypoxia (10% O₂) + 1 µM TTX	1.7 ± 0.3 [b]	40

[a] [³H]CA released during 20 min incubation with veratridine and [b] during 10 min incubation with 10% O₂. Data are expressed as times basal.

To investigate the contribution of Na^+ channels to the physiological response of type I cells to the hypoxic stimulus, we have studied the effect of TTX on the release of $[^3H]CA$ evoked by a mild hypoxic stimulus (Table I). Pairs of CBs were incubated for 10 min in mild hypoxic solution ($PO_2 \approx 70$ mm Hg) in the presence or absence of 1 μM TTX. Table I shows that TTX inhibited the release of $[^3H]CA$ induced by moderate hypoxia by 40%.

DISCUSSION

Taking into account that veratridine modifies Na^+ channels only in their open state (Barnes & Hille, 1988), our findings would suggest that type I cells in basal conditions exhibit spontaneous action potentials. This notion is reinforced by the fact that the time course, dose-, Na^+- and Ca^{2+}- dependence and sensitivity to TTX of the action of veratridine in the CB are similar to those described for adrenomedullary cells (Kirpekar & Prat, 1979) which are known to exhibit spontaneous action potentials (Kidokoro & Ritchie, 1980). This suggestion is further supported by the observation that dialysed type I cells from adult animals generate Na^+-dependent action potentials (Lopez-Lopez et al., 1989).

In the other hand, it is known that type I cells from neonatal animals lack TTX-sensitive Na^+ currents (Peers & Green, 1991) or have very small ones (Stea & Nurse, 1991), and yet they respond to hypoxia as it does the intact neonatal CB (Blanco et al., 1984). These facts may lend to suggest that Na^+ channels are not necessary for the hypoxic transduction. The data of the present work indicate that Na^+ channels provide some kind of amplification mechanism for the response elicited by mild hypoxia and allow the suggestion that the requirement of very intense hypoxia to activate neonatal CBs may be related to the absence of Na^+ channels in neonatal type I cells.

Work supported by DGICYT, grant PB92/0267.

REFERENCES

Barnes, S. & Hille, B. (1988) Veratridine modifies open sodium channels. J. Gen. Physiol. 91: 421-443.

Biscoe, T.J. & Duchen, M.R. (1990) Monitoring PO_2 by the carotid chemoreceptor. News in Physiol. Sci. 5: 229-233.

Blanco, C.E., Dawes, G.S., Hanson, M.A. & McCooke, H.B. (1984) The response to hypoxia of arterial chemoreceptors in fetal sheep and new-born lambs. J. Physiol.(Lond.) 351: 25-37.

Duchen, M.R., Caddy, K.W.T., Kirby, G.C., Patterson, D.L., Ponte, J. & Biscoe, T.J. (1988) Biophysical studies of the cellular elements of the rabbit carotid body. Neuroscience 26: 291-311.

Gonzalez, C., Almaraz, L., Obeso, A. & Rigual, R. (1992) Oxygen and acid chemoreception in the carotid body chemoreceptors. Trends in Neurosci. 15: 146-153.

Kidokoro, Y. & Ritchie, A. (1980) Chromaffin cell action potentials and their possible role in adrenaline secretion from rat adrenal medulla. J. Physiol. (Lond.) 307: 199-216.

Kirpekar, S.M. & Prat, J.C. (1979) Release of catecholamines from perfused cat adrenal gland by veratridine. Proc. Nat. Acad. Sci. USA 76: 2081-2083.

Lopez-Barneo, J., Lopez-Lopez, J.R., Ureña, J. & Gonzalez, C. (1988) Chemotransduction in the carotid body: K^+ current modulated by pO_2 in type I chemoreceptor cells. Science 241: 580-582.

Lopez-Lopez, J., Gonzalez, C., Ureña, J. & Lopez-Barneo, J. (1989) Low pO_2 selectively inhibits K^+ channel activity in chemoreceptor cells of the mammalian carotid body. J. Gen. Physiol. 93: 1001-1014.

Obeso, A., Rocher, A., Fidone, S. & Gonzalez, C. (1992) The role of dihydropyridine-sensitive Ca^{2+} channels in stimulus-evoked catecholamine release from chemoreceptor cells of the carotid body. Neuroscience 47: 463-472.

Peers, C. & Green, F.K. (1991) Inhibition of Ca^{2+}-activated K^+-currents by intracellular acidosis in isolated type I cells of the neonatal rat carotid body. J. Physiol.(Lond.) 437: 589-602.

Rocher, A., Obeso, A., Herreros, B. & Gonzalez, C. (1988) Activation of the release of dopamine in the carotid body by veratridine. Evidence for the presence of voltage-dependent Na^+ channels in type I cells. Neurosci. Lett. 94: 274-278.

Stea, A. & Nurse, C.A. (1991) Whole-cell and perforated-patch recordings from O_2-sensitive rat carotid body cells grown in short- and long-term culture. Pflug. Arch. 418: 93-101.

ACTIVATION OF GTP-BINDING PROTEINS BY ALUMINUM FLUORIDE MODULATES CATECHOLAMINE RELEASE IN THE RABBIT CAROTID BODY

M.T.G. Cachero, A. Rocher, R.J. Rigual and C. Gonzalez

Departamento de Bioquímica, Biología Molecular y Fisiología, Facultad de Medicina. Universidad de Valladolid. Valladolid, Spain

INTRODUCTION

The involvement of GTP-binding proteins (G proteins) in the regulation of stimulus-secretion coupling is extensively documented in a great number of preparations (Gomperts, 1990), and an important regulatory role for G proteins has been described in the transduction process of gustatory and olfactory chemoreceptors (Lancet, 1986; Bruch, 1990). However in the carotid body (CB) chemoreceptor cells, no attempts have been made to clarify the nature and the function of G proteins, although the involvement of second messenger systems in the release of catecholamines (CA) and in the chemoreceptor response (Pérez-García et al., 1991; Gómez-Niño et al., 1992) suggest a modulatory role for G proteins in the transduction-transmission processes in the arterial chemoreceptors.

A common feature of G proteins is their direct activation by fluoroaluminate (AlF_4^-) which is able to interact with the GDP located on the α-subunit of G proteins and by mimicking the γ-phosphate group of GTP, causes the dissociation of the α and $\beta\gamma$-subunits. It is accepted that the modification of a cell function by the AlF_4^- implies the participation of G proteins in the process (Gilman, 1987).

In the present paper we have explored the involvement of G proteins in the stimulus-secretion coupling process of the CB chemoreceptors by studying the effects of AlF_4^- on the release of CA.

METHODS

CBs were isolated from adult New Zealand rabbits. Protocols and analytical procedures to measure the release of CA by CB *in vitro* have been described (Perez-Garcia et al., 1991). In brief, the CA stores were labelled by incubating with ^{3}H-tyrosine, and CBs transferred to vials containing precursor-free solution (in mM: NaCl, 116; KCl, 5; $CaCl_2$, 2.2; $MgCl_2$, 1.1; HEPES, 10; glucose, 5; $NaHCO_3$, 24; equilibrated with 5% CO_2, 20% O_2 and 75% N_2, pH 7.40) for 2h to wash out the precursor; thereafter, the incubation solutions were collected every 10 minutes and their ^{3}H-CA content analyzed by adsorption into alumina. Positive identification was made by HPLC (Gonzalez-Guerrero et al., 1992), and dopamine (DA) plus DOPAC represented more than 90% of CA released. 20 μM AlCl$_3$ was added to all NaF containing solutions.

RESULTS

Fig. 1A shows a single experiment representative of a total of six in which one CB was incubated in a medium containing 10 mM NaF for 70 min. ^{3}H-CA release was increased by AlF$_4^-$. Part B of the figure represents the average of the ^{3}H-CA evoked release responses obtained from 6 CBs subjected to 50 min of incubation in a medium containing 5, 10, or 20 mM NaF. There is a dose-dependent effect of AlF$_4^-$ on ^{3}H-CA release.

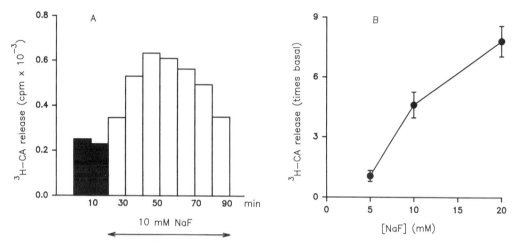

Figure 1. Effects of AlF$_4^-$ on ^{3}H-CA release by CB. A. Single experiment in which 10 mM NaF was applied as figure shows. B. Total ^{3}H-CA release evoked by 50 min of 5, 10 and 20 mM NaF treatment. Data are means ± S.E.M. from 8 CBs. 20 μM AlCl$_3$ was added to NaF solutions.

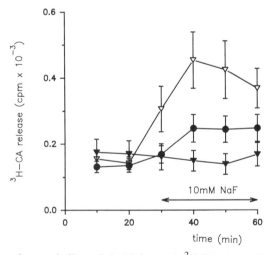

Figure 2. Calcium dependence and effects of nisoldipine on the ^{3}H-CA release elicited by AlF$_4^-$. CBs were incubated in: control solution (unfilled triangles), Ca^{2+}-free solution (filled triangles) or 1 μM nisoldipine (filled circles). 10 mM NaF was present in the medium during the last 40 min. Nisoldipine was added to the control solution 10 min prior to and during the application of 10 mM NaF. 20 μM AlCl$_3$ was added to NaF solutions. Data are means ± S.E.M. of 6 experiments.

Fig. 2 shows the ^{3}H-CA outflow from 6 CBs incubated for 40 min with 10 mM NaF in the presence of 2 mM CaCl$_2$ or in nominally Ca^{2+} free solution; in the last condition release of ^{3}H-CA induced by AlF$_4^-$ was almost abolished (> 95%). To explore the mechanisms involved in the secretory response evoked by AlF$_4^-$, 1 μM nisoldipine, a dihydropyridine antagonist of L-type voltage dependent Ca^{2+}-channels (L-type VOCCs), was applied 10 min prior to and during the AlF$_4^-$ application period. Fig. 2 also shows that nisoldipine inhibited (≈ 60%) the ^{3}H-CA release response evoked by 10 mM NaF.

DISCUSSION

Measurements of ^{3}H-CA outflow from the *in vitro* rabbit CB have been extensively used as an index of the chemoreceptor/secretory activity of the chemoreceptor cells (Fidone et al., 1990). AlF$_4^-$ is a general activator of G proteins (Gilman 1987). Consequently in the CB, the increase of CA release induced by AlF$_4^-$ implies that the mechanisms involved in the transduction-secretion process are controlled or modulated by G proteins.

The Ca$^{2+}_e$ dependence of the increase in ^{3}H-CA release induced by AlF$_4^-$ indicates that entry of Ca^{2+} is a relevant step in the activation sequence and suggest that intracellular Ca^{2+} stores do not contribute as a triggering mechanism in the secretory response induced by AlF$_4^-$. The sensitivity to nisoldipine suggests that L-type VOCCs are pathways for Ca^{2+} entry; direct activation or depolarization could be responsible of L-type VOCCs activation promoted by AlF$_4^-$. Other mechanisms for Ca^{2+} entry must not be excluded. Thus, in chromaffin cells AlF$_4^-$ activates Na$^+$/H$^+$ exchanger by stimulating phosphoinositide metabolism and activation of Na$^+$/H$^+$ exchanger drives the entry of Ca^{2+} through the Na$^+$/Ca^{2+} exchanger (Ito et al., 1991). Notice that activation of L-type VOCCs and the sequential activation of a Na$^+$/H$^+$ and Na$^+$/Ca^{2+} antiporters are the mechanisms proposed for the increase in Ca$^{2+}_i$ previous to the CA release in the hypoxic and the acidic transduction cascades in the CB, respectively (González et al., 1992).

In conclusion, the increase in the release of ^{3}H-CA induced by AlF$_4^-$ should be the net result of the activation of all the G proteins expressed in the CB chemoreceptors cells. The G proteins activated by AlF$_4^-$ might include G proteins involved directly in the transduction processes and/or coupled to autoreceptors to neurotransmitters. In this regard, the presence of several autoreceptor types in chemoreceptor cells, probably coupled to G proteins, is well documented (see Fidone et al., 1990). Several steps of the secretory process have been suggested as possible targets for G proteins, including ionic channels and antiporters. The modulation showed could be exerted by direct and/or via second messenger systems.

We thank M. Bravo for technical assistance. This work was supported by DGICYT grant PB92/0267.

REFERENCES

Bruch, R.C. (1990) Signal transduction in olfaction and taste. In "G-Proteins". R. Iyengar & L. Birnbaumer, eds., Acad. Press Inc., San Diego, USA.

Fidone, S.J., González, C., Obeso, A., Gómez-Niño, A. & Dinger, B. (1990) Biogenic amine and neuropeptide transmitters in carotid body chemotransmission: Experimental findings and perspectives. In "Hypoxia: the adaptations" J. Sutton, G. Coates & J. Remmers, eds., Marcel Decker Inc., Toronto.

Gilman, A.G. (1987) G-Proteins: Transducers of receptor-generated signals. Ann. Rev. Biochem. 56: 615-649.

Gómez-Niño, A., Almaraz, L. & González, C. (1992) Potentiation by cyclooxygenase inhibitors of the release of catecholamines from the rabbit carotid body and its reversal by prostaglandin E_2. Neurosci. Lett. 140: 1-4.

Gomperts, B.D. (1990) GTP-Bindings proteins and exocytotic secretion. In "G-Proteins" R. Iyengar & L. Birnbaumer, eds., Acad Press Inc., San Diego, USA.

González, C., Almaraz, L., Obeso, A. & Rigual, R. (1992) Oxygen and acid chemoreception in the carotid body chemoreceptors. Trends in Neurosci. 15: 146-153.

González-Guerrero, P.R., Rigual, R. & González, C. (1993) Opioid peptides in the rabbit carotid body. Identification and evidence for co-utilization and interactions with dopamine. J. Neurochem. 60: 1762-1768.

Ito, S., Negishi, M., Mochizuki-Oda, N., Yokohama, H. & Hayaishi, O. (1991) Sodium fluoride mimics the effect of protaglandin E_2 on catecholamine release from bovine adrenal chromaffin cells. J. Neurochem. 56: 44-51.

Lancet, D. (1986) Vertebrate olfactory reception. Ann. Rev. Neurosci. 9: 329-355.

Pérez-García, M.T., Almaraz, L. & González, C. (1991) Cyclic AMP modulates differentially the release of dopamine induced by hypoxia and other stimuli and increases dopamine synthesis in the rabbit carotid body. J. Neurochem. 57: 1992-2000.

CATECHOLAMINES IN THE RABBIT CAROTID BODY : CONTENT AND SECRETION

L.-M. Leitner[1] and J.-M. Cottet-Emard[2]

[1]Université Paul Sabatier, Faculté de Médecine, URA CNRS 649,
133, Route de Narbonne - 31062 - Toulouse-Cedex - France
[2]Université de Lyon I, URA CNRS 1195, 8, Avenue Rockefeller,
69373 - Lyon-Cedex-08 - France

INTRODUCTION

Catecholamines (mainly dopamine and noradrenaline) are present in the carotid body of numerous species and speculations about their role in chemoreception have grown extensively. Although no direct evidence was found for an inhibitory action on chemoafferent discharges (Zapata, 1975) this idea recurrently appears in the literature. This is in contrast with findings indicating that dopamine is released by the hypoxic carotid body, and the larger the hypoxia, the greater the release; yet everybody agrees that hypoxia is an exquisite stimulus to chemoafferent discharges. Although the role of catecholamines as a transmitter between the receptor (type I cells) and the chemoafferent endings is still a matter of controversy, their importance in the chemoreception process is crucial, as exemplified by experiments on reserpinised carotid bodies both in the rabbit and in the cat (Leitner & Roumy, 1986). It is thus important to see if the secretion of catecholamines, already measured indirectly by the tritiated precursor technique, follows the exquisite stimuli (slight hypoxia, hypercapnia, acidity) when measured directly in the effluent of the superfused carotid body.

METHODS

In the first series of experiments rabbit carotid bodies were carefully dissected and put in micro-chambers (volume 1 µl) superfused with a flow rate of 60 µl/min by Locke's solution. Since it is known that the catecholamine content of this preparation is stable between 1 h and 5 h of superfusion, hypoxia (10 % O_2 in N_2), hypercapnia (8 % CO_2, 21 % O_2, 71 % N_2), acidity (acetate 10 mM) and alkalinity (benzylamine 10 mM) were applied to the CB for 1 h and the resulting change was measured every 20 min in order to know the minimum period of time necessary to evaluate the secretion of dopamine (DA), noradrenaline (NA) and 3,4-dihydroxyphenylacetic-acid (DOPAC) : a period of 15 min was found adequate. All measurements were made with high performance liquid chromatography with electrochemical detection (HPLC-ED). In the case of secretion a preliminary processing with alumina was used to concentrate DA, NA and DOPAC. Results were treated with non parametric Mann-Whitney U-test for catecholamine contents and with Wilcoxon paired-test for secretions.

RESULTS

Effect of natural stimuli on DA, NA and DOPAC contents

After 1 h of hypoxic superfusion the content of DA decreased significantly by 50% together with NA whereas DOPAC increased (perhaps a consequence of DA catabolism by MAO). These effects were not sensitive to absence of Ca^{2+} accomplished by adding EGTA (1 mM) to the superfusing medium , except that the NA decrease was more pronounced in the Ca^{2+}-deprived medium. Hypercapnia lead also to a significant decrease in DA, NA and an increase in DOPAC and none of these changes were calcium-dependent. The change in internal pH induced by acetate elicited a significant (50%) decrease in DA and NA, abolished by the absence of Ca^{2+} in the superfusate. DOPAC increased as expected since the optimal pH of MAO is acid. Benzylamine increased internal pH and decreased DA, NA and DOPAC content dramatically and this last phenomenon was probably due to a reduced activity of MAO at alkaline pH. These changes were not dependent on the presence of calcium.

Table 1. DA, NA and DOPAC secretion from superfused carotid bodies during hypoxia, with and without extracellular Ca^{2+}, and before and after sympathectomy

	A		B	
	Hypoxia	Hypoxia $0Ca^{2+}$	Hypoxia	Hypoxia $0Ca^{2+}$
DA	102	90	130	352*
NA	132	75	116	113
DOPAC	75	77	155	505*

Values are % control, A before sympathectomy, B after sympathectomy
* different from control, p < 0.05, Wilcoxon paired - test.

Effects of natural stimuli on DA, NA and DOPAC secretion

The superfusate was collected in 2 ml vials for 15 min and the following experimental sequence was used: control, stimulus without Ca^{2+} but with EGTA (1 mM), stimulus alone. The experiment was done in the dark and the 2 ml vials contained 100 µl of EDTA (200 µM) as antioxidant to obviate any degradation of DA and NA. Immediately after each sequence, vials were deep frozen at -80°C, and eventually processed with alumina before measurements made with HPLC-ED.

A total of 235 control samples were measured and yielded the following amounts of DA, NA and DOPAC (median) : 0.216, 0.426, 0.155 pmole/15 min. It should be noticed that the spontaneous secretion of NA was twice that of DA although the content of DA was, in vivo, about 5 times that of NA (246 and 49 pmol/CB respectively).

Hypoxia did not change the secretion of DA, NA or DOPAC in intact carotid bodies; however after sympathectomy DA secretion increased and even more after Ca^{2+} deprivation whereas NA remained unchanged. DOPAC increased only after sympathectomy and calcium deprivation (Table 1).

Hypercapnia yielded different results: DA increased substantially from 0.35 pmole/15 min to 2.72 pmol/15 min in CO_2 medium deprived of calcium and this effect was not changed by sympathectomy. DOPAC also increased slightly but significantly in the Ca^{2+}-deprived medium whereas the amount of NA released remained unchanged whatever the experimental situation.

Acidification of the internal medium did not significantly modify the secretion of DA, NA or DOPAC except that the values were higher in Ca^{2+}-deprived media. Benzylamine increased tremendously DA and NA secretion and even more after Ca^{2+} removal whereas DOPAC secretion was decreased.

DISCUSSION

The effect of hypoxia, hypercapnia, acidity or alkalinity on DA, NA and DOPAC content was mostly expected and was in keeping with previous results of secretion obtained with the use of tritiated precursor technique (Fidone et al., 1982). However, apparently unexpected was the change occurring with benzylamine, i.e. the tremendous increase in secretion caused by the alkalinization of type I cells; actually this is less surprising if we suppose that the proton gradient which maintains catecholamines within the dense-cored vesicles is abolished by alkalinization and that catecholamines pour out of the vesicles. Such a result is incompatible with the contention that chemoafferent discharges evoked by natural stimuli are induced by catecholamine secretion from type I cells; indeed, alkalinization of the chemoreceptor cells decreases the chemoafferent discharges.

Another discrepancy with previously published results is the role of Ca^{2+} in the secretory process. Although care was taken to present the stimulus without Ca^{2+} before the normal stimulus because, as already observed the amount of catecholamine secreted decreases with time, the absence of Ca^{2+} improved the secretion of DA and NA . Nevertheless this phenomenon was expected from the results concerning the changes in catecholamine content.

In conclusion, natural stimuli but also and mainly alkalinization of the internal medium increased secretion of DA and NA from the superfused carotid body. This observation together with the fact that secretion decreases with time are not in favour of a direct relation between chemoafferent activity and catecholamine release.

We thank Ms C. Fortun for typing the manuscript.

REFERENCES

Fidone, S., Gonzalez, C., Yoshizaki, K. (1982) Effects of low oxygen on the release of dopamine from the rabbit carotid body. J. Physiol. (London) 333 : 93-110.

Leitner, L.-M., Roumy, M. (1986) Chemoreceptor response to hypoxia and hypercapnia in catecholamine depleted rabbit and cat carotid bodies in vitro. Pflügers Arch. 406 : 419-423.

Zapata, P. (1975) Effects of dopamine on carotid chemo- and baroreceptors in vitro.
J. Physiol. (London) 244 : 235-251.

CHOLINERGIC ASPECTS OF CAROTID BODY CHEMOTRANSDUCTION

Robert S. Fitzgerald[1,2,3], Machiko Shirahata[1,4], and Tohru Ide[1]

Departments of Environmental Health Sciences[1], Physiology[2], Medicine[3],
and Anesthesiology/Critical Care Medicine[4]
The Johns Hopkins Medical Institutions
Baltimore, Maryland 21205, USA

INTRODUCTION

Neurotransmitters have always been seen as an integral part of the carotid body transducing hypoxia, hypercapnia, and acidosis into increased neural output. Acetylcholine (ACh) was one of the first to be delivered exogenously with a resultant increase in neural output. Hence, ACh was proposed as the principal excitatory neurotransmitter during physiological challenges. A significant amount of data supported this notion, especially studies from Sweden. However, data from other studies was not consistent with this hypothesis. It was reported, for example, that though cholinergic blockers could reduce or abolish an increase in ventilation due to exogenously delivered ACh, they did not block the increase due to hypoxia.

It seemed worthwhile to test again the hypothesis that ACh is an excitatory neurotransmitter in carotid body chemotransduction with a different technique. As an operating model we propose ganglionic transmission, addressing both the muscarinic and nicotinic dimensions of the cholinergic effect. We propose that ACh is released from the Type I cell ("presynaptic unit") and binds to nicotinic and muscarinic receptors on the apposed dendrite ("postsynaptic unit"). Hence, we try to block the excitatory effect of hypoxia, first, with a mixture of muscarinic and nicotinic blockers. Next, acknowledging that the ganglion's M_1 and M_2 receptors are responsible for the slow excitatory postsynaptic potential (sEPSP) and slow inhibitory postsynaptic potential (sIPSP) respectively, we try to influence the carotid body response to hypoxia by blocking either the M_1 or the M_2 receptor individually. The technique is to provide the blockers only to the carotid body region.

METHODS

The common carotid artery of anesthetized, paralyzed, artificially ventilated cats was fitted with a loop having a 3-way stopcock. The lingual artery was fitted with a collecting cannula and the external carotid artery rostral to it was patent while the remaining arterial branches were ligated. During 95% of the experiment the carotid body was perfused with its own arterial blood. When Krebs Ringer bicarbonate solution (KRB) at 37⁰ C was to be perfused, snares around the common and external carotid arteries were drawn tight and the stopcock turned arresting blood flow to the region, and KRB with/without the blockers perfused the region, exiting via the lingual artery and the carotid body venous system. Whole nerve activity in the carotid sinus nerve was recorded; baroreceptor activity was removed by mechanical/thermal treatment of the carotid sinus area.

Three protocols were followed: (1) The carotid body was exposed to hypoxic blood after it had been "prepared" for three minutes by either a blocker-free KRB or KRB containing the mixture of nicotinic-muscarinic blockers. (2) After exposure to hypoxic blood for three minutes the carotid body was perfused for two minutes with either a blocker-free hypoxic KRB or hypoxic KRB containing the above mix of blockers. (3) The normoxic carotid body was exposed to one minute of hypoxic KRB followed immediately by one minute of hypoxic KRB containing either an M_1 or M_2 receptor blocker.

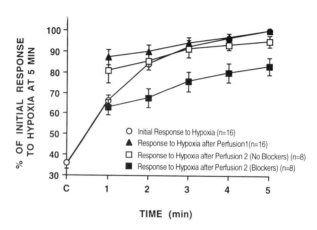

Fig. 1. Response of the carotid body to hypoxic blood, to hypoxic blood after a perfusion of blocker-free KRB, or to hypoxic blood containing (μM) 1.1 alpha bungarotoxin, 67 mecamylamine, 157 atropine. The first two blockers are nicotinic; the third, muscarinic.

RESULTS

(1) Figure 1 shows the initial output of the carotid body was about 37% of its response to hypoxic blood at 5 minutes. While the cat remained hypoxic, a perfusion of blocker-free KRB was made after which hypoxic blood again perfused the carotid body for five minutes; the response was recorded. A second time KRB was perfused, being either blocker-free like the first or blocker-containing. The response to hypoxic blood after the blocker-containing KRB was significantly less than the other responses to hypoxic blood. The response to an intra-arterial injection of 1 μg nicotine was reduced by 30% after the blockers compared to the pre-blocker response to nicotine.

(2) The initial exposure to hypoxia was reduced to three minutes and perfusion durations were shortened to two minutes. The perfused KRB was as hypoxic as the blood, and was either blocker-free or contained concentrations of the blockers at 2X, 6X, and 10X the values in the legend above (except for alpha bungarotoxin, kept at 2X). The

reduction in the response to hypoxic KRB was dose-dependent. After two minutes of perfusion the carotid body response to: (a) blocker-free hypoxic KRB was 100% of the pre-perfusion response to hypoxic blood; (b) hypoxic KRB with 2X blockers was 58% of the pre-perfusion response; (c) to hypoxic KRB with 6X blockers was completely abolished; and (d) hypoxic blood with 10X blockers dropped below the pre-hypoxic blood control value. Recovery from the blockers over three minutes was also dose-dependent.

(3) Switching from the first reservoir of hypoxic KRB after one minute of perfusion to a second reservoir containing equally hypoxic KRB not unexpectedly maintained the increased neural output. However, switching from the first reservoir to one containing hypoxic KRB with 300uM gallamine (M_2 receptor blocker) elevated the neural output by 40%. Whereas switching from the first reservoir to one containing hypoxic KRB with 300uM pirenzepine (M_1 receptor blocker) reduced the neural response by 30%.

DISCUSSION

The data from the first two protocols suggest an excitatory role for ACh in the chemotransduction of hypoxia in that cholinergic blockade reduces in a dose-dependent fashion the response to hypoxia. Further, the data suggests that there may be some similarity between ganglionic transmission and carotid body sensing of hypoxia in that blocking of both nicotinic and muscarinic pathways proved to be a very effective technique for depressing the response to hypoxia. The third set of data suggested that there was indeed a differential muscarinic effect depending upon the blocker, and indicating that perhaps M_1 and M_2 receptors were involved. For the blocking of the M_2, reducing or eliminating the sIPSP would make the postsynaptic element more excitable to ACh, and blocking the M_1 should make this element less excitable. The results, then, are consistent with the operating model. However, data can be fitted to a wide variety of models. And it does seem that the model of ganglionic transmission could well be overly simplistic when other data demonstrating roles for other neurotransmitters are considered. Nonetheless, the data do support the hypothesis and this model.

The failure of earlier efforts using cholinergic blockers to reduce the carotid body response to hypoxia is difficult to explain. Perhaps their giving of the blockers systemically did not allow a sufficiently high concentration of the blocker to infiltrate the carotid body. It is not always clear how much time elapsed between the administration of the blocker and the hypoxic challenge. If the blocker was absorbed more quickly and steadily into other tissues, it is conceivable that the concentration at the carotid body was too low to offset the endogenously released ACh, which could reach very high micromolar concentrations in the synaptic cleft. Whatever the explanation, at this point, on the basis of the above data, it seems a bit premature to discount an excitatory role for ACh in the carotid body's chemotransduction of hypoxia.

This work was supported by HL 10342, HL 50712, and HL 47044.

LOW PO$_2$ DEPENDENCY OF NEUTRAL ENDOPEPTIDASE AND ACETYLCHOLINESTERASE ACTIVITIES OF THE RAT CAROTID BODY

Ganesh K. Kumar[1,2], Nanduri R. Prabhakar[2,3], Kingman P. Strohl[2,3], Agnes Thomas[2] and Pat A. Cragg[2]

Departments of Biochemistry[1], Medicine[2] and Biophysics & Physiology[3],Case Western Reserve University, Cleveland, OH 44106 USA

INTRODUCTION

Multiple neurochemicals contribute to the chemosensory response of the carotid body to hypoxia. In addition to biogenic amines, the mammalian carotid body contains several neuropeptides which include enkephalins (Enk), and substance P (SP) (Fidone & Gonzalez, 1986; Prabhakar et al., 1989). Several studies have demonstrated that hypoxia influences catecholamine metabolism in the carotid body by affecting their synthesis, re-uptake or degradation pathways (Fidone & Gonzalez, 1986; Wang et al., 1990). Few studies have addressed the effects of hypoxia on the neuropeptides in the carotid body (Prabhakar et al., 1989; Hansen et al., 1986). One hour of sustained, moderate hypoxia increased SP (Prabhakar et al., 1989) in the cat carotid body whereas intermittent hypoxia decreased the tissue content of SP and Enk in the rabbit carotid body (Hansen et al., 1986). After two weeks of hypoxic exposure, SP-like immunoreactivity of the type I cells significantly decreased in the cat carotid body (Wang et al., 1990). These results suggest that the effects of hypoxia on neuropeptides are complex and may arise either from enhanced *in vivo* peptide synthesis or decreased degradation.

In other systems, the enzyme, neutral endopeptidase (NEP; E.C.3.4.24.11) is involved in the inactivation of several neuropeptides (Erdos & Skidgel, 1989). Previously, we presented evidence for the occurrence of relatively abundant NEP-like activity in the cat chemoreceptor tissue (Kumar et al., 1990a) and by *in vitro* studies demonstrated that NEP is involved in the hydrolysis of SP in the carotid body (Kumar et al., 1990b). If the alterations in peptide levels of the carotid body caused by hypoxia are due to its direct effect on their degradation via peptidases, given the fact that the premier peptidase of the carotid body is NEP, then it is conceivable that NEP activity in the carotid body may be altered in response to low PO$_2$.

We tested the above possibility using rats that were exposed to various durations of hypobaric hypoxia (0.4 ATM). NEP activity was determined in the carotid body and also in the adrenal glands which served as a control. The enzyme specific effects of hypoxia were also assessed by comparing the activity of NEP with acetylcholinesterase (AChE) activity in both the tissues.

MATERIALS AND METHODS

Experiments were performed on Sprague-Dawley rats of either sex (n = 24). The experimental groups (n = 4 for each exposure) were exposed to hypoxia in a hypobaric chamber (0.4 ATM) for the following durations: 1 hour, 1 week and 2 weeks. Equal numbers of age matched control groups breathed room air (21% O_2 balanced with N_2) for similar durations. The animals from control and experimental groups were anaesthetized with urethane (i.p.; 1.4 - 1.6 g/kg) and allowed to breathe spontaneously appropriate gas mixtures during dissection of the carotid bodies and adrenal glands. The tissues were frozen and stored in liquid nitrogen until they were further analyzed for enzyme activities.

Cell-free extracts of the carotid body and the adrenal gland of the rat were made in 100 mM HEPES buffer, pH 7.4 containing 0.1 mM PMSF as described previously (Kumar et al., 1990a). NEP activity in the cell-free extracts of the tissues was determined by a modification of the procedure described by Sonnenberg et al. (1988). For AChE activity the procedure of Ellman et al (1961) was followed. Enzyme activity is expressed in units which are defined as the amount of product formed per minute at 37°C. Specific activity is expressed in units/mg protein. Protein concentration was determined by the colloidal gold method (Stoscheck, 1987) using bovine serum albumin as the standard. Specificity of NEP and AChE was assessed using controls incubated with phosphoramidon or prostigmine respectively prior to enzyme assay.

Results are expressed as mean ± SEM. Standard statistical methods, including Student's unpaired t test and one way and two-way analysis of variance (ANOVA), were used where appropriate. $P < 0.05$ was considered significant.

RESULTS AND DISCUSSION

Measurement of NEP activity in individual rat carotid body within a given animal yielded identical values. For example, NEP activity of the right carotid body averaged 15.2 ± 0.3 pmol.min^{-1}.mg^{-1} whereas for the left carotid body it was 14.8 ± 0.6 pmol.min^{-1}.mg^{-1}. With the onset of hypoxia, NEP activity of the carotid body was altered in a biphasic manner with an initial decrease followed by a marked increase (Table 1). Exposing animals to one hour of hypoxia decreased NEP activity by 30% (Table 1). This decrease in NEP activity was significant (P<0.05). NEP activity of the carotid body after 2 weeks of hypoxia was 24.1 ± 1.0 pmol.min^{-1}.mg^{-1} protein which corresponded to a ~ 56% increase in the enzyme activity.

Table 1. Effects of hypoxia on NEP and AChE activities of the rat carotid body

Enzyme	Duration of hypoxia			
	Control	1 hour	1 week	2 weeks
NEP (pmol.min^{-1}.mg^{-1})	15.2 ± 0.3	9.9 ± 0.4	21.2 ± 0.5	24.1 ± 1.0
AChE (μmol.min^{-1}.mg^{-1})	13.0 ± 0.8	13.1 ± 1.2	9.6 ± 0.9	8.9 ± 1.0

NEP activity of the adrenal glands was determined to assess possible tissue specific effects of hypoxia and the results are presented in Table 2. NEP activity of the adrenal gland was 53.7 ± 4.5 pmol.min^{-1}.mg^{-1} protein which was ~ 3.5 fold higher than the activity found in the carotid body. In contrast to the carotid body, the NEP activity of the adrenal gland was unaffected during 1 hour of hypoxia but decreased to ~ 45 % and ~ 52 % of the normoxic value by 1 week and 2 weeks of hypoxia respectively.

Is the effect of hypoxia limited to NEP activity? We addressed this issue by determining the effect of hypoxia on AChE, the enzyme that degrades acetylcholine and certain neuropeptides. AChE activity of the carotid body was higher by several orders of magnitude than the activity of adrenal glands. In both tissues, AChE activity was unaltered after 1 hour exposure to hypoxia. In response to extended hypoxia, the AChE activity of the carotid body and adrenal glands decreased by ~ 32 % and ~ 45 % respectively.

Table 2. Effects of hypoxia on NEP and AChE activities of the rat adrenal glands

Enzyme	Duration of hypoxia			
	Control	1 hour	1 week	2 weeks
NEP (pmol.min^{-1}.mg^{-1})	53.7 ± 4.5	51.8 ± 1.8	29.6 ± 2.2	26.0 ± 3.2
AChE (nmol.min^{-1}.mg^{-1})	16.6 ± 0.8	15.8 ± 0.9	11.3 ± 0.8	9.1 ± 1.0

The results suggest that in the rat carotid body NEP and AChE activities are not regulated in a co-ordinated fashion but rather via independent mechanisms. By contrast, in the adrenal glands these activities are regulated by hypoxia in a co-ordinated manner suggesting a tight coupling of these neurochemical mediated mechanisms.

REFERENCES

Ellman, G.L., K.D. Courtney, V. Andres, Jr. & R. M Featherstone (1961) A new and rapid colorimetric determination of acetylcholinesterase activity. Biochem. Pharmacol. 7:88-95.

Erdos, E.G., & R.A. Skidgel (1989) Neutral endopeptidase 24.11 (enkephalinase) and related regulators of peptide hormones. FASEB J. 3:145-151.

Fidone, S., & C. Gonzalez (1986) Initiation and control of chemoreceptor activity in the carotid body, in: "Handbook of Physiology, Section 3: The respiratory System", N.S.Cherniack and J.G. Widdicombe, eds., American Physiological Society, Bethesda, pp 267-312.

Hansen, G., L. Jones & S. Fidone (1986) Physiological chemoreceptor stimulation decreases enkephalin and substance P in the carotid body. Peptides 7:767-769.

Kumar, G.K., M. Runold, R.D. Ghai, N.S. Cherniack & N.R. Prabhakar (1990a) Occurrence of neutral endopeptidase activity in the cat carotid body and its significance in chemoreception. Brain Res. 517:341-343.

Kumar, G.K., N.R. Prabhakar & N.S. Cherniack, (1990b) In vitro degradation of substance P by the carotid body proteases. In: "Arterial chemoreception", C. Eyzaguirre, S.J. Fidone, R.S. Fitzgerald, S. Lahiri and D.M. McDonald, eds., Springer-Verlag, New York pp 137-141.

Prabhakar, N.R., S. Landis, G.K. Kumar, D. Mullikin-Kilpatrick, N.S. Cherniack, & S.E. Leeman (1989) Substance P and neurokinin A in the cat carotid body: localization, exogenous effects and changes in content in response to arterial PO_2. Brain Res. 481:205-214

Sonnenberg, J.L., Y. Sakane, A.Y. Jeng, J.A. Koehn, J.A. Ansell, L.P. Wennogle & R.D. Ghai (1988) Identification of protease 3.4.24.11 as the major atrial natriuretic factor degrading enzyme in the rat kidney. Peptides 9:173-180.

Stoscheck, C.M. (1987) Protein assay sensitive at nanogram levels. Anal. Biochem. 160:301-305.

Wang, Z.-Z., B. Dinger, S.J. Fidone & L.J. Stensaas. (1990) An immunocytochemical study of biogenic amines and neuropeptides in the hypoxic cat carotid body. Soc. Neurosci. 16:363.3

NITRIC OXIDE SYNTHASE OCCURS IN NEURONS AND NERVE FIBERS OF THE CAROTID BODY

P.A. Grimes[1], S. Lahiri[2], R. Stone[1], A. Mokashi[2] and D. Chug[2]

[1]Department of Ophthalmology and Scheie Eye Institute and [2]Department of Physiology, University of Pennsylvania School of Medicine, Philadelphia, PA 19104

INTRODUCTION

Nitric oxide (NO), a free radical, can be produced by vascular endothelial cells and certain neurons of the central and peripheral nervous systems upon activation of its biosynthetic enzyme, nitric oxide synthase (NOS). NO may function as a non-conventional neurotransmitter in the nervous system, and either NO or an NO-producing compound is believed to be the endothelium-derived relaxing factor of the vascular system. An antiserum recognizing the molecular form of NOS present in brain has been used to localize the enzyme in brain and peripheral tissues (Bredt et al., 1990). NOS containing neurons also display intense NADPH-diaphorase activity (Dawson et al., 1991; Hope et al., 1991), and this histochemical reaction, though less specific than immunohistochemistry, provides a label for NOS activity in both central and peripheral neurons.

Because of accumulating evidence of a physiological role of NO in O_2 chemoreception (Hague et al., 1993; Wang et al., 1993; Katayama et al., 1993), we sought to localize NOS in the cat carotid body using immunocytochemistry and diaphorase histochemistry.

METHODS

Carotid bodies with a connecting segment of carotid artery were removed from anesthetized cats and fixed *in vitro* by intra-arterial perfusion with either 4% paraformaldehyde or periodate-lysine-paraformaldehyde (PLP). The tissues were post-fixed by immersion for another two hours in the same fixatives, cryoprotected with 30% sucrose, frozen, and sectioned in a cryostat at 16 μm thickness. Portions of the glossopharyngeal nerve including the petrosal ganglion, fixed by immersion in either solution for two hours, were similarly processed and sectioned.

Sections of PLP fixed tissues were incubated with a rabbit polyclonal antibody against NOS (Bredt et al., 1990); immunoreactivity was localized with a biotinylated secondary antibody and a streptavidin-Texas red conjugate. Specificity of immunostaining was established by omitting the primary antiserum from the incubation procedure.

The histochemical reaction for NADPH-diaphorase was applied to both paraformaldehyde and PLP fixed tissues. Sections were incubated for 45-60 minutes at

37°C in a solution containing 1.5 mM ß-NADPH, 0.2 mM nitro blue tetrazolium and 0.2% Triton X-100 in 0.05 M Tris buffer (pH 7.6). Portions of the carotid sinus nerve near the carotid body also were processed for diaphorase histochemistry as whole mount preparations.

RESULTS

NOS-like immunoreactive (NOS-LI) nerve fibers and ganglion cells were present in all carotid bodies examined (Figure 1). Positively stained nerve fibers, both smooth and varicose, coursed throughout the structure, usually in connective tissue septa and in association with blood vessels. Occasionally NOS-LI nerves appeared to lie close to or among Type I glomus cells, but specific innervation of these cells could not be detected. Some part of the NOS-LI innervation of the carotid body derived from endogenous NOS-positive ganglion cells. The number of positive ganglion cells seen in a carotid body and its closely adjacent tissues ranged from 10 to 30 depending on the animal examined; not all of the ganglion cells within the a given organ were NOS-positive. Small nerve bundles of unknown origin in the proximity of the carotid body often contained several NOS-positive axons. The main trunk of the glossopharyngeal nerve distal to the petrosal ganglion also contained a small population of immunoreactive axons, though examination of a limited number of sections from 2 petrosal ganglia demonstrated no positive ganglion cells.

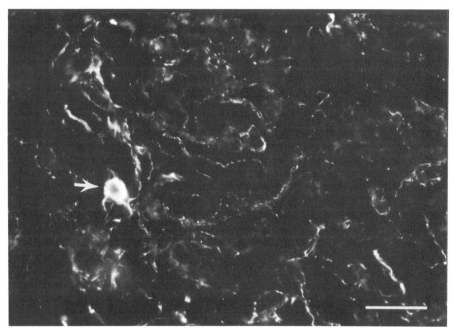

Figure 1. NOS-LI nerve fibers, both smooth and varicose, are dispersed throughout the carotid body. Some endogenous ganglion cells (arrow) are also NOS-positive. Type I glomus cells show faint, non-specific staining. Magnification bar, 50 μm.

The distribution of NADPH-diaphorase activity in the carotid body was the same as that of NOS immunoreactivity (Figure 2). Smooth and varicose nerve fibers and some ganglion cells were intensely stained; other components of the tissue were unstained or showed very weak activity. Application of the histochemical method to whole preparations of portions of the carotid sinus nerve demonstrated that some diaphorase positive axons traversed the nerve and its branches entering the carotid body.

DISCUSSION

In the carotid body, NOS immunoreactivity and NADPH-diaphorase activity are detected only in nerve fibers and in some endogenous ganglion cells. The nerve fibers are prominently associated with blood vessels and presumably function in vasoregulation. Other fibers dispersed through the tissue occasionally approach the Type I glomus cells, but termination of stained nerves on the chemoreceptor cells could not be detected.

The origin of the NOS-positive nerves in the carotid body is not yet known. Some undoubtedly derive from the NOS-positive ganglion cells scattered within the structure and in adjacent tissue. In the rat, NOS is not detected in sympathetic neurons of the superior cervical ganglion but is present and often coexists with vasoactive intestinal polypeptide in parasympathetic ganglion cells projecting to blood vessels (Nazaki et al., 1993; Yamamoto

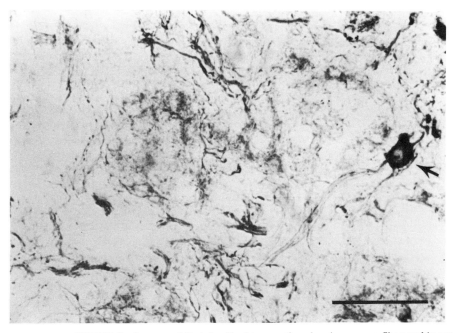

Figure 2. Intense NADPH diaphorase activity is localized in smooth and varicose nerve fibers and in some ganglion cells (arrow) of the carotid body. Type I glomus cells are only weakly stained. Magnification bar, 50 μm.

et al., 1993). Thus, NOS-positive ganglion cells in the cat carotid body, like VIP-positive ganglion cells (Wharton et al., 1980), probably are dispersed parasympathetic ganglion cells. Positively stained axons of unknown origin located in the glossopharyngeal and carotid sinus nerves and in other unidentified nerves in the vicinity of the carotid body also contribute to the innervation.

Identification of NOS in carotid body nerves indicates that NO can be produced from neural sources in the chemoreceptor organ and may affect glomus cell activity either directly by diffusion from nearby nerves or indirectly by NO-induced vascular changes.

We thank Drs. David Bredt and Solomon Snyder for the generous supply of NOS antiserum. Supported by NIH grants EY-05454 and HL-43413 and a grant from the Nina and Paul Mackall trust.

REFERENCES

Bredt, D.S., Hwang, P.M., & Snyder, S.H. (1990) Localization of nitric oxide synthase indicating a neuronal role for nitric oxide. Nature 347:768.

Dawson, T.M., Bredt, D.S., Fotuhi, P.M., Hwang, P.M., & Snyder, S.H. (1991) Nitric oxide synthase and neuronal NADPH diaphorase are identical in brain & peripheral tissue. Proc. Natl. Acad. Sci. USA 88:7797.

Hague, U., Agani, F., Chang, C.H., & Prabhakar, N.R. (1993) NO, a novel chemical messenger in carotid body. FASEB J. 7:A431.

Hope, B.T., Michael, G.J., Knigge, K.M., & Vincent, S.R. (1991) Neuronal NADPH diaphorase is a nitric oxide synthase. Proc. Natl. Acad. Sci. USA 88:2881.

Katayama, M., Chug, D., Mosaki, A., Ray, D., Bebont, D., & Lahiri, S. (1993) NO mimics O_2 in the carotid body chemoreception. This volume

Nazaki, K., Moskowitz, M.A., Maynard, K.I., Koketsu, N., Dawson, T., Bredt, D.S., & Snyder, S.H. (1993) Possible origins and distribution of immunoreactive nitric oxide synthase-containing nerve fibers in cerebral arteries. J. Cereb. Blood Flow Metab. 13:70.

Wharton, J., Polak, J.M., Will, J.A., Bisgard, G.E., Bryant, M.G., McGregor, G.P., Emson, P.C., & Bloom, S.R. (1980) Enkephalin-, vasoactive intestinal polypeptide- and substance P-like immunoreactivity in the cat carotid body. J. Endocrinol. 85:40P.

Wang, Z.Z., Dinger, B., Fidone, S.J., & Stensas, L.J. (1993) Physiological role of nitric oxide (NO) in the cat carotid body. FASEB J. 7:A431.

Yamamoto, R., Bredt, D.S., Snyder, S.H., & Stone, R.A. (1993) The localization of nitric oxide synthase in the rat eye and related cranial ganglia. Neuroscience 54:189.

NO MIMICS O$_2$ IN THE CAROTID BODY CHEMORECEPTION

Masao Katayama, Deepak K. Chugh, Anil Mokashi, Dilip K. Ray, Donald E. Bebout and Sukhamay Lahiri

Department of Physiology, University of Pennsylvania School of Medicine
Philadelphia, PA 19104, USA

INTRODUCTION

Nitric oxide (NO) by virtue of its chemical binding with biological heme compounds in competition with O$_2$ (Martin et al., 1986), can mimic carotid body responses to PO_2 changes. That NO is produced endogenously (Palmer et al., 1987) and that its application dilates blood vessels and improved coronary blood flow have long been known (Amezcua et al., 1989). More recently nitric oxide synthase (NOS) which generates NO from L-arginine has been localized in many tissues including blood vessels (Moncada et al., 1991), peripheral nerves (Gillespie et al., 1990) neurons in the central nervous system (CNS) and ganglia (Ross et al., 1990; Garthwaite, 1990; Bredt et al., 1990). The consensus is that the mechanism of effects of NO is due to its reaction with soluble guanylate cyclase, a heme compound, and an increased production of cGMP which mediates the physiological responses (Bredt & Snyder, 1992)

The carotid body, a major O$_2$ chemoreceptor, is an ideal testing organ for the NOS-NO pathways because of its extensive vasculature and innervation. Numerous nerve fibers in the carotid body have been shown to contain NOS (Grimes et al., 1993). Based on this, it was hypothesized that blockade of NO production would stimulate carotid chemosensory nerve discharge.

METHODS

Eighteen carotid bodies (CB) from ten cats were studied in vitro. The carotid bodies in anesthetized cats (40 mg/kg pentobarbital) were vascularly isolated and carotid artery, proximal to carotid sinus, was cannulated. The CB was flushed with oxygenated and heparinized perfusate, and excised with most of the length of the carotid sinus nerve. Modified tyrode containing CO$_2$-HCO$_3^-$ (pH = 7.38-7.40 at 37 °C) was used for perfusion and superfusion of the CB preparation, as described previously (Iturriaga et al., 1991).

To study the effect of NO, we used NOS inhibitor L-nitro-arginine-methylester (L-NAME), decreasing endogenous NO production, and sodium nitroprusside (SNP), raising exogenous NO supply. Following protocols were used: (a) perfusion with L-NAME (25-200 μM) during normoxia; (b) mixture of L-arginine (50-500 μM) and L-NAME (50 μM and 100 μM) during normoxia; (c) administration of hyperoxic perfusate during L-NAME induced excitation; (d) SNP (0.5-10 μM) during L-NAME administration; (e) SNP perfusion (0.5-10 μM) with and without hypoxia, and (f) interruption of perfusate flow with and without SNP (1-2 μM) to test if NO blocked the response to severe hypoxia.

Separate perfusates were placed in separate bottles, and equilibrated with continuous flow of gases (O_2, CO_2 and N_2). Perfusate flow was by gravity at a pressure difference of 80-100 Torr, through water jacketed glass tubing at 37 °C. PO_2, PCO_2 and pH were checked using a blood gas analyzer at 37 °C (PHM 73, Radiometer Inc.).

RESULTS AND DISCUSSION

Figure 1 shows the effects of L-NAME (50 μM) during normoxia (PO_2 = 145 Torr) on the chemosensory activity. Following L-NAME perfusion, after a delay, there was a gradual rise of chemosensory activity. With 100 μM L-NAME the chemosensory nerve response increased from a baseline activity of 87.98 ± 13.26 (mean ± SEM) to 406.74 ± 41.85. The latency was 2.2 ± 0.34 min and time to peak response was 5.49 ± 0.97 min The slow development of excitation is consistent with the competitive displacement of L-arginine by L-NAME at the same site in NOS. This also indicates that a basal release of NO in the carotid body is a part of the regulation of chemosensory nerve activity. The peak activity during L-NAME administration showed a dose response effect over a range of L-NAME concentrations (25-200 μM).

On testing the mixture of L-NAME (50 μM) and L-arginine (500 μM), there were oscillations in the sensory activity.

On transition from a normoxic (PO_2 ~ 145 Torr) to a hyperoxic perfusate ($PO_2 \geq 400$ Torr) during L-NAME administration, the activity diminished promptly and remained low for about 3 min. Thus L-NAME appears to exaggerate the chemosensory response to hypoxia.

SNP (0.5-10 μM), an exogenous source of NO, consistently blocked the stimulatory effect of L-NAME, both during normoxia as well as during hyperoxia. Presumably this means that cGMP production was augmented. Administration of SNP during hypoxia decreased the response, as compared to hypoxia alone. But SNP did not abolish the response to extreme hypoxia as shown by an almost equal response to perfusate interruption with and without SNP. This leads to the assumption that cGMP is not the critical mediator of O_2 chemoreception. It seems that cGMP level in the carotid body is normally high, which keeps the sensory activity low.

In a separate study on the cat carotid body, using immunohistochemistry and diaphorase staining, we (Grimes et al., 1993) found that NOS was mostly localized in the nerves as well as in and around the blood vessels. It is possible that NO stimulates dopamine release in the carotid body as it has been observed to release insulin from pancreatic beta cells (Schmidt et al., 1992). NO induced increased efferent inhibition seems to be a possibility in chronic hypoxia.

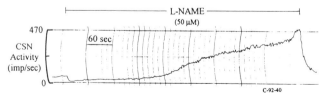

Figure 1. Example of an excitatory effect of L-NAME (50μM) on carotid chemosensory activity. The effect developed slowly and withdrawal of L-NAME was followed by a decrease in the activity.

Taken together the results suggest the following sequence. The free NO production in the carotid body is a normal occurrence and the carotid body P_{O_2} plays a role.

Supported in part by HL-43413-05. The grant T32-HL-07027-18 provided a research training fellowship to D.K. Chugh and D.K. Ray.

REFERENCES

Amezcua, J.L., Palmer, R.M.J., de Souza, B.M. & Moncada, S. (1989) Nitric oxide synthesized from L-arginine regulates vascular tone in the coronary circulation of the rabbit. Br. J. Pharmacol. 97:1119-1124.

Bredt, D.S., Hwang, P.M. & Snyder, S.H. (1990) Localization of nitric oxide synthase indicating a neural role for nitric oxide Nature 347:768-770.

Bredt, D.S. & Snyder, S.H. (1992) Nitric oxide, a novel neural messenger Neuron 8:3-11.

Garthwaite, J. (1990) Nitric oxide synthesis linked to activation of excitatory neurotransmitter receptors in the brain. In:"Nitric oxide from L-arginine: A Bioregulatory System," S. Moncada & E.A. Higgs, ed., Elsevier, Amsterdam, pp. 115-137.

Gillespie, J.S., Liu, X. & Martin, W. (1990) The neurotransmitter of the non-adrenergic non-cholinergic inhibitory nerves to smooth muscle of the genital system, in: "Nitric oxide from L-arginine: A Bioregulatory System," S. Moncada & E.A. Higgs, ed., Elsevier, Amsterdam, pp. 147-164.

Grimes, P., Lahiri S., Mokashi A., Chugh D. & Stone R. (1993). Nitric oxide synthase occurs in neurons and nerve fibers of the cat carotid body. This volume.

Iturriaga, R., Rumsey W. L., Mokashi A., Spergel D., Wilson D. F. & Lahiri, S. (1991) In-vitro perfused and superfused cat carotid body for physiological and pharmacological studies. J. Appl. Physiol. 70:1393-1400.

Martin, W., Smith, J.A. & White, D.G. (1986) The mechanisms by which haemoglobin inhibits the relaxation of rabbit aorta induced by nitrovasodilators, nitric oxide, or bovine retractor penis inhibitory factor. Br. J. Pharmacol. 89:563-571.

Moncada, S., Palmer, R. M. V. & Higgs, E. A.(1991). Nitric oxide: physiology, pathophysiology and pharmacology. Pharm. Revs. 43:109-142.

Palmer, R.M.J., Ferrige, A.G. & Moncada, S. (1987) Nitric oxide release accounts for the biological activity of endothelium derived relaxing factor. Nature 327:524-526.

Ross, C.A., Bredt, D. & Snyder, S.H. (1990) Messenger molecules in the cerebellum, Trends in Neurosci. 13:216-222

Schmidt, H.H.H.W., Warner, T.D., Ishi, K., Sheng, H. & Murad, F. (1992) Insulin secretion from pancreatic beta cells caused by L-Arginine-derived nitrogen oxide. Science 255:721-723.

MECHANISMS OF CAROTID BODY INHIBITION

Z.-Z. Wang[1], L.J. Stensaas[1], D.S. Bredt[2], B.G. Dinger[1] and S.J. Fidone[1]

[1]Department of Physiology, University of Utah School of Medicine,
410 Chipeta Way, Research Park, Salt Lake City, Utah 84108 U.S.A.
[2]Department of Neuroscience, Johns Hopkins University School of Medicine,
Baltimore, Maryland 21205 U.S.A.

INTRODUCTION

Some 25 years ago, Neil & O'Regan (1969, 1971) and Fidone & Sato (1970) demonstrated that electrical stimulation of the peripheral cut end of the carotid sinus nerve (CSN) inhibited spontaneous chemoreceptor activity recorded from nerve filaments split off from the main CSN trunk. These findings complemented the contemporary studies of Biscoe & Sampson (1968), who recorded spontaneous centrifugal neural activity from the central stump of the nerve, indicating the likely presence of an efferent or motor pathway in the CSN. Except for the finding that "efferent inhibition" of chemoreceptor discharge was mediated by unmyelinated, or C-fibers (Fidone & Sato, 1970), very little information has been forthcoming regarding the identity of the neurons or their mechanism of action in mediating this physiological phenomenon (O'Regan & Majcherczyk, 1983). McDonald & Mitchell (1981) postulated that efferent inhibition of the chemoreceptors was mediated by antidromic activity in afferent petrosal ganglion neurons, because the inhibitory effects persisted following chronic decentralization and sympathectomy. However, it was later pointed out that these careful surgical procedures would not have eliminated a group of presumptive autonomic neurons, first described by de Castro in 1926, which are present within the carotid body and along the CSN (see O'Regan & Majcherczyk, 1983, for review).

Recent studies in our laboratory have examined several cellular and neurochemical mechanisms which may mediate inhibition of chemoreceptor activity. A principal finding from these studies is that the cyclic nucleotide second messenger, cyclic GMP (cGMP), may be a key mediator of chemoreceptor inhibition. We have observed that cell permeant analogs of cGMP inhibit the CSN response to hypoxia and nicotine (Wang et al., 1993a), and moreover, that atrial natriuretic peptide (ANP), a substance linked to cGMP production in other tissues, can be immunocytochemically localized to carotid body type I cells (Wang et al., 1991b). Application of submicromolar concentrations of ANP or its analogs greatly elevates cGMP levels in type I cells, while profoundly inhibiting the stimulus-evoked chemosensory activity (Wang et al., 1992,1993a). In other systems, it has been found that ANP is released from the tissues by calcitonin gene-related peptide (CGRP; Yamamoto et al., 1988); consequently, the discovery that CGRP-positive neurons from the petrosal ganglion innervate type I cell lobules (Kondo et al., 1988; Kummer et al., 1990) suggests the possible involvement of ANP, and cGMP, as mediators of chemosensory inhibition (Wang et al., 1991b,1993a).

Nitric oxide (NO) is another novel substance capable of activating guanylate cyclase, the enzyme responsible for cGMP production (Bredt & Snyder, 1989,1992). In the study reported here, we have used a multidisciplinary approach to investigate the possible involvement of NO in chemosensory inhibition. Our immunocytochemical experiments have demonstrated an extensive plexus of fibers in the carotid body containing nitric oxide synthase (NOS). These fibers originate from two anatomically and neurochemically distinct neuronal populations, innervating the carotid body vasculature and the type I cell lobules, respectively. In addition, we have found that the NO precursor, L-arginine, inhibits, and that NOS blockers enhance, CSN activity. Moreover, electrical stimulation of the CSN greatly augments the production of NO in the carotid body, and increases cGMP immunostaining in type I cells. These effects are accompanied by inhibition of chemoreceptor activity, which is likewise reversed by NOS blockers. Details of the experimental methods can be found in Wang et al. (1993b,1993c).

RESULTS

NOS Immunoreactivity in the Carotid Body, CSN and Petrosal Ganglion

The immunocytochemical data presented in Figure 1 summarizes our findings from more detailed studies published elsewhere (Wang et al., 1993b,1993c). An extensive plexus of NOS-IR fibers penetrates the parenchyma of the cat and rat carotid body and innervates blood vessels and lobules of type I cells (Fig. 1). It consists of small caliber axons (≤ 1 μm, presumably non-myelinated), which branch to give rise to even thinner, sinuous processes with multiple, bead-like enlargements or varicosities. Some of these axons branch within the parenchymal cell lobules to encircle type I cells (Fig. 1A), while others can be observed in proximity to both large ($\approx$30-100 μm) and small ($\approx$10-30 μm) blood vessels, where they lie in association with the vascular adventitial layer (Fig. 1B). NOS immunoreactivity can occasionally be observed in endothelial cells lining the larger vessels, but is not seen in the sinusoidal capillaries surrounding the lobules. Parenchymal type I cells, as well as sustentacular type II cells, fibroblasts and vascular smooth muscle cells are devoid of NOS immunoreactivity.

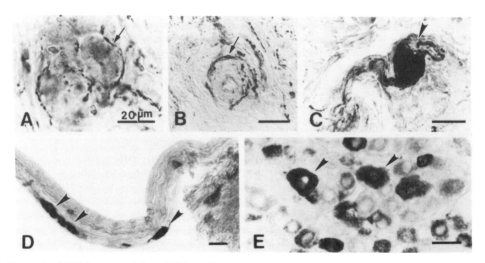

Figure 1. NOS immunostaining. NOS-positive nerve fibers penetrate parenchymal cell lobule (A) and surround blood vessel (B; arrows) in cat carotid body. Neurons containing NOS are located in the periphery of the carotid body (C), along the carotid sinus nerve (D), and in the petrosal ganglion (E; arrowheads).

High levels of NOS immunoreactivity are found in some large neurons (≈15-30 μm) located near the connective tissue capsule at the periphery of the organ in both the cat and rat carotid body (Fig. 1C). Similar neurons are found dispersed along the CSN and are particularly numerous near the CSN/glossopharyngeal nerve branch point (Fig. 1D). The somata of these neurons show short dendritic, tapering processes which resemble autonomic microganglial neurons, as first described by de Castro in 1926. These neurons also display a single NOS-IR axon which projects towards the carotid body.

The majority of NOS-IR nerve fibers in the CSN arise from neurons concentrated near the proximal (central) end of the petrosal ganglion. Unlike the strongly immunoreactive autonomic neurons described above, levels of NOS-IR in petrosal ganglial cells vary considerably (Fig. 1E). The spectrum of immunoreactivity ranged from almost undetectable to extremely high levels. Most NOS-IR petrosal neurons were small cells (15-20 μm), lacking dendrites and having the smooth contour of sensory neurons. Such elements are absent from the superior cervical ganglion, where NOS immunoreactivity is confined exclusively to preganglionic sympathetic axons (not illustrated).

Effects of NOS Substrate and Antagonist on Chemoreceptor Activity

Basal chemoreceptor activity was established *in vitro* in superfusion media equilibrated with 100% O_2 (see Fig. 2). Under these 'resting' conditions, the NO precursor, L-arginine, did not affect CSN discharge; however, the chemoreceptor response in low O_2 (20%) superfusion media was markedly delayed in the presence of L-arginine, and both the peak and sustained discharge were reduced (Fig. 2A). This inhibition of stimulus-evoked CSN activity by L-arginine was dose related and preparations bathed in basic amino acids which are not substrates for NOS (e.g., D-arginine [1 mM] and L-lysine [1 mM]) displayed normal responses to low O_2 stimuli. Furthermore, the inhibitory effects of L-arginine were completely reversed by the competitive NOS inhibitor, L-N^G-nitroarginine methylester (L-NAME, 1 mM; not shown), suggesting that the inhibition is NOS/NO related, and not due to non-specific metabolic effects.

Additional experiments demonstrated that L-NAME alone, even at relatively low concentrations (0.01 mM, Fig. 2B), augmented the chemosensory response to moderate low O_2 stimuli (40% O_2-equilibrated media, 5 min). This excitatory effect was dose-related and could be reversed by simultaneous administration of excess L-arginine (1 mM). Basal chemoreceptor discharge in 100% O_2-equilibrated superfusion media was slightly enhanced by L-NAME at concentrations up to 1 mM. These experiments suggest that NO may be an endogenous neuroactive agent which tonically inhibits the chemoreceptor response to hypoxia.

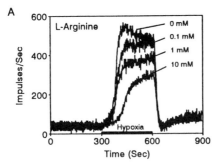
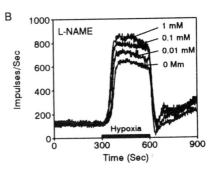

Figure 2. Effect of L-arginine (A) and L-NAME (B) on chemoreceptor activity evoked by hypoxia in superfused cat carotid body.

The Effect of CSN Stimulation on NO Production

The possibility that NOS mediates efferent chemosensory inhibition was further studied in experiments which examined NO production during electrical stimulation of the CSN in superfused carotid body preparations. Because NO is a highly diffusible gas, it is difficult to monitor directly (Bredt & Snyder, 1992). Consequently, we measured instead the production of ^{3}H-citrulline, the by-product of NO synthesis from ^{3}H-arginine (Bredt & Snyder, 1989). The results presented in Table 1 demonstrate that NO production is elevated by electrical stimulation of the CSN (5 V, 1 msec, 20 Hz). Monitoring the stimulus-evoked compound action potentials from the CSN confirmed the activation of C-fibers. In contrast, activation of only CSN A-fibers failed to alter ^{3}H-citrulline formation. Finally, C-fiber activation in the absence of Ca^{2+} also failed to elevate ^{3}H-citrulline production, a finding consistent with the known Ca^{2+} dependency of the NOS enzyme.

Table 1. Effects of CSN Stimulation on NO Synthesis in the Cat Carotid Body

	[^{3}H]Citrulline Formation (dpm/h/mg tissue)	n
Control	777 ± 41	6
A-fiber	808 ± 67	4
C-fiber	1503 ± 133 *	6
C-fiber/Zero Ca^{++}	679 ± 58	4

n represents the number of carotid bodies. * represents $p < 0.01$ vs. control

NO, cGMP and Efferent Inhibition in the Carotid Body

Experiments designed to assess the role of NO in mediating chemosensory inhibition utilized a modification of the perfused/superfused preparation described by Belmonte & Eyzaguirre (1974). Figure 3 presents typical records of multiple chemoreceptor units obtained from nerve filaments split-off from the main CSN trunk. When the low O_2 stimulus was delivered simultaneously with electrical stimulation of the CSN trunk, there was no diminution of the hypoxic response (not shown). However, delivering the low O_2 stimulus 5-10 min after the start of electrical CSN stimulation significantly attenuated both the basal chemoreceptor discharge and the response to low O_2 (compare Fig. 3A with 3B and 3C). Multiple experiments showed that the magnitude of the integrated response to low O_2 was inversely proportional to the length of the preceding period of CSN stimulation. Furthermore, moderate concentrations (0.1 mM) of the NOS antagonist, L-NAME, completely reversed the effects of CSN electrical stimulation (Fig. 3D). Similar experimental trials involving only superfusion of the carotid body revealed that prolonged electrical stimulation of the CSN inhibited the low O_2 response without modifying basal chemoreceptor discharge. These findings suggest that basal chemoreceptor activity measured in perfused/superfused preparations is greatly influenced by the organ's vasculature, while NO appears to exert its effects on the low O_2 response via innervation of the type I cell lobules by NOS-IR afferent fibers.

In parallel experiments, we assessed changes in carotid body cGMP levels evoked by electrical stimulation of the CSN. Our immunocytochemical data demonstrated that brief (1 min) periods of CSN stimulation enhanced cGMP staining primarily in smooth muscle cells surrounding arterioles (compare Fig. 4A and B). Prolonged nerve stimulation (10 or 15 min; Fig. 4C), on the other hand, elevated cGMP levels in type I cells as well. These findings correlate well with the inhibition of basal and low O_2-evoked chemoreceptor activity presented in Figure 3. Furthermore, the changes in cGMP evoked by CSN stimulation could be prevented by the addition of 0.1 mM L-NAME to the bathing media (Fig. 4D), and these effects of L-NAME could be reversed by competing concentrations of L-arginine (1 mM; not shown).

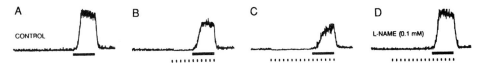

Figure 3. Effect of electrical stimulation (5 V, 1 msec, 20 Hz) of main carotid sinus nerve (CSN) trunk on basal and evoked activity recorded in multiple filaments split off from the CSN. Perfused/superfused cat preparation. (A) Control response to 5 min hypoxic stimulus (solid bar). (B and C) The hypoxic response is inhibited and basal activity depressed by CSN stimulation (dashed line). (D) The inhibition is reversed in the presence of 0.1 mM L-NAME.

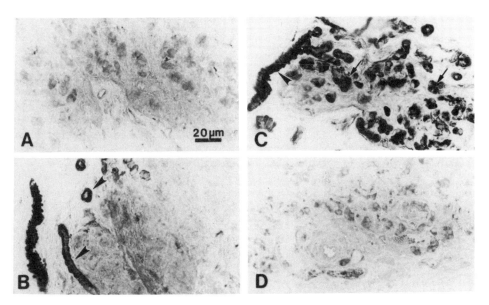

Figure 4. cGMP immunostaining. (A) Levels of cGMP are undetectable in unstimulated cat carotid body. (B) Following C-fiber activation of the CSN for 1 min, cGMP levels are high in vascular smooth muscle (arrowheads) but not in chemosensitive lobules. (C) Nerve stimulation for 15 min elevates cGMP in type I cells (arrows) and small arterioles (arrowheads). (D) In the presence of L-NAME, cGMP levels remain low following 15 min of C-fiber activation.

DISCUSSION

The findings presented here favor the hypothesis that NO mediates CSN inhibition via two neural pathways, which separately modulate blood flow and type I cell activity, respectively. In support of this view are additional immunocytochemical findings showing that NOS-IR neurons located in the periphery of the organ also contain choline acetyltransferase (ChAT), and display dendritic spines and a single axon which projects to the center of the organ (Wang et al., 1993b). Our earlier studies demonstrated that the

NOS-IR innervation of the carotid body vasculature remained largely intact following chronic transection of the CSN and chronic sympathectomy (removal of the superior cervical ganglion; Wang et al., 1993b, 1993c). Together such findings suggest that these NOS-IR neurons are autonomic ganglionic elements which innervate small to medium sized arterioles in the chemosensory tissue.

In contrast, the NOS-IR nerve fibers which penetrate the chemosensory lobules and encircle type I cells disappear following chronic CSN transection (Wang et al., 1993b,1993c). The morphological characteristics of NOS-IR petrosal ganglion neurons, including their smooth, rounded somal surfaces and the absence of dendrites, suggest these are sensory ganglion cells, a conclusion supported by earlier ultrastructural studies which demonstrated the absence of autonomic neurons from this ganglion (Stensaas & Fidone, 1977). In addition, we have shown that NOS-IR petrosal ganglion neurons are `back-labeled' by a fluorescent retrograde tracer applied to the central end of the transected CSN, thus confirming their innervation to the carotid body (Wang et al., 1993b).

The morphological data demonstrating that separate and distinct NOS pathways in the carotid body innervate the vasculature and chemosensory lobules, respectively, is consonant with our pharmacological and physiological observations. In superfused preparations, the chemoreceptor response to hypoxia is inhibited by the NOS substrate, L-arginine, while the NOS antagonist, L-NAME, enhances the response. Furthermore, the elevation of basal chemoreceptor discharge by L-NAME in superfused preparations is potentiated 3-4 fold when the preparation is both perfused/superfused, suggesting that the vascular effects of NO greatly influence basal chemoreceptor activity (Wang et al., 1993c). Likewise, endogenous NO produced by C-fiber activation rapidly depresses basal chemoreceptor discharge in perfused, but not in superfused preparations. The chemoreceptor response to hypoxia is inhibited only by prolonged (>5 min) C-fiber activation, and the time course and magnitude of this effect is similar in both perfused and superfused preparations. Furthermore, the effect is completely reversed in the presence of specific NO antagonists. Collectively, these findings suggest that NO released from autonomic (presumably parasympathetic) fibers mediate vasodilation in the carotid body, which indirectly modulates the steady state activity of type I cells. NO produced and released from afferent fibers, on the other hand, behaves as a retrogradely-acting transmitter, which influences the dynamic response to hypoxia. The distinctly different time course for chemoreceptor inhibition produced by these two NO pathways is reflected by the changes in cGMP which are observable in vascular smooth muscle versus chemosensory type I cells. Moreover, such increases in cGMP evoked by C-fiber stimulation can be reversed by L-NAME.

In conclusion, our data suggest that NO is yet another participant in the dynamic balance between multiple excitatory and inhibitory agents known to influence chemoreceptor activity. NO acts both on the carotid body vasculature and on the chemosensory lobules, and like ANP, its effects are mediated by cGMP. The presence of both ANP and NO within the primary chemoreceptor apparatus suggests that powerful inhibitory mechanisms are important physiological components contributing to the moment-to-moment regulation of chemosensory activity.

REFERENCES

Belmonte, C. & Eyzaguirre, C. (1974) Efferent influences on carotid body chemoreceptors. J. Neurophysiol. 37:1131-1143.

Biscoe, T.J. & Sampson, S.R. (1968) Rhythmical and non-rhythmical spontaneous activity recorded from the central cut end of the sinus nerve. J. Physiol. (Lond.) 196:327-338.

Bredt, D.S. & Snyder, S.H. (1989) Nitric oxide mediates glutamate-linked enhancement of cGMP levels in the cerebellum. Proc. Natl. Acad. Sci. USA 86:9030-9033.

Bredt, D.S. & Snyder, S.H. (1992) Nitric oxide, a novel neuronal messenger. Neuron 8:3-11.

De Castro, F. (1926) Sur la structure el l'innervation de la glande intercarotidienne (glomus caroticum) de l'homme et des mammiferes, et sur un nouveau systeme d'innervation autonome du nerf glosopharyngien. Trabajos Lab. Invest. Biol. Univ. Madrid 24:365-432.

Fidone, S.J. & Sato, A. (1970) Efferent inhibition and antidromic depression of chemoreceptor A-fibers from the cat carotid body. Brain Res. 22:181-193.

Kondo, H. & Yamamoto, M. (1988) Occurrence, ontogeny, ultrastructure and some plasticity of CGRP (calcitonin gene-related peptide)-immunoreactive nerves in the carotid body of rats. Brain Res. 473:283-293.

Kummer, W. & Fischer, A. (1990) Tachykininergic axons in the guinea pig carotid body: origin, ultra-structure and coexistence with other peptides. In "Arterial Chemoreception," C. Eyzaguirre, S.J. Fidone, R.S. Fitzgerald, S. Lahiri & D.M. McDonald, Springer-Verlag, New York, pp. 229-234.

McDonald, D.M. & Mitchell, R.A. (1981) The neural pathway involved in "efferent inhibition" of chemo-receptors in the cat carotid body. J. Comp. Neurol. 201:457-476.

Neil, E. & O'Regan R.G. (1969) Effects of sinus and aortic nerve efferents on arterial chemoreceptor function. J. Physiol. (Lond.) 200:69P-71P.

Neil, E. & O'Regan R.G. (1971) The effects of electrical stimulation of the distal end of the carotid sinus and aortic nerve on peripheral arterial chemoreceptor activity in the cat. J. Physiol. (Lond.) 215:15-32.

O'Regan, R.G. & Majcherczyk, S. (1983) Control of peripheral chemoreceptors by efferent nerves. In "Physiology of the Peripheral Arterial Chemoreceptors." H. Acker & R.G. O'Regan, eds., Elsevier, pp. 257-298.

Stensaas, L.J. & Fidone, S.J. (1977) An ultrastructural study of cat petrosal ganglia: a search for autonomic ganglion cells. Brain Res. 124:29-39.

Wang, W.-J., Cheng, G.-F., Yoshizaki, K., Dinger, B. & Fidone, S. (1991a) The role of cyclic AMP in chemoreception in the rabbit carotid body. Brain Res. 540:96-104.

Wang, W.-J., He, L., Chen, J, Dinger, B. & Fidone, S. (1993a) Mechanisms underlying chemoreceptor inhibition induced by atrial natriuretic peptide in rabbit carotid body. J. Physiol. 460:427-441.

Wang, Z.-Z., Bredt, D.S., Fidone, S.J. & Stensaas, L.J. (1993b) Neurons synthesizing nitric oxide innervating the carotid body. J. Comp. Neurol. 336:419-432.

Wang, Z.-Z., Bredt, D.S., Dinger, B.G., Fidone, S.J. & Stensaas, L.J. (1993c) Localization and actions of nitric oxide in the cat carotid body. Neurosci. (in press).

Wang, Z.-Z., He, L., Stensaas, L.J., Dinger, B.G. & Fidone, S.J. (1991b) Localization and in vitro actions of atrial natriuretic peptide in the cat carotid body. J. Appl. Physiol. 70:942-946.

Wang, Z.-Z., Stensaas, L.J., Wang, W.-J., Dinger, B., de Vente, J. and Fidone, S.J. (1992) Atrial natriuretic peptide increases cyclic guanosine monophosphate immunoreactivity in the carotid body. Neurosci. 49:479-486.

Yamamoto, A., Kimura, S., Hasui, K., Fujisawa, Y., Tamaki, T., Fukui, K., Iwao, H. & Yonichi, A. (1988) Calcitonin gene-related peptide (CGRP) stimulates the release of atrial natriuretic peptide (ANP) from isolated rat atria. Biochem. Biophys. Res. Comm. 155:1452-1458.

PROPORTIONAL SENSITIVITY OF ARTERIAL CHEMORECEPTORS TO CO_2

P. Kumar,[1] P.C.G. Nye,[2] and R.W. Torrance[3]

[1] Department of Physiology, University of Birmingham B15 2TJ
[2] University Laboratory of Physiology, Oxford OX1 3PT
[3] St John's College, Oxford OX1 3JP

INTRODUCTION

It is still discussed whether the arterial chemoreceptors behave as rate receptors (Linton & Band, 1988) or as adapting proportional receptors (Black et al., 1971) in their response to CO_2. The question arises because the amplitude of their response to an oscillating CO_2 stimulus (Goodman et al., 1974) is much greater than would be expected if they were proportional receptors which do no more than follow the appropriate straight CO_2 response line of a Fitzgerald and Parks (1971) fan. To test this we have made the CO_2 stimulus vary over a fourfold range of rates by making it follow a symmetrical sawtooth cycle which repeatedly rose and fell linearly. The cycle length was 5, 10, 20 or 40s but its amplitude was usually the same so the rate of change of stimulus varied eightfold. If then the response is determined by the rate of change of stimulus the response should have alternated between two steady levels and the amplitude of the alternation should have varied over a eightfold range.

METHODS AND RESULTS

We used the ventilator and methods of dissection of Kumar et al. (1988). In open chest cats under pentobarbitone the alveolar PCO_2 or PO_2 was made to follow a sawtooth cycle with the mean P_ACO_2 and P_AO_2 at about 40 Torr and 65 Torr respectively. The cycles of discharge thus produced in single or few-fibre preparations of the sinus nerve were recorded and then summed over several cycles.

The shape of the cycles of discharge was broadly sawtooth with the rise and fall of equal but opposite slopes. Discharge did not alternate between two steady levels. The amplitude of the oscillations in discharge decreased when the rate of change of the stimulus was increased by reducing the length of the stimulus cycle (Fig. 1).

Sometimes the cycles of stimulus were not all of equal amplitude and so the overall response amplitudes could not be compared. Instead the change of response per change of stimulus half way through the rise or fall of the sawtooth was measured to give the slope of the CO_2 response curve. It was greater in the slower cycles than in the fast ones. The slope of build up of the CO_2 response in the long 40s cycles might decrease late in the build up.

The response to a cycle of PO_2 was like a catenary: it changed more rapidly when it was near to its peak. This is to be expected because the Po_2 was changed linearly but the response curve to PO_2 is hyperbolic.

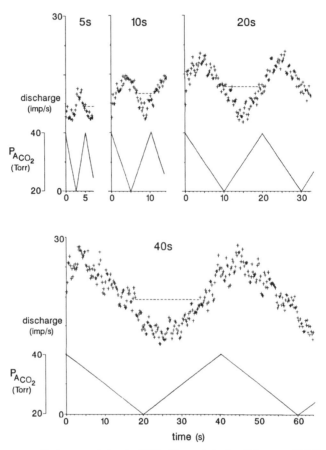

Figure 1. Chemoreceptor discharge and alveolar PCO_2 (drawn in by hand) in an artificially ventilated cat. Sawtooth stimuli given at four different cycle durations reveal no hint of rate sensitivity of discharge. Mean discharge at each cycle duration is shown by the dashed horizontal lines.

CONCLUSIONS

The response of chemoreceptors to a sawtooth of PO_2 is that to be expected from the steady-state responses to PO_2. The response to a sawtooth of PCO_2 is not that of a rate receptor but rather that of an adapting proportional receptor which its responses to step changes of stimulus had shown it to be (Black et al., 1971). It does not adapt quickly enough to make it approximate to a rate receptor during respiratory changes of PCO_2.

This work was supported by the Medical Research Council.

REFERENCES

Black, A.M.S., McCloskey, D.I. & Torrance, R.W. (1971). The responses of peripheral chemoreceptors in the cat to sudden changes of hypercapnic and hypoxic stimuli. Respir. Physiol. 13:36-49.

Fitzgerald, R.S. & Parks, D.C. (1971). Effect of hypoxia on carotid chemoreceptor response to carbon dioxide in cats. Resp. Physiol. 12:218-229.

Goodman, N.W., Nail, B.S. & Torrance, R.W. (1974). Oscillations in the discharge of single carotid chemoreceptor fibres of the cat. Respir. Physiol. 20:251-269.

Kumar, P., Nye, P.C.G. & Torrance, R.W. (1988). Do oxygen tension variations contribute to the respiratory oscillations of chemoreceptor discharge in the cat? J. Physiol. 395:531-552.

Linton, R.A.F. & Band, D.M. (1988). The relationship between arterial pH and chemoreceptor firing in anaesthetized cats. Resp. Physiol. 74:49-54.

EFFECTS OF EXPIRATORY DURATION ON CHEMORECEPTOR OSCILLATIONS

R. W. Torrance, R. Iturriaga and P. Zapata

Laboratory of Neurobiology, Catholic University of Chile, Santiago, Chile

INTRODUCTION

We have studied the effect of suddenly altering the duration of expiration (T_E) on the variations in the frequency of chemosensory discharges (f_x) with respiration.

Linton and Band (1988) have asserted that the amplitude of the respiratory oscillations in the discharge of arterial chemoreceptors may be independent of the frequency of alveolar ventilation between 14 and 20 cycles/min, and so of T_E. From this, they have argued that the chemoreceptors should be regarded as responding to the rate of change of their stimulus within the time-scale of a breath rather than to its actual value, since it is the rate of change of the stimulus during expiration that is independent of T_E, whereas the amplitude of the change, in contrast, is linearly dependent on T_E.

We (Goodman et al., 1974), however, and others have found that the amplitude of the oscillation in discharge is greater when respiratory frequency is reduced and so T_E is increased. Also we found that the time course of discharge within one cycle matched the actual course of the alveolar stimulus rather than its rate of change (Kumar et al., 1988).

The rise in the oscillation in discharge is attributed to the rise in the stimulus during expiration. If, then, in a regularly ventilated cat, a single expiration were lengthened by delaying an inflation of the lungs, the discharge of a proportional receptor would show an increased amplitude of its oscillation for one breath, whereas a differential one, such as Linton and Band (1988) assert, would show an unchanged amplitude.

METHODS AND OBSERVATIONS

We recorded f_x in carotid nerve multifibre preparations from cats anesthetized with pentobarbitone, paralysed with alcuronium, thermostabilized at 38.0°C, tracheally intubated and ventilated with positive pressure pumps, providing constant durations of inspiration (T_I). Ventilation was recorded by means of a pneumotachograph.

One type of experiment consisted in ventilating with a pump providing $T_I = T_E$ and which could be disconnected from the cat for one or more inflations. With one inflation omitted, discharge built up for longer and reached a higher peak. Since $T_E = T_I$, omitting one inflation trebled T_E. Peaks in chemosensory discharge were proportionally higher with 2 to 5 inflations omitted (Fig. 1A).

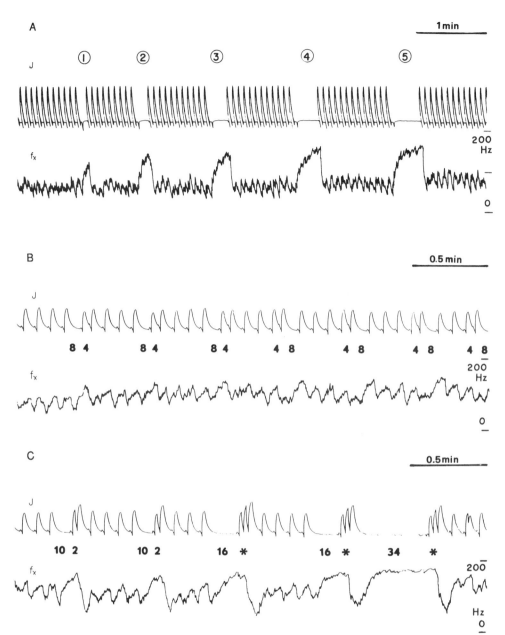

Figure 1. Recordings of ventilatory flow (J) and instantaneous frequency of carotid chemosensory discharges (f_X; scales = 0-200 Hz). **A.** Cat ventilated at 14 cycles/min, with $T_I = T_E$. Effects of omitting forced inspirations from 1 to 5 cycles (encircled numbers). **B,C.** Cat ventilated by directing a stream of air into the tracheal tube for 1 s (T_I), interspersed by periods in which the tube was open to room air (T_E). Effects of variations in T_E by advancing or postponing the 1-s period of lung inflation. Total length of ventilatory cycles = 6 s, except those indicated by numbers underneath. Prolonged cycles (16 and 34 s) followed by twin compensatory cycles (asterisks) of 2-s lengths.

The other type of experiment consisted in producing inflations by directing a steady stream of air into the lungs for 1 s. A single inflation within the regular series was brought in early or late, making T_E shorter or longer, for one cycle. With T_E lengthened, discharge continued rising longer and it reached a higher level (Fig. 1B,C). If T_E was shortened, the rise was less (Fig. 1B). With T_E much longer, the rise slowed (ca. 5 s) and reached a plateau (ca. 15 s) (Fig. 1C).

DISCUSSION

The time course within one breath of regular respiratory oscillations in chemoreceptor discharge is easily explained if the receptor responds proportionally. The present results with acute changes in the time course of a single breath agree with this. When T_E was lengthened and so alveolar gas tensions approached asymptotically venous level, discharge rose for longer and then plateaued. It did not fall even though the rate of rise of the stimulus must have decreased markedly late in expiration with a long T_E.

Two things contribute to the discharge plateau: (1) the stimulus tends to a plateau when T_E is long; (2) the receptor adapts to CO_2 with a half time of 5-10 s.

The oscillation in discharge with spontaneous respiration is great because the stimulus cycle lasts only a few seconds in normal respiration. The degree of adaptation therefore changes little during one breath and so the response follows a steep transient curve rather than a flatter steady state one. Only with distinctly slower changes of stimulus than those within one breath do changes in the degree of adaptation determine the course of responses enough to make the receptor approximate to a rate receptor.

This work was supported by grant 1930645 from FONDECYT, Chile.

REFERENCES

Goodman, N.W., Nail, B.S. & Torrance, R.W. (1974). Oscillations in the discharge of single carotid chemoreceptor fibres in the cat. Respir. Physiol. 20:251-270.

Kumar, P., Nye, P.C.G. & Torrance, R.W. (1988). Do oxygen variations contribute to the respiratory oscillations of chemoreceptor discharge in the cat? J. Physiol. (Lond.) 395:531-552.

Linton, R.A.F. & Band, D.M. (1988). The relationship between arterial pH and chemoreceptor firing in anaesthetized cats. Respir. Physiol. 74:49-54.

EFFECTS OF INTRAVENOUS INFUSIONS OF KCl AND LACTIC ACID ON CHEMORECEPTOR DISCHARGE IN ANAESTHETIZED CATS

P. McLoughlin[2], R. A. F. Linton[1] and D. M. Band[1].

[1]Laboratory of Applied Physiology, United Medical and Dental School, St. Thomas's Hospital, Lambeth Palace Road, London SE1 7EH, UK; [2]Department of Human Anatomy and Physiology, University College, Earlsfort Terrace, Dublin 2, Ireland

INTRODUCTION

We have previously reported that infusion of KCl and lactic acid together led to a greater increase in ventilation, in anaesthetized cats, than infusion of lactic acid alone (McLoughlin et al., 1993). A similar interaction may provide an important drive to ventilation during heavy exercise, which causes both metabolic acidosis and arterial hyperkalaemia (McLoughlin et al., 1990). Increasing $[K^+]_a$ stimulates ventilation solely through its action on the peripheral chemoreceptors (Linton & Band, 1985). Metabolic acidosis also stimulates ventilation through an action on the peripheral chemoreceptors (Bainton, 1978). It seems likely, therefore, that the interactive effect of the two stimuli on ventilation is mediated via these receptors.

The present series of experiments was undertaken to compare the effect on carotid chemoreceptor discharge of intravenous infusion of lactic acid alone with that of infusion of lactic acid in combination with KCl, in anaesthetized, artificially ventilated cats.

METHODS

Six cats (weight 2.2 - 3.5 kg) were anaesthetized with intraperitoneal pentobarbitone (40 mg/kg) plus intravenous supplementation as required. The animals' temperature was maintained at 37.0°C. They were paralysed with alcuronium and ventilated (Ideal Respiration Pump, Palmer London) to maintain $P_{ET}CO_2$ constant (14 breaths/min). Air flow was monitored with a pneumotachograph (Fleisch) and strain gauge pressure transducer (Statham). The resultant flow signal was electrically integrated to give tidal volume. End-tidal gas composition was measured by a mass spectrometer (BOC Medishield). Cannulae were inserted into the jugular veins for infusion of drugs and solutions. Blood pressure was monitored using a strain gauge pressure transducer (Bell and Howell) connected to a cannula introduced into the brachial artery. This cannula was also used for intermittent sampling of arterial blood. A H^+ selective catheter electrode was placed in the abdominal aorta through a femoral artery. An external silver/silver chloride reference electrode was connected to a saline filled catheter which was introduced into the inferior vena cava via a

Arterial Chemoreceptors: Cell to System
Edited by R. O'Regan *et al*, Plenum Press, New York, 1994

femoral vein. The tip of this electrode lay in the inferior vena cava at the same level as the ion selective electrode. Afferent chemoreceptor activity was recorded from a few fibre preparation (2 - 4 fibres) of the cut right carotid sinus nerve. All signal outputs were recorded on paper (Gould Elecrostatic ES1000) for later analysis.

Two infusion protocols were completed in each cat. Following a control period of one minute, lactic acid (0.5 mmol/kg in 5 ml of distilled water) was infused over a period of one minute either alone or together with KCl (0.15 mmol/kg). The order of the infusions was randomised. A minimum of thirty minutes elapsed between each infusion and $NaHCO_3$ was administered as required to correct the metabolic acidosis. $[K^+]_a$ was allowed to return to control values spontaneously. Arterial blood samples were taken during the control periods and between seconds 40 - 50 of the infusions.

Ventilation, $P_{ET}CO_2$ and pH_a were measured breath by breath throughout each experiment. The mean discharge rate and the amplitude of oscillations in chemoreceptor discharge throughout the respiratory cycle were described by best fit, least squares, sine waves (Band et al., 1978). In the control period all breaths were included in the sine wave fitting. During the infusion protocols the mean carotid sinus discharge rate had, in all experiments, achieved greater than 90% of its maximum 17 s after the beginning of the infusion. Therefore, respiratory cycles beginning after this time were included in the fitting of sine waves. Because chemoreceptor activity was recorded from multi-fibre preparations which had differing baseline firing rates, the changes produced in the mean discharge rates and in the amplitude of oscillations during the experimental protocols were expressed as ratios (mean experimental discharge/mean control discharge and mean experimental amplitude/mean control amplitude).

RESULTS

Mean pH_a, P_aCO_2, P_aO_2 and $[K^+]_a$, measured by sampling of blood during the control periods were similar. Infusion of KCl together with lactic acid caused $[K^+]_a$ to increase from a mean ($\pm$ S.E.M.) control value of 3.0 ($\pm$ 0.1) mmol/l to 5.5 ($\pm$ 0.1) mmol/l. Mean pH_a (7.235 $\pm$ 0.004 vs 7.241 $\pm$ 0.006), P_aCO_2 (37.4 $\pm$ 0.9 vs 36.4 $\pm$ 0.6 mmHg) and P_aO_2 (114.1 $\pm$ 3.2 vs 113.3 $\pm$ 2.3 mmHg) measured at the end of the combined infusion protocol were not significantly different from the mean values during the lactic acid alone infusion (P > 0.05, Paired t test).

The mean (range) and amplitude of chemoreceptor discharge for the group (n = 6), during the control period prior to infusion of lactic acid alone, were 3.0 (1.7 - 4.1) imp/s and 2.0 (1.2 -3.2) imp/s respectively. These values did not differ significantly (P > 0.05, Wilcoxon Signed-Rank test) from the mean, 3.5 (1.9 - 7.8) imp/s, and amplitude, 2.0 (1.2 - 3.2) imp/s, prior to the infusion of lactic acid and KCl together. Infusion of lactic acid alone caused the mean firing rate (range) to increase to 1.9 (1.6 -2.3) times the control value while the combined infusion of lactic acid and KCl led to an increase of 2.2 (1.8 -2.7) times control (P < 0.05, Wilcoxon Signed-Rank test). The amplitude of oscillation of chemoreceptor discharge rose by a factor of 2.1 (1.3 - 3.2) times the control value during the infusion of lactic acid alone while the combined infusion protocol produced an increase of 3.3 (2.2 - 5.1) times the control value (P < 0.05, Wilcoxon Signed-Rank test).

DISCUSSION

When KCl was infused together with lactic acid both the increase in mean firing and in the amplitude of the oscillations in firing were greater than when lactic acid alone was infused. The lactic acid infusions caused an increase in carbon dioxide production (double resting value), a fall in pH_a and a slight rise in P_aCO_2. Reductions in pH_a and elevations of P_aCO_2 stimulate the peripheral arterial chemoreceptors (Lahiri et al., 1983), while increased carbon dioxide production alters the pattern of chemoreceptor discharge (Linton & Band,

1988). The simultaneous elevation of $[K^+]_a$ may have interacted with each of these effects of lactic acid administration and led to the altered chemoreceptor response observed.

Band and Linton (1989), using an extracorporeal gas exchanger, have previously shown, in anaesthetized cats, that elevation of $[K^+]_a$ increases both the mean and the amplitude of oscillation of carotid chemoreceptor discharge in response to intravenous CO_2 loading. The increases in $[K^+]_a$ and carbon dioxide production during the infusions of lactic acid reported here were similar to those observed during the intravenous CO_2 loading reported by Band and Linton. The changes in the mean and amplitude of oscillation of chemoreceptor discharge were also similar. This suggests that an interaction between increased $[K^+]_a$ and the increased CO_2 production due to the infusion of lactic acid may have contributed importantly to the alteration in chemoreceptor discharge observed in the present series of experiments.

The magnitude of the changes in pH_a and $[K^+]_a$ and BE produced in these experiments is similar to that observed in exercising humans (McLoughlin et al., 1990). It is important to note that the approximate doubling of resting carbon dioxide production, caused by these lactic acid infusions, is a small change compared to the 20 - 30 fold increases seen in heavy exercise. An interactive effect of changing pH_a, $[K^+]_a$ and carbon dioxide production on peripheral chemoreceptor discharge, similar to that demonstrated in these anaesthetized animals, may provide an important drive to ventilation during heavy exercise.

We are grateful to the Wellcome Trust for supporting this work. P. McLoughlin was a Wellcome Trust Research Fellow.

REFERENCES

Bainton, C.R. (1978). Canine ventilation after acid-base infusions, exercise, and carotid body denervation. J. Appl. Physiol. 44: 28-35.

Band, D.M., M. McClelland, D.L. Phillips, K.B. Saunders & C. B. Wolff. (1978). Sensitivity of the carotid body to within-breath changes in arterial PCO_2. J. Appl. Physiol. 45: 768-777.

Lahiri, S., N.J. Smatresk & E. Mulligan. (1983). Responses of peripheral chemoreceptors to natural stimuli. In. "Physiology of the peripheral arterial chemoreceptors". H. Acker & R.G. O'Regan, eds., Elsevier Science Publications, Amsterdam.

Linton, R.A.F. & D.M. Band. (1985). The effect of potassium on carotid chemoreceptor activity and ventilation in the cat. Respir. Physiol. 59: 65-70.

Linton, R.A.F. & D.M. Band. (1988). The relationship between arterial pH and chemoreceptor firing in anaesthetized cats. Respir. Physiol. 74: 49-54.

McLoughlin, P., P. Popham, R.C.H. Bruce, R.A.F. Linton & D.M. Band. (1990). Plasma potassium and the ventilatory threshold in man. J. Physiol. 427: 44P.

McLoughlin, P., R.A.F. Linton & D.M. Band. (1991). The effect of potassium and lactic acid on ventilation in anaesthetized cats. Respir. Physiol. 95(2):171-180.

THE EFFECT OF INTRAVENOUS INFUSION OF LACTIC ACID ON CAROTID CHEMORECEPTOR DISCHARGE IN ANAESTHETIZED CATS VENTILATED WITH ROOM AIR OR 100% O$_2$

P. McLoughlin[2,] R. A. F. Linton[1] and D. M. Band.[1]

[1] Laboratory of Applied Physiology, United Medical and Dental School,
St. Thomas's Hospital, Lambeth Palace Road, London SE1 7EH, UK;
[2] Department of Human Anatomy and Physiology, University College,
Earlsfort Terrace, Dublin 2, Ireland

INTRODUCTION

It has been suggested that the responses of the peripheral arterial chemoreceptors to physiological stimuli are effectively abolished at high P_aO_2 (Cunningham 1987; Dejours 1962; Ward & Bellville 1983). Consequently, inspiration of hyperoxic gas mixtures has been widely used to silence the peripheral chemoreceptors in order to assess their contribution to the control of ventilation (e.g. Conway & Petersen 1987; Holtby et al., 1988; Rausch et al., 1991). More recently, Dahan et al. (1990) have suggested that 100% O$_2$ does not silence the peripheral chemoreceptor response to increases in P_aCO_2 in man. Furthermore, Kozlowski et al. (1971) reported that lesser degrees of hyperoxia do not abolish peripheral chemoreceptor drives. These findings call into question the hypothesis that hyperoxia abolishes the peripheral arterial chemoreceptor responses to physiological stimuli. In particular, the response of these receptors to metabolic acidosis, such as occurs during heavy exercise, may not be silenced.

The experiments reported here were undertaken to examine the effect on carotid chemoreceptor discharge of infusions of lactic acid in anaesthetized cats, ventilated with either room air or 100% O$_2$. $P_{ET}CO_2$ was maintained constant throughout the experiments. The infusion protocols were designed to produce changes in pH_a similar, in both magnitude and time course, to those seen during the onset of heavy exercise in humans.

METHODS

Six cats (weight 2.6 - 3.5 kg) were anaesthetized with intraperitoneal pentobarbitone (40 mg/kg) plus intravenous supplementation as required. The animals' temperature was maintained at 37.0°C. They were paralysed with alcuronium and ventilated (Ideal Respiration Pump, Palmer London) to maintain $P_{ET}CO_2$ constant (14 breaths/min). Air flow was monitored with a pneumotachograph (Fleisch) and strain gauge pressure transducer (Statham). The resultant flow signal was electrically integrated to give tidal volume. Ventilation was calculated breath by breath. End-tidal gas composition was measured by mass spectrometer (BOC Medishield). Cannulae were inserted into the jugular veins for infusion of drugs and solutions. Blood pressure was monitored using a strain gauge pressure transducer (Bell and Howell) connected to a cannula introduced into the brachial artery. This cannula was also used for intermittent sampling of arterial blood. A H^+ selective catheter electrode was placed in the abdominal aorta through a femoral artery. An external silver/silver chloride reference electrode was connected to a saline filled catheter which was introduced into the inferior vena cava via a femoral vein. The tip of this electrode lay in the inferior vena cava at the same level as the ion selective electrode. Afferent chemoreceptor activity was recorded from a few fibre preparation (2 - 4 fibres) of the cut right carotid sinus nerve. All signal outputs were recorded on paper (Gould Electrostatic ES1000) for later analysis.

Two infusion protocols were completed in each cat. Following a control period of one minute, lactic acid (0.5 mmol/kg in 5 ml of distilled water) was infused into the vena cava over a period of one minute while the cat was ventilated with room air or 100% O_2. The order of the infusions was randomised. Ventilation with 100% O_2 was begun 5 minutes before the start of the acid infusion in the hyperoxic trials. A minimum of thirty minutes elapsed between each infusion and $NaHCO_3$ was administered as required to correct the metabolic acidosis. Arterial blood samples were taken during the control periods and between seconds 40 - 50 of the infusions.

Throughout each experiment average discharge rates of the chemoreceptor fibres were determined breath by breath (number of discharge spikes/duration of breath in seconds). Since chemoreceptor afferents were recorded from multi-fibre preparations, the baseline discharge rates differed between preparations. Thus discharge rates were standardised, before further analysis was undertaken, by expressing firing during the experimental period as a ratio, value during each breath/average discharge rate while ventilated with room air during the one minute period immediately prior to the experimental protocol (i.e. when animals were ventilated with air, the average discharge rate during the 1 minute before acid infusion and when animals were ventilated with 100% O_2 the average discharge rate, while breathing air, immediately before switching to 100% O_2). The average of the resultant standardised values was determined, in each animal, for the one minute period prior to the infusion and over the last 30 s of the infusion protocol. The mean (range) of the individual average discharge rates was determined for the group (n = 6) during ventilation with 100% O_2 before acid infusion and during both acid infusion protocols.

RESULTS

Results of analyses of blood samples are presented as means (± S.E.M.). pH_a, P_aCO_2, and $[K^+]_a$, measured while the cats were ventilated with air or 100% O_2, before acid infusion, were similar. At the end of the acid infusions there was still no significant difference, depending on whether the cats were ventilated with air ($P_aO_2 = 115 \pm 2$ mmHg) or 100% O_2 ($P_aO_2 = 568 \pm 45$ mmHg), between the respective values of pH_a (7.211 ± 0.018 vs 7.202 ± 0.023), P_aCO_2 (36.1 ±0.9 vs 35.4 ± 2.1 mmHg) and $[K^+]_a$ (3.1 ± 0.1 vs 3.1 ± 0.1 mmol/l)

The mean (range) discharge rate for the group (n = 6) during the last 30 s of the acid infusion, while the cats were ventilated with air, rose significantly (P < 0.05, Wilcoxon Signed-Rank Test) to 2.39 (1.75 - 2.90) times the control rate in air. Ventilation with 100% O_2, before acid infusion, caused chemoreceptor discharge to fall significantly (P < 0.05, Wilcoxon Signed-Rank Test) to a mean of 0.19 (0.12 - 0.4) times the control value in air. Subsequent infusion of lactic acid led to an increase to 1.54 (0.75 - 3.46) times the control value. This discharge rate was significantly greater than that prior to acid infusion while ventilated with 100% O_2 (P < 0.05, Wilcoxon Signed-Rank Test).

In 5 of the 6 cats standardised chemoreceptor discharge during each breath was plotted against pH_a measured by the intravascular electrode. In one animal this was not possible due to technical difficulties with the pH electrode. The mean ($\pm$ S.E.M) slope in air (-12.2 $\pm$ 2.1) was similar (P > 0.05, Paired t Test) to that in hyperoxia (-11.0 $\pm$ 3.0).

DISCUSSION

Rapid isocapnic changes in pH_a, produced by infusion of lactic acid, caused significant increases in carotid chemoreceptor discharge in these anaesthetized cats when ventilated with either air or 100% O_2. Furthermore, the similarity of the slopes of the plots of chemoreceptor discharge against pH_a in both air and hyperoxia suggests that the sensitivity of the chemoreceptor to alterations in pH_a is similar in both circumstances, although the absolute discharge rate at a given pH_a is less in hyperoxia. It is important to note that these plots do not represent steady state responses. However, since the infusion protocols used under the two different experimental conditions were the same and produced similar patterns of change in pHa, use of the fitted regression lines allows valid comparisons under the present experimental conditions.

Hornbein and Roos (1963) and Pokorski and Lahiri (1983) have previously demonstrated that the peripheral chemoreceptors respond to isocapnic acidosis in hyperoxia. However, both groups examined steady state responses, several minutes after the administration of acid or alkali. The present series of experiments demonstrates significant responses to rapid changes in pH_a, similar to those seen in human subjects during heavy exercise. If human peripheral chemoreceptors are similarly responsive to metabolic acidosis, then inhalation of 100% O_2 (or lesser degrees of hyperoxia) clearly would not abolish their contribution to ventilatory drive in heavy exercise.

We are grateful to the Wellcome Trust for supporting this work. P. McLoughlin was a Wellcome Trust Research Fellow.

REFERENCES

Conway, M. A. & E. S. Petersen. (1987). Effects of beta-adrenergic blockade on the ventilatory responses to hypoxic and hyperoxic exercise in man. J. Physiol. (Lond.). 393: 43-55.

Cunningham, D. J. C. (1987). Studies on arterial chemoreceptors in man. J. Physiol. 384: 1-26.

Dahan, A., J. DeGoede, A. Berkenbosch & I. C. Olievier. (1990). The influence of oxygen on the ventilatory response to carbon dioxide in man. J. Physiol (Lond.). 428: 485-99.

Dejours, P. (1962). Chemoreflexes in breathing. Physiol. Rev. 42: 335-358.

Holtby, S. G., D. J. Berezanski & N. R. Anthonisen. (1988). Effect of 100% O_2 on hypoxic eucapnic ventilation. J Appl. Physiol. 65(3): 1157-62.

Hornbein, T. F. & A. Roos. (1963). Specificity of H^+ ion concentration as a carotid chemoreceptor stimulus. J. Appl. Physiol. 18: 580-584.

Kozlowski, S., B. Rasmussen & W. G. Wilkoff. (1971). The effect of high oxygen tensions on ventilation during severe exercise. Acta Physiol. Scand. 81: 385-395.

Pokorski, M. & S. Lahiri. (1983). Aortic and carotid chemoreceptor responses to metabolic acidosis in the cat. Am. J. Physiol. 244: 652-8.

Rausch, S. M., B. J. Whipp, K. Wasserman & A. Huszczuk. (1991). Role of the carotid bodies in the respiratory compensation for the metabolic acidosis of exercise in humans. J. Physiol (Lond.). 444: 567-578.

Ward, S. A. & J. W. Bellville. (1983). Peripheral chemoreceptor suppression by hyperoxia during moderate exercise in man, in:: "Modelling and control of breathing." B. J. Whipp and D. M. Wiberg, eds. Elsevier Science Publishing, New York.

THE CAROTID BODIES AS THERMOSENSORS: EXPERIMENTS *IN VITRO* AND *IN SITU*, AND IMPORTANCE FOR VENTILATORY REGULATION

P. Zapata, C. Larraín, R. Iturriaga and J. Alcayaga

Laboratory of Neurobiology, Catholic University of Chile, Santiago, Chile

INTRODUCTION

The carotid bodies are not only sensitive to changes in the chemical composition of the blood, but also to changes in flow, osmolality and temperature (Eyzaguirre & Zapata, 1984). We have been searching for the capability of carotid body chemoreceptors to detect thermal changes within or close to the physiological range and the possibility that they could contribute to the ventilatory adjustments to hyperthermic conditions.

THERMOSENSITIVITY OF CAROTID BODIES *IN VITRO*

Experiments with cat carotid bodies superfused *in vitro* demonstrate that the frequency of chemosensory discharges (f_x) is highly dependent on bath temperature, as shown by the high energies of apparent activation (μ) and high thermal coefficients (Q_{10}) exhibited by these receptors (Gallego et al., 1979). When exposed to nearly rectangular thermal variations, the carotid bodies exhibit both dynamic and static components in their fx responses (Eyzaguirre & Zapata, 1984).

We (Alcayaga et al., 1993) have recently studied the f_x of carotid bodies superfused at different steady state temperatures. Their thermal sensitivity was dependent on the oxygenation and flow rate of the superfusing saline (Fig. 1A). The results obtained indicate that the basal mean f_x is capable of detecting 0.5°C differences in temperature between 36.0 and 38.5°C. Furthermore, the larger gains for the dependency of f_x levels on temperature degrees were obtained close to the range of fluctuations of the cat's core body temperature (T_b).

In summary, experiments *in vitro* demonstrate that the carotid bodies may be considered as potential thermosensors and that higher thermal modulation of their chemosensory discharges is attained within a range close to physiological conditions.

THERMOSENSITIVITY OF CAROTID BODIES *IN SITU*

Increasing the temperature of the blood perfusing the vascularly isolated carotid bifurcations of dogs induces transient hyperventilation (Bernthal & Weeks, 1939). Later recordings of carotid (sinus) nerves during local warming of the blood circulating through cat's carotid bifurcations confirmed transient increases in f_x (McQueen & Eyzaguirre, 1974).

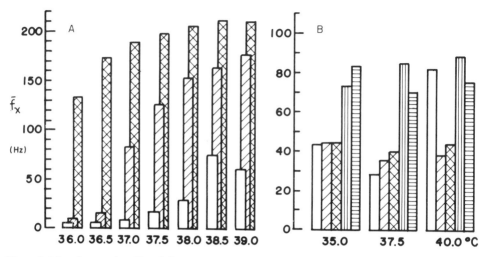

Figure 1. Mean frequencies of basal chemosensory discharges (fx). **A.** One carotid body superfused in vitro with saline equilibrated with 100% O_2 at 3 different flows (open bars, 1.5 ml/min; hatched bars, 1.0 ml/min; cross-hatched bars, 0.4 ml/min) maintained at different bath temperatures. Consistent increases in fx were obtained while raising temperature. **B.** Carotid bodies in situ from 5 different cats under controlled artificial ventilation ($P_{ET}CO_2$ kept ca 35 Torr) at 3 different Tb's. There are no significant changes in fx between different thermal conditions.

In pentobarbitone-anaesthetized cats, we (Loyola et al., 1991) observed that raising Tb from 35 to 40°C induced mild increases in f_x in some cats, more commonly after severing the contralateral carotid nerve. We assumed that fx could be enhanced by the increased T_b, but depressed by the reduced levels of chemical stimuli resulting from hyperthermic hyperventilation.

The above observations led us to study f_x in artificially ventilated cats, in which the end tidal pressure of carbon dioxide ($P_{ET}CO_2$) was allowed to fluctuate with changes in T_b or kept constant by modifying the rate of the ventilator. Animals maintained sequentially at hypothermic (ca 35.0°C), normothermic (ca 37.5°C) and hyperthermic (ca 40.0°C) levels showed proportional rises in $P_{ET}CO_2$ and f_x, but if $P_{ET}CO_2$ was kept constant no significant changes in f_x were observed (Fig. 1B). Thus, although the carotid bodies may subserve the role of thermosensors, their discharges are not consistently modified by hyperthermia when changes in levels of chemical stimuli are compensated by modifying alveolar ventilation.

IMPORTANCE FOR VENTILATORY REGULATION

The depth and rate of ventilation are increased when the T_b of pentobarbitone anaesthetized, spontaneously ventilating cats is raised from 37 to 40°C (Fadic et al., 1991).

Therefore, we studied whether the ventilatory output was modified by changing T_b in pentobarbitone anaesthetized, paralyzed, artificially ventilated cats, in which the ventilator setting could be adjusted to maintain $P_{ET}CO_2$ within the normal range. Recording the integrated electroneurogram (IENG) of one phrenic branch revealed that the inspiratory burst duration was reduced as Tb was raised from 35 to 40°C; the phrenic IENG amplitude was also reduced at 40°C, as compared to 37.5°C. Otherwise, brief exposures to 100% O_2

breathing showed transient falls in f_x and phrenic ENG amplitude at hypothermic, normothermic and hyperthermic levels, an indication that the chemosensory drive of ventilation is preserved under the three conditions. Furthermore, i.v. injections of NaCN augmented f_x and phrenic IENG amplitude in a dose-related manner, but the response of phrenic discharges did not increase during hyperthermia. Thus, relationships between f_x and IENG were not modified during normocapnic hyperthermia.

Summing up, although the carotid bodies have the intrinsic properties of dynamic and tonic thermosensors, they play a minor role in the ventilatory adaptive reactions to sustained hyperthermia.

Work supported by grants 92-0652 and 1930645 from FONDECYT.

REFERENCES

Alcayaga, J., Sanhueza, Y. & Zapata, P. (1993). Thermal dependence of chemosensory activity in the carotid body superfused in vitro. Brain Res. 600:103-111.

Bernthal, T. & Weeks, W.F. (1939). Respiratory and vasomotor effects of variations in carotid body temperature. Am. J. Physiol. 127:94-105.

Eyzaguirre, C. & Zapata, P. (1984). Perspectives in carotid body research. J. Appl. Physiol. 57:931-957.

Fadic, R., Larrain, C. & Zapata, P. (1991). Thermal effects on ventilation in cats. Participation of carotid body chemoreceptors. Respir. Physiol. 86:51-63.

Gallego, R., Eyzaguirre, C. & Monti-Bloch, L. (1979). Thermal and osmotic responses of arterial receptors. J. Neurophysiol. 42:665-680.

Loyola, H., Fadic, R., Cardenas, H., Larrain, C. & Zapata, P. (1991). Effects of body temperature on chemosensory activity of the cat carotid body in situ. Neurosci. Lett. 132: 251-254.

McQueen, D.S. & Eyzaguirre, C. (1974). Effects of temperature on carotid chemoreceptor and baroreceptor activity. J. Neurophysiol. 37:1287-1296.

INHIBITION OF VENTILATION BY CAROTID BODY HYPOCAPNIA DURING SLEEP

Curtis A. Smith, Kurt W. Saupe, Kathleen S. Henderson,
and Jerome A. Dempsey

The John Rankin Laboratory of Pulmonary Medicine, University of
Wisconsin, School of Medicine, 504 North Walnut Street, Madison,
Wisconsin, 53705-2368 U.S.A.

INTRODUCTION

Apneas and hypopneas during sleep, however caused, are typically preceded by hyperventilation and concomitant hypocapnia (Dempsey & Skatrud, 1986). This hypocapnia is a transient event and would most likely be sensed primarily by the carotid body chemoreceptors. We asked, therefore, whether hypocapnia isolated to the carotid body would inhibit ventilation and, if so, whether this inhibition would be dependent on state of consciousness. To answer this question we studied unanesthetized dogs during normal sleep and wakefulness using a preparation in which blood gases in the perfusate supplying the carotid sinus region could be controlled in isolation from the systemic circulation.

METHODS

Seven mixed-breed, female dogs were studied. Four to six days prior to study each dog was prepared surgically for extracorporeal perfusion of an isolated carotid sinus region. Our technique is a modification of that developed by Busch et al. (1985). Briefly, on the dog's right side all arterial branches between the cranial thyroid artery and the facial artery are ligated. A Silastic arterio-venous shunt is inserted between the external carotid artery and the jugular vein. On the left side the carotid body is denervated but the arteries are left intact. On both sides the cranial thyroid artery is cannulated for the measurement of carotid sinus (right) and systemic (left) blood pressures. On days of study, the A-V shunt is attached to an extracorporeal oxygenator (Terumo 350). By means of valves the normal A-V flow can be switched abruptly (<2 sec) to retrograde perfusion of the carotid sinus region *via* the extracorporeal circuit. The extracorporeal circuit is replenished by drawing blood from the venous half of the A-V shunt. PO_2 and PCO_2 of the extracorporeal circuit can be controlled by varying the composition of the gas supplied to it.

Protocols consisted of: a) Perfusion of the isolated carotid sinus region with extracorporeal circuit blood matched to each dog's normal P_aCO_2 and P_aO_2. b) Before and during the control perfusion, intravenous NaCN (40 µg/kg) was administered as a bolus. c) Two-minute perfusions of the isolated carotid sinus region with normoxic and hypocapnic

(-10 to -14 Torr relative to eupnea) blood during wakefulness, NREM sleep, and REM sleep. d) Some dogs were exposed to two-minute perfusions with normoxic blood with a relative hypocapnia of -5 Torr. e) Some dogs were exposed to two-minute perfusions with normocapnic and hyperoxic (PO_2 > 500 Torr) blood. In all cases the ventilatory responses were calculated on a breath-by-breath basis.

RESULTS

Perfusion of the isolated carotid sinus region with normoxic, normocapnic blood had no significant effect on ventilation or systemic arterial blood pressure and heart rate. Cyanide tests before and during perfusion showed that all dogs had a viable carotid body on the isolated carotid sinus region side, complete denervation of the contralateral carotid body, and no detectable response from aortic chemoreceptors.

During wakefulness, NREM sleep, and REM sleep carotid body hypocapnia between -10 and -14 Torr (relative to eupnea) inhibited ventilation immediately by 25-33% due mostly to 25-29% decreases in V_T although occasional prolongations of T_E were observed. Ventilation remained inhibited throughout the two-minute period resulting in systemic CO_2 retention of 2-4 Torr. In 3 dogs in which -5 Torr carotid body hypocapnia was imposed, a qualitatively similar response occurred but with less inhibition of V_T. In 3 dogs in which the carotid body was exposed to hyperoxia (> 500 Torr), ventilatory inhibition was qualitatively and quantitatively similar to that observed during -10 to -14 Torr carotid body hypocapnia.

DISCUSSION

Our results have several implications for carotid body function and the control of breathing during sleep:

1) Carotid body hypocapnia is a potent inhibitor of ventilation. Short-term carotid body hypocapnia of magnitudes achievable following hyperpneic episodes during sleep must have caused a marked reduction of carotid body chemoreceptor afferent traffic. We reach this conclusion because the changes in ventilation observed with carotid body hypocapnia were very similar in magnitude to those observed with carotid body hyperoxia, which is known to reduce carotid body chemoreceptor afferent traffic to residual levels.

2) Carotid body hypocapnia caused hypopnea but its role in apnea is unclear. Abrupt reduction in carotid body chemoreceptor afferent traffic by means of hypocapnia caused marked reductions in V_T and hypoventilation which persisted throughout the duration of carotid body hypocapnia. Prolongation of T_E was variable but the data suggest there may be a transient prolongation of T_E following the onset of hypocapnia. Thus, carotid body hypocapnia results in clear hypopnea but not apnea. Apneas may require longer term hypocapnia at the carotid body and/or CNS. Unstable breathing has been observed in awake goats with long-term (10-30 min) isolated hypocapnic (-11 Torr) perfusion of the carotid body (Daristotle et al., 1990) despite significant systemic CO_2 retention. Therefore the profound central apneas caused by decreased P_aCO_2 in the sleeping animal or human must result to a small extent from carotid body hypocapnia but primarily from decreased medullary PCO_2. In turn, this would mean that hypocapnic-induced apnea in sleep would probably require sustained periods of hypocapnia to ensure sufficient alkalinization of the central chemoreceptors.

3) Sleep state appeared to have no effect on the ventilatory response to carotid body hypocapnia. The overall level of ventilation during NREM and REM sleep was reduced relative to wakefulness but the response to carotid body hypocapnia was similar in all states despite the increased variability in REM sleep.

Supported by NHLBI.

REFERENCES

Busch, M.A., Bisgard, G.E. & Forster, H.V. (1985). Ventilatory acclimatization to hypoxia is not dependent on arterial hypoxemia. J. Appl. Physiol. 58:1874-1880.

Daristotle, L., Berssenbrugge, A.D., Engwall, M.J. & Bisgard, G.E. (1990). The effects of carotid body hypocapnia on ventilation in goats. Respir. Physiol. 79:123-136.

Dempsey, J.A. & Skatrud, J.B. (1986). A sleep-induced apneic threshold and its consequences. Am. Rev. Resp. Dis. 133:1163-1170.

METABOLIC ACID-BASE STATUS AND THE ROLE OF CAROTID CHEMORECEPTORS IN HYPEROXIC BREATHING

Heidrun Kiwull-Schöne, Sabine Bungart, and Peter Kiwull

Department of Physiology, Ruhr-University, 44780 Bochum, Germany

INTRODUCTION

There is controversy as to how much the peripheral chemoreceptors may contribute to pulmonary ventilation during hyperoxia under normocapnic and hypercapnic conditions. Whereas cutting the carotid sinus nerves (CSN) is reported to considerably depress ventilation in cats (Katsaros, 1968, Berkenbosch et al., 1979), we did not find any significant effect of cutting or cooling the CSN in rabbits (Kiwull et al., 1972). It has to be questioned, whether the metabolic acid-base status under otherwise normal blood-gas conditions could be responsible for these discrepancies. To exclude feedback effects of spontaneous breathing, this study was carried out with artificial ventilation.

METHODS

The experiments were performed in 11 anaesthetized, vagotomized, paralysed and mechanically ventilated rabbits (average weight 3.6 ±0.1 kg, pentobarbital sodium i.v. induction 50.7 ±1.4 mg/kg, continuous maintenance 6.4 ±0.2 mg/kg/h). The following variables were recorded: Blood pressure, tracheal pressure, end-tidal CO_2-pressure ($P_{ET}CO_2$) and integrated phrenic nerve activity (IPNA) with inspiratory and expiratory times (T_I, T_E). Under steady state conditions, arterial blood samples were taken and analysed for pHa, P_aCO_2, $HCO_3^-{}_a$ and $HCO_3^-{}_{st}$ by means of the two-gas equilibration method and for PaO_2 by electrode (Radiometer). The animals were ventilated with oxygen-enriched air ($F_IO_2 \sim 0.5$) to achieve arterial PO_2-levels of >150 mmHg.

First, the control level of $P_{ET}CO_2$ was adjusted to that during spontaneous breathing (35.9 ±1.1 mmHg). To reach the apneic threshold of phrenic nerve activity, the PCO_2 was lowered by hyperventilation. When phasic nerve discharge ceased and became tonic, arterial blood was analysed immediately. The PCO_2 was then elevated by reduced ventilation and later CO_2-inhalation up to 30 mmHg above threshold-P_aCO_2, to achieve complete CO_2-responses of tidal IPNA, respiratory frequency (f) and minute phrenic activity (IPNA·f). Maximum values of IPNA during hypercapnia were normalized to 100 arbitrary units. The whole procedure was repeated after cutting both carotid sinus nerves.

Arterial Chemoreceptors: Cell to System
Edited by R. O'Regan *et al*, Plenum Press, New York, 1994

RESULTS

The metabolic acid-base condition was taken into account by dividing the total of investigated rabbits into a more alkaline and a more acid group with initial standard bicarbonate concentrations ($HCO_3^-{}_{st}$) above and below 24 mM (Table 1). There were slight but significant changes towards normality in both groups during the course of experiments.

In the more <u>alkaline group</u>, cutting the carotid sinus nerves had no significant effect, neither on the threshold values of $P_{ET}CO_2$, P_aCO_2 or pH, nor on the initial slope (up to 5 mmHg above threshold), nor on the maximum level of the $IPNA \cdot f$ to P_aCO_2 response. In the more <u>acid group</u>, both threshold $P_{ET}CO_2$ and P_aCO_2 were significantly enhanced by cutting the CSN, and, although there was again no significant effect on the initial slope, the plateau of the CO_2-response was now significantly enhanced (by about 25%).

Table 1. Significance of the metabolic acid-base status for the contribution of carotid chemoreflexes to the respiratory CO_2-response during hyperoxia in rabbits.

	$HCO_3^-{}_{st}$ > 24 mM		$HCO_3^-{}_{st}$ < 24 mM	
	CSN intact	CSN cut	CSN intact	CSN cut
Apneic threshold				
$P_{ET}CO_2$ [mmHg]	26.4 ±1.1	28.1 ±1.8	25.8 ±1.6	29.9 ±1.3*
P_aCO_2 [mmHg]	31.3 ±1.1	32.3 ±1.3	28.4 ±1.2	33.8 ±1.5*
pH_a	7.512 ±0.011	7.491 ±0.008	7.465 ±0.014	7.448 ±0.019
$HCO_3^-{}_{st}$ [mM]	26.4 ±0.3	25.7 ±0.4*	22.6 ±0.3	24.0 ±0.5*
$IPNA \cdot f / P_aCO_2$-response				
slope [units·min^{-1}·mmHg^{-1}]	553 ±94.8	454 ±33.8	438 ±55.7	360 ±88.4
plateau [units·min^{-1}]	4581 ±248.0	4264 ±120.5	4122 ±234	5172 ±218.2*

Mean values ±SEM in rabbits with initial standard bicarbonate levels either below (N=5) or above (N=6) 24 mM. P_aO_2 >150 mmHg. Characteristics of the response of phrenic minute activity ($IPNA \cdot f$) to P_aCO_2 between apneic threshold and up to 30 mmHg above.
* Significant effect of cutting the carotid sinus nerves, paired t-test, P <0.05.

DISCUSSION

A significant contribution of carotid chemoreflexes to respiration during hyperoxia becomes evident in artificially ventilated rabbits, a phenomenon which is probably masked by feedback control during spontaneous breathing (Kiwull et al., 1972). This chemoreflex contribution strikingly depends on the prevailing respiratory and metabolic acid-base condition. Thereby, chemoreflex activation predominates during metabolic acidosis and in the hypocapnic sub-normal, near-threshold range. Although chemoreceptor activation by H^+ besides CO_2 has been directly shown only for cats (Pokorski & Lahiri, 1983) and not for rabbits, it is most likely to explain the present findings. On the other hand, there is a growing inhibitory effect on carotid chemoreflexes during combined metabolic acidosis and hypercapnia. Inhibitory control of carotid chemoreceptors by sinus nerve efferents in response to changes in arterial gas tensions and pH is still puzzling (O'Regan & Majcherczyk, 1983), so that it is difficult to interpret the attenuation of the maximum hypercapnic response mediated by intact CSN during metabolic acidosis.

Since the metabolic acid-base status appears to be of great importance, one may hypothesize that natural species differences in this respect may be responsible for the differences in the chemoreflex contribution to hyperoxic breathing. For that reason, literature data for cats dealing with $P_{ET}CO_2$-thresholds over a wide range of acid-base changes

(Kuwana and Natsui, 1981) were compared with the present data in rabbits (Fig. 1). The normal metabolic acid-base status is considerably more alkaline in rabbits (herbivores) than in cats (carnivores) and is accompanied by a smaller effect of cutting the CSN on threshold PCO_2. This behaviour can be mimicked by alkaline infusion in cats. Likewise, the more acid rabbit group is noticeably shifted towards the cats' control group. Thus, the observed species differences in chemoreflex contribution to normal non-hypoxic breathing may sufficiently be explained by acid-base differences due to specific nutrition in cats and rabbits.

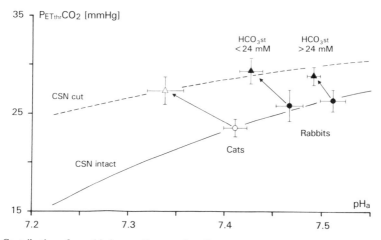

Figure 1. Contribution of carotid chemoreflexes to the adjustment of apneic threshold PCO_2 in rabbits and cats under different metabolic acid-base conditions.
End-tidal threshold PCO_2 as a function of arterial pH. Means ± SEM of rabbits with intact (●) or cut (▲) carotid sinus nerves (CSN) at higher (● n=8, ▲ n=14) and lower (● n=6, ▲ n=9) levels of $HCO_3^-{}_{st}$. For comparison, data of cats (unfilled symbols) were adapted from Kuwana and Natsui, 1981: Means ± SEM under normal acid-base conditions (O n=11 CSN intact, △ n=7 CSN cut) as well as regression lines obtained during acid and base infusions. Note: Rabbit values are predicted by cats' regression lines upon base infusion.

The expert assistance and drawings by S. Adler and C. Bräuer are highly appreciated.

REFERENCES

Berkenbosch, A., van Dissel, J., Olievier, C.N., De Goede, J., & Heeringa, J. (1979). The contribution of the peripheral chemoreceptors to the ventilatory response to CO_2 in anaesthetized cats during hyperoxia. Respir. Physiol. 37:381-390.

Katsaros, B. (1968). Evidence for the existence of a respiratory drive of unknown origin conducted in the carotid sinus nerves. In "Arterial Chemoreceptors." R.W. Torrance, ed., Blackwell, Oxford-Edinburgh.

Kiwull, P., Wiemer, W. & Schöne, H. (1972). The role of the carotid chemoreceptors in the CO_2-hyperpnea under hyperoxia. Pflügers Arch. 336:171-186.

O'Regan, R.G. & Majcherczyk, St. (1983). Control of peripheral chemoreceptors by efferent nerves. In "Physiology of the Peripheral Chemoreceptors." H. Acker & R.G. O'Regan, eds., Elsevier, Amsterdam.

Kuwana, S. & Natsui, T. (1981). Effect of arterial [H^+] on threshold PCO_2 of the respiratory system in vagotomized and carotid sinus nerve denervated cats. J. Physiol. (Lond.) 318:223-237.

Pokorski, M. & Lahiri, S. (1983). Aortic and carotid chemoreceptor responses to metabolic acidosis in the cat. Am. J. Physiol. 244:R652-R658

VENTILATORY RESPONSES TO HISTOTOXIC CHEMOSTIMULATION IN HYPOXIA ADAPTED RATS

Denise Lagneaux

Department of Physiology, University of Liège, 17 Place Delcour, B-4020, Liège, Belgium

INTRODUCTION

Rats adapted to prolonged hypobaric hypoxia present a blunted hypoxic ventilatory response (HVR) when stimulated by steady state (Wach et al., 1989) or transient acute hypoxia (Lagneaux & Lecomte, 1991). The origin of this post-acclimatization blunted HVR remains controversial. Central or peripheral mechanisms, alone or in association must be investigated. In large animals, the site of inhibition can be detected by comparison between simultaneous recordings of carotid sinus nerve activity and ventilatory responses to the hypoxic stimulus. This technique is difficult to manage in the rat and an alternative approach must be used to identify the site of the blunted mechanism: glomic chemosensitivity or transduction at central level.

In our acclimatized animals, we have chosen to study, in the same rats, besides the ventilatory responses to acute transient hypoxia, the effects of stimuli acting on glomic cells in a manner different from low PO_2. Sodium cyanide and almitrine bismesylate, respectively short and long acting agents, were examined in this respect, as they act by an inhibition of the mitochondrial electron transfer and not by a reduction of local PO_2

METHODS

Experiments were performed on rats of a Wistar strain (300-400 g). From 6 litters, 12 rats were submitted to hypobaric conditions (simulated altitude 5.500m, 2 weeks) and 12 were maintained as control in normobaria. On the day of the experiments, chronically hypoxic rats were studied 1 to 1.5 hours after their return to sea level conditions. All the rats were anesthetized with pentobarbital (40 mg.kg^{-1}, i.p.) and tracheotomized. A catheter was inserted via a femoral vein into the posterior vena cava for administration of drugs . After heparinization (10 mg.kg^{-1}), a second catheter was introduced into a femoral artery in order to record blood pressure by electromanometry. The tracheal cannula was inserted into a "T" joint, with a home made Fleisch pneumotachograph (PTG) in its axial arm and the tip of a gas sampling capillary to a mass spectrometer for gas analysis. The stem of the "T" was flushed by a constant flow of air (4 l.min^{-1}). The PTG was connected to a differential pressure transducer (Validyne DP 45) with a CD 101 demodulator and an analogue integrator (Pneumometer Elema) in order to obtain flow rate and tidal volume (VT). The

Arterial Chemoreceptors: Cell to System
Edited by R. O'Regan *et al*, Plenum Press, New York, 1994

outputs of the manometers and of the mass spectrometer were fed into an ink-jet multichannel recorder (Mingograph EEG) for continuous monitoring. In addition, flow and gas signals were processed by a computer (IBM PS2/30) at a sampling rate of 200 Hz. Data were stored in the computer for periods of 80 s. Then automated treatment of the data was performed breath by breath to obtain ventilatory parameters and alveolar partial pressure of gas (P_ACO_2 and P_AO_2) used to estimate the blood gas levels.

Transient acute hypoxia (N_2 test) was produced by the inhalation of 2 to 6 V_T of N_2 and the ventilatory response was quantified as total hyperventilation (Excess V) above pre-test values, expressed in % of basal ventilation. Ventilatory responses after i.v. administration of NaCN (160 and 300 $\mu g.kg^{-1}$) were similarly calculated. After i.v. bolus of almitrine bismesylate (ALM: 1 $mg.kg^{-1}$), ventilatory variations were averaged from minute to minute during the first 7.5 min.

Values were expressed as mean ± SEM. A Student paired t-test was used to determine if a significant difference was obtained during stimulations. Differences between normoxic and chronically hypoxic rats were compared using a t-test for unpaired values. A P value of 0.05 or less was considered significant.

RESULTS

The relation between inhaled volume of N_2 (ml) and hyperventilation (Excess V * 100/control V) was represented by linear regression lines, respectively: y = 166 x -450 (r=0.75; n=41) in normoxic rats and y = 59* x - 126 (r=0.71; n=51; * indicates the coefficient is statistically significantly different from normoxic rats) in chronically hypoxic rats. The blunting of the response was depending on a reduction in amplitude and duration. This smoothed ventilatory response delayed P_AO_2 return to control conditions: 5 s after the onset of the response, P_AO_2 was at - 2.26* ± 0.29 in chronically hypoxic rats compared with - 0.72 ± 0.40 kPa in normoxic rats. This short hypoxemic hypoxia induced little systemic hypotension in the 2 groups of rats.

Hyperventilation induced by iv administration of NaCN was not significantly different in normoxic and chronically hypoxic rats: respectively 3.882 ± 425 compared with 3.750 ± 796 for 160 $\mu g.kg-1$ and 5.410 ± 467 compared with 5.817 ± 613 for 320 $\mu g.kg-1$. No differences were found in the related maximum hypocapnia and hyperoxia.

In the two groups, hyperventilation induced by ALM was identical from 1 to 7.30 min: i.e. 194 ± 16 and 195 ± 14 % at the 5th min, with a reduction of P_ACO_2 = -1.93 ± 0.15 and - 1.65 ± 0.33 kPa and an increase of P_AO_2 = 3.09 ± 0.21 and 2.79 ± 0.90 kPa, respectively.

DISCUSSION

Anesthetized rats previously adapted to hypobaric hypoxia maintained a vigorous ventilatory response to i.v. administration of NaCN and of ALM in contrast with the blunted HVR to transient hypoxemic hypoxia. This transient N_2 stimulus avoids the central inhibiting effect of prolonged hypoxia whose importance after chronic hypoxia is unknown. Another interference from baroreflex origin was also avoided: the CO_2 uncompensated steady state hypoxia induces larger systemic hypotension in normoxic rats than in altitude adapted rats (Wach et al. 1989), transient hypoxia avoids this problem. Althought, a blunted ventilatory response to N_2 tests is present after chronic hypoxia, the normal responses to cyanide and ALM indicate an intact glomic sensitivity to mitochondrial electron transfer inhibitors. Moreover, central transducing mechanisms from peripheral chemoreceptors inputs appear unmodified. As stressed by Gonzalez et al. (1992), mechanisms of action of metabolic poisoning and of low PO_2 are not equivalent and possibly not similarly modified by chronic hypoxia. So we hypothesize that in altitude adapted rats, low PO_2 glomic sensitivity is selectively perturbed, localizing at this level the origin of the blunted HVR in chronically hypoxic rats.

REFERENCES

Gonzalez, C., Almaraz, L., Obeso, A. & Rigual, R. (1992). Oxygen and acid chemoreception in the carotid body chemoreceptors. Trends in Neurosci. 15: 146-153.

Lagneaux, D. & Lecomte, J. (1991). D2-receptors blockade and blunted hypoxic ventilatory response in rats soon after chronic hypobaric hypoxia. Arch. int. Physiol. Bioch. 100: P10.

Wach, R.A., Bee, D. & Barer, G.R. (1989). Dopamine and ventilatory effects of hypoxia and almitrine in chronically hypoxic rats. J. Appl. Physiol. 67: 186-192.

CHEMOREFLEX SENSITIZATION AUGMENTS SYMPATHETIC VASOMOTOR OUTFLOW IN AWAKE HUMANS

Barbara J. Morgan[1], David Crabtree[2], and James B. Skatrud[2]

Departments of [1]Kinesiology and [2]Medicine, University of Wisconsin and Middleton Memorial Veterans Hospital, Madison, Wisconsin, USA

INTRODUCTION

Prolonged exposure to a steady state of hypoxia causes a time-dependent increase in ventilation which persists even after return to normoxia (Dempsey & Forster, 1982). Although the precise mechanism is unknown, this persistent elevation in ventilation is critically dependent on an intact carotid chemoreflex (Forster et al., 1981; Lahiri et al., 1982; Smith et al., 1986). The goal of this research was to determine whether carotid chemoreflex control of sympathetic vasomotor outflow is similarly sensitized by short-term exposure to intermittent asphyxia. We measured ventilation, arterial pressure, and sympathetic outflow to skeletal muscle before, during, and after 20 minutes of intermittent asphyxia (combined hypoxia-hypercapnia) in healthy, awake humans.

METHODS

Seven men, aged 27-47 years (mean $\pm$ SD = 38 $\pm$ 7), served as subjects. All subjects were free from cardiovascular and pulmonary disease as evaluated by history and physical examination. The experimental protocol was approved by the institution's Human Subjects Committee and all subjects provided informed consent.

Subjects were studied supine in the postabsorptive state. Tidal volume, arterial oxygen saturation, and arterial pressure were measured using a pneumotachograph, pulse oximeter, and automated cuff, respectively. End-tidal O_2 and CO_2 tensions were measured using medical gas analyzers. Recordings of postganglionic sympathetic nerve activity in the peroneal nerve were made by the technique of Vallbo et al. (1979) as previously described (Morgan et al., 1993).

After stable baseline recordings were obtained, subjects were exposed to 20 minutes of intermittent asphyxia (combined hypoxia-hypercapnia) administered by nasal mask. Intermittent asphyxia was produced by addition of N_2 and CO_2 so that $S_aO_2 = 80\%$ and $P_{ET}CO_2 = +3\text{-}5$ mmHg for thirty seconds of each minute. Observations were continued for 30 minutes following the asphyxic exposure.

Arterial Chemoreceptors: Cell to System
Edited by R. O'Regan *et al*, Plenum Press, New York, 1994

RESULTS

Exposure to intermittent asphyxia caused a significant decrease in $P_{ET}O_2$ (-30 Torr) and increase in $P_{ET}CO_2$ (+2 Torr) (both $p < 0.05$). This intervention caused a 2-fold increase in minute ventilation which promptly subsided after restoration of normoxia. Arterial pressure rose above the baseline level only in the first five minutes of asphyxia (+ 6 ± 2 mmHg, $p < 0.05$).

During intermittent asphyxia, sympathetic nerve activity increased to 123 ± 10% of baseline at 5 minutes and 165 ± 14% of baseline at 20 minutes (both $p < 0.05$). Sympathetic nerve activity remained elevated after return to room air breathing (155 ± 7% of baseline after 20 minutes of normoxia, $p < 0.05$) despite the return of chemical stimuli and ventilation to control levels. No change in any of the variables of interest was noted during time control experiments.

DISCUSSION

We studied the neurocirculatory responses to intermittent asphyxia in healthy, awake humans. The major findings are 2-fold. First, 20-minute exposure to intermittent asphyxia caused a substantial increase in sympathetic outflow to skeletal muscle. This increase in sympathetic activity was progressive over the course of the 20-minute intervention, even though the average levels of chemical stimuli remained constant. Second, this asphyxia-induced sympathetic activation persisted even after return of chemical stimuli to baseline levels. In contrast, sympathetic nerve activity did not change during 20-minute room air control experiments.

In spite of a sustained increase in sympathetic vasomotor outflow, arterial pressure was only transiently elevated during the asphyxic exposure. One possible explanation for this observation is that the magnitude of the sympathetic activation was insufficient to overcome the local vasodilatory effects of hypoxia (Chalmers et al., 1967) and hypercapnia (Richardson et al., 1961). In addition, we have measured sympathetic outflow to only one of many vascular beds which contribute to total peripheral vascular resistance. It is possible that the asphyxia-induced increase in sympathetic outflow to skeletal muscle was counterbalanced by simultaneous decreases in sympathetic outflow to other regional circulations.

What is the mechanism by which brief intermittent asphyxia causes persistent elevation of sympathetic nerve activity? In subsequent experiments performed in our laboratory, hyperoxic hypercapnia alone caused an increase in sympathetic outflow which was similar in magnitude to that caused by asphyxia. The hypercapnia-induced sympathetic activation was also maintained following removal of the stimulus. Apparently, hypoxia per se was not required to produce this after-effect of chemostimulation on sympathetic nerve activity. Our findings to date do not allow us to identify the site at which asphyxia exerts this effect (i.e. the carotid chemoreceptor, the central nervous system, or both).

In conclusion, we have demonstrated that a relatively brief period of chemoreceptor stimulation causes a substantial augmentation of sympathetic vasomotor outflow which outlasts the chemical stimuli. We postulate that the intermittent asphyxia which occurs during sleep disordered breathing contributes to persistently elevated sympathetic nervous system activity in patients with clinically significant apneas and hypopneas.

This research was supported by the American Heart Association of Wisconsin, the National Heart Lung and Blood Institute, and the Veterans Administration Research Service. A preliminary report of this work was presented at the 1993 American Lung Association/American Thoracic Society International Conference. The authors are indebted to Mr. Domenic Puleo and Ms. Mary Lowenberg for technical assistance and to Ms. Pat Mecum for secretarial assistance.

REFERENCES

Chalmers, J.P., Korner, P.I. & White, S.W. (1967). Distribution of peripheral blood flow in primary tissue hypoxia induced by inhalation of carbon monoxide. J. Physiol. (Lond.) 192:549-559.

Dempsey, J.A. & Forster, H.V. (1982). Mediation of ventilatory adaptions. Physiol. Rev. 62:262-346.

Forster, H.V., Bisgard, G.E. & Klein, J.P. (1981). Effect of peripheral chemoreceptor denervation on acclimatization of goats during hypoxia. J. Appl. Physiol. 50:392-398.

Lahiri, S., Edelman, N.H., Cherniack, N.S. & Fishman, A.P. (1982). Role of carotid chemoreflex in respiratory acclimatization to hypoxemia on goat and sheep. Respir. Physiol. 46:367-382

Morgan, B.J., Denahan, T. & Ebert, T.J. (1993). Neurocirculatory consequences of negative intrathoracic pressure vs. asphyxia during voluntary apnea. J. Appl. Physiol. 74:2969-2975.

Richardson, D.W., Wasserman, A.J. & Patterson, J.L. (1961). General and regional circulatory responses to change in blood pH and carbon dioxide tension. J. Clin. Invest. 40:31-43.

Smith, C.A., Bisgard, G.E., Nielsen, A.M., Daristotle, L., Kressin, N., Forster, H.V. & Dempsey, J.A. (1986). Carotid bodies are required for ventilatory acclimatization to moderate and severe chronic hypoxemia. J. Appl. Physiol. 60:1003-1010.

Vallbo, A.B., Hagbarth, K.E., Torebjörk & Wallin, B.G. (1979). Somatosensory, proprioceptive, and sympathetic activity in human peripheral nerves. Physiol. Rev. 59:919-957.

CAROTID CHEMORECEPTOR CONTROL OF VASCULAR RESISTANCE IN RESTING AND CONTRACTING SKELETAL MUSCLE

M. de Burgh Daly and M.N.Cook

Department of Physiology
Royal Free Hospital School of Medicine
Rowland Hill Street
London NW3 2PF, UK

INTRODUCTION

Selective stimulation of the carotid body chemoreceptors causes vasoconstriction in resting skeletal muscle (Daly & Scott, 1962). Their excitation is also known to contribute to the increased systemic vascular resistance that occurs in apnoeic asphyxia and in the asphyxial stage of the response to breath-hold diving in which a conspicuous increase in activity of the carotid chemoreceptors has been demonstrated (see Daly, 1986). The present experiments were undertaken to determine whether the reflex vasoconstrictor response in resting muscle was in any way modified during simulated exercise when vasodilator metabolites would be expected to oppose it.

METHODS

Cats were used of either sex and anaesthetized with a mixture of 2% alpha-chloralose (52 mg kg^{-1}) and 20% urethane (520 mg kg^{-1}) administered intra-peritoneally. Respiration was spontaneous, tidal volume being recorded by a pneumotachograph. Some animals were ventilated artificially with an open pneumothorax. The superior laryngeal nerves were dissected, cut peripherally and their central ends mounted on stimulating electrodes. The right hindlimb, and sometimes the left, were vascularly isolated and perfused with arterial blood at constant flow so that changes in perfusion pressure indicated similar directional changes in vascular resistance. In some experiments the skin was removed and the limb tied at the level of the ankle joint, so that the territory perfused consisted largely of muscle. The limb muscles were stimulated electrically via needles inserted into the muscles or through their motor nerves L6, L7 and S1 in the cauda equina. In the latter case, the corresponding sensory roots were also cut. Heparin was administered to render the blood incoagulable.

The procedure was to carry out all tests of carotid body stimulation during a 20s period of apnoea evoked by electrical stimulation of the superior laryngeal nerves. In this way, the primary cardiac (bradycardia) and systemic vascular (vasoconstrictor) responses resulting from excitation of the carotid bodies were uncomplicated by alterations in respiration (see Daly, 1986). In those animals in which ventilation was controlled, the respiration pump was switched off during the period of stimulation of the superior laryngeal nerves to exclude changes in lung stretch afferent activity.

RESULTS

Typical responses are shown in Fig.1. When the results of 11 such series of observations in 6 experiments were averaged, stimulation of the carotid bodies increased the right hindlimb perfusion pressure by 24.2 ± 2.0 (SEM) mm Hg, but only by 6.0 ± 1.7 mm Hg immediately after a 30s period of stimulation of the muscle, the difference being a statistically highly significant (P<0.001). The control level of pressure in the two states was 113.0 ±5.2 and 82.2 ± 9.3 mm Hg respectively, the difference representing the fall in pressure due to stimulation of the muscle (P<0.001). The increases in pulse interval and arterial blood pressure occurring on stimulation of the carotid chemoreceptors were, however, similar in the two conditions.

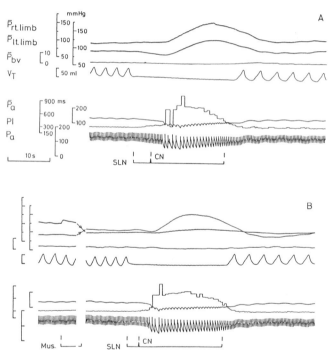

Figure 1. Spontaneously breathing cat. A and B, stimulation of both carotid bodies by the intracarotid injection of 5 µg kg^{-1} sodium cyanide (CN) during a period of reflexly induced apnoea evoked by electrical stimulation of the superior laryngeal nerves (SLN), 2.5 V, 2 ms pulse duration, 20 Hz. In B, start of direct electrical stimulation of right limb muscles at 12 Hz which continued during break in records for a total of 30 s (Mus). Recording commenced 10 s after cessation of stimulation. Records from above downwards: P rt. limb, P lt. limb, right and left hindlimb mean perfusion pressures; P_{bv}, brachial vein mean pressure; V_T, tidal volume; P_a, P_a, mean and phasic arterial pressure; PI, pulse interval. Time calibration 10 s. Note (1), the reduction in right hindlimb perfusion pressure, indicating vasodilatation, due to stimulation of the muscle and (2) the striking reduction in the vasoconstrictor response in the right hindlimb, but not in the left, to stimulation of the carotid bodies in (B) immediately following the period of excitation of the muscle. Final control test of stimulation of the carotid chemoreceptors made 15 min after (B) evoked a rise in right hindlimb perfusion pressure quantitatively similar to that in (A) (not shown).

In contrast to the reduced vasoconstrictor response occurring on stimulation of the carotid bodies in the stimulated muscle, the increased perfusion pressure in the contralateral non-stimulated limb was unaffected (Fig.1).

In the artificially ventilated animal in which the muscles of the right skinned limb were stimulated through the cut motor roots of L6, L7 and S1 in the cauda equina, increasing the frequency of stimulation in steps up to 16 Hz resulted in a progressive vasodilatation and a progressive reduction in the size of the carotid chemoreceptor vasoconstrictor response. The increase in hindlimb perfusion pressure to excitation of the carotid bodies in the unstimulated limb was 27.0 ± 3.5 mm Hg and in the limb stimulated at 16 Hz was 8.0 ± 3.9 mm Hg, the difference being statistically significant ($P<0.001$). Similar results were obtained when perfusion of the muscle was made at constant pressure.

After neuromuscular blockade, the vasodilator response to stimulation of the motor roots was abolished, while the size of the chemoreceptor vasoconstrictor response that occurred without stimulation of the motor roots remained the same at all frequencies of stimulation. Guanethidine abolished the chemoreceptor vasoconstrictor responses.

DISCUSSION

It has been shown that stimulation of the carotid body chemoreceptor caused vasoconstriction in the muscle in the non-stimulated state. With increasing frequency of stimulation of the muscle, either directly or through the motor roots, which produced a progressive vasodilatation, the chemoreceptor vasoconstrictor response was progressively reduced in size, and in some experiments, abolished altogether. The mechanism responsible for this inhibition cannot have been centrally mediated because the chemoreceptor vasoconstrictor response occurring in the contralateral non-stimulated limb remained unaffected, and furthermore, the sensory innervation to the muscles was interrupted. It must therefore be due to events occurring in the active muscle itself.

The carotid chemoreceptor vasoconstrictor response is the result of activation of sympathetic noradrenergic fibres and its inhibition by stimulation of the motor nerves to the skeletal muscle is dependent on the muscles actually contracting. This suggests that activation of the sympathetic supply is antagonized by the metabolic products of muscular contraction.

These findings are consistent with observations indicating that simulated exercise reduces the vasoconstrictor response to noradrenaline and to sympathetic nerve stimulation (Rein, 1930; Janczewska et al 1980), and indicate that local metabolic factors in muscle predominate over the effects of sympathetic activity evoked reflexly by stimulation of the carotid bodies.

This work was supported by the British Heart Foundation.

REFERENCES

Daly, M. de B. (1986). Interactions between respiration and circulation. In: Handbook of Physiology, sect.3, The Respiratory System, vol. 2, Control of Breathing, Part II.,N.S. Cherniack and J.G. Widdicombe, eds., pp. 529-594. Bethesda, MD, USA, American Physiological Society.

Daly, M. de B. & Scott, M.J. (1962). An analysis of the primary cardiovascular reflex effects of stimulation of the carotid body chemoreceptors in the dog. J. Physiol. (Lond.) 162:555-573.

Janczewska, H., Bogdanski, W. & Trzebski, A. (1980). Influence of alpha and beta adrenergic receptors blockade on the adrenolytic effect of muscular work. Acta Physiol. Pol. 31:469-474.

Rein, H. (1930). Der Interferenz der Vasomotorischen Regulationen. Klin. Wochenschr. 9:1485-1489.

SUBSTANCE P INHIBITS VENTILATION IN THE GOAT

G.E. Bisgard, J. Pizarro, M. Ryan, and M. Hedrick

Department of Comparative Biosciences
University of Wisconsin
Madison, Wisconsin 53706

INTRODUCTION

Substance P (SP) has been established as an excitatory neuromodulator in the cat carotid body (CB) (Prabhakar et al., 1987; 1989). These workers have suggested that SP may be an important link between the transduction mechanism for hypoxia and the production of afferent neural discharge.

The purpose of this study was to determine if SP was excitatory to the CB of the goat. Such a finding would strengthen the case for SP as an excitatory neuromodulator in the CB.

METHODS

Six adult goats of various breeds were prepared for study by surgical translocation of both common carotid arteries to a subcutaneous location to enable ease of percutaneous catheterization. One CB was denervated. These procedures were carried out using aseptic methods and under general anesthesia (halothane, nitrous oxide and oxygen). The unilateral CB denervation allowed agents to be infused into either the CB intact common carotid artery or the opposite common carotid artery (CB denervated side) as control.

For each study, the common carotid arteries were cannulated and a muzzle mask was placed on the goat for measuring inspired ventilation via pneumotachograph. Ventilation, expired CO_2 and arterial blood pressure were measured continuously. The goats were studied awake and unsedated.

Because of the potential effects of SP induced bronchoconstriction on ventilatory measurements two additional goats were studied under general anesthesia (intravenous chloralose). In these animals one 6th cervical phrenic nerve was surgically exposed and recorded using bipolar electrodes. Integrated phrenic nerve activity, arterial blood pressure and expired CO_2 were continuously monitored. The goats were paralyzed (pancuronium and metubine) and artificially ventilated in order to maintain constant arterial blood gases. Airway pressure was measured via the tracheal cannula as an index of bronchoconstriction.

In awake goats SP (Sigma) was infused at the rate of up to 6 μ/kg/min for a period of one minute. In some awake animals and in both anesthetized goats bolus intracarotid injections of 3 or 6 μg/kg of SP were given. Studies were conducted with the animals breathing room air under normoxic conditions.

Arterial Chemoreceptors: Cell to System
Edited by R. O'Regan *et al*, Plenum Press, New York, 1994

RESULTS

Intracarotid infusions of SP at a dose as low as 1 µg/kg/min produced a mean reduction in ventilation in awake goats, but the reduction was only significant at a dose of 6 µg/kg/min (P <0.05, Fig. 1). The reduction in ventilation occurred when SP was injected into either the CB intact or CB denervated carotid arteries (Fig. 1). The mean reduction was 28% on the intact side and 15% on the denervated side. These reductions were not different from each other. The decreased ventilation reached its minimum during the period between 15 and 45 seconds of the one minute infusion. The decrease in ventilation was due to non-significant decreases in tidal volume and respiratory frequency. In 3 of the 6 animals a transient increase in ventilation was noted after termination of SP infusion. This was thought to be related to a rising PCO_2 during the preceding ventilatory inhibition. Arterial blood pressure was increased by an average of 25 mmHg in awake goats during the SP infusion. Bolus intracarotid injections of SP gave results similar to the effects of one minute infusions in awake goats.

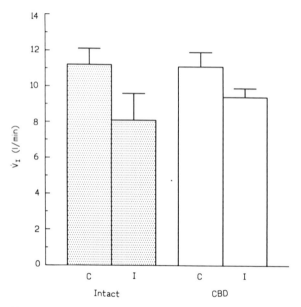

Figure 1. The effect of intracarotid infusion of SP (6 µg/kg/min) on ventilation in awake goats. Shaded bars indicate infusion into the carotid body intact side and open bars into the carotid body denervated side. C indicates control, I indicates infusion of SP.

In both anesthetized goats a decrease in integrated phrenic activity was found that was qualitatively similar to that occurring in the awake animals. In one of the animals a clear cut increase in frequency and amplitude of phrenic activity followed the phrenic inhibition even though blood gases were clamped. In both anesthetized goats mean arterial blood pressure decreased following SP infusion by 20 to 40 mmHg. All of these changes persisted after cutting the carotid sinus nerves.

In one anesthetized goat no increased airway pressure was noted following SP injections. In the other one an increase in airway pressure (3 -5 mmHg) was noted, but the rise in airway pressure followed the initial fall in phrenic amplitude by 20 seconds. These data suggest a dissociation between bronchoconstriction and the inhibition of phrenic nerve activity.

DISCUSSION

The results of these studies indicate that intracarotid infusion or bolus injection of SP causes inhibition of ventilation. This is not mediated by the carotid body or carotid baroreceptors because the inhibition of breathing is found after injection of SP into either the CB intact or denervated side and after cutting the carotid sinus nerve in anesthetized goats. Data from two anesthetized goats indicate that ventilatory inhibition is not caused by bronchoconstriction (Lundberg & Saria, 1987).

In one anesthetized goat an increase in phrenic amplitude and frequency occurred following the inhibition of phrenic activity. This suggests that there may be two possible mechanisms of the late excitation of ventilation observed in the awake goats, that due to an elevated PCO_2 from ventilatory inhibition and a true increase in central neural drive.

An unexpected finding was an increased arterial blood pressure during SP infusion in awake goats. Vasodilation is commonly observed with SP infusion (Pernow, 1983) as was noted in our anesthetized goats; however, CNS application of SP causes an increase in blood pressure (Brattstrom & Seidenbecher, 1992).

We conclude that there is no evidence in these studies to indicate that SP is an excitatory agent in the CB of the goat suggesting that SP is probably not a required component in the response of the CB to stimulation. The cause for ventilatory inhibition by SP is unknown. CNS effects are possible, but local injection of SP into various regions of the brain stem are more likely to produce ventilatory stimulation rather than inhibition (Chen et al., 1990).

The authors thank G. Johnson and Li Quimin for their assistance in these studies. This research was supported by NIH grant HL15473.

REFERENCES

Brattstrom, A. & Seidenbecher, T. (1992). Central substance P increased blood pressure, heart rate and splanchnic nerve activity in anaesthetized rats without impairment of the baroreflex regulation. Neuropeptides 23:81-86.

Chen, Z, Hedner, J. & Hedner, T. Substance P in the ventrolateral medulla oblongata regulates ventilatory responses. (1990). J. Appl. Physiol. 68:2631-2639.

Lundberg, J.M. & Saria, A. (1987). Polypeptide containing neurons in airway smooth muscle. Ann. Rev. Physiol. 49:555-572.

Pernow, B. (1983). Substance P. Pharmacological Rev. 35:85-141.

Prabhakar, N.R., Landis, S.C., Kumar, G.K., Mullikin-Kilpatrick, D., Cherniack, N.S. & Leeman, S. (1989). Substance P and neurokinin A in the cat carotid body: localization, exogenous effects and changes in content in response to arterial PO_2. Brain Res. 481:205-214.

Prabhakar, N.R., Mitra, J. & Cherniack, N.S. (1987). Role of substance P in hypercapnic excitation of carotid chemoreceptors. J. Appl. Physiol. 63:2418-2425.

CENTRAL GLUTAMATE AND SUBSTANCE-P IN THE HYPOXIC VENTILATORY RESPONSE

Homayoun Kazemi and Ivan Soto-Arape

Department of Medicine, (Pulmonary and Critical Care Unit)
Massachusetts General Hospital and Harvard Medical School
Boston, Massachusetts 02114, U.S.A.

INTRODUCTION

In acute sustained hypoxia there is a rise in ventilation during the first few minutes, then the ventilation declines, but remains above prehypoxic levels (Vizek, et al., 1987) A diverse group of factors are involved in this biphasic response, among them are neurotransmitters and neuropeptides in the brain that are released during hypoxia (Dempsey et al., 1986) which affect ventilation.   Two excitatory neurochemicals of significance are the amino acid neurotransmitter glutamate (Kazemi & Hoop, 1991; Ang et al.,1992) and the neuropeptide substance-P (SP) (Kawanno & Chiba, 1984).   Glutamate and SP may be co-localized and co-released in the CNS (Kangra & Randic, 1990) and one exerts a modulatory influence on the other.   The hypothesis of the present study was that the hyperventilatory response to hypoxia is mediated by glutamate release centrally and further modulated by substance-P and that the ventral medullary surface (VMS) is structurally important in this response.

METHODS

18 male Sprague-Dawley rats (300-350 gms) were anesthetized with continuous inhalation of 2.5% of isoflurane and mechanically ventilated through a cervical tracheostomy (Harvard Apparatus rodent ventilator). Abdominal aorta was cannulated. Body temperature was maintained at 37.5°C. The ventrolateral medullary surface (VMS) was exposed and covered with a pool of CSF. A phrenic nerve was exposed and connected to a bipolar AgCl electrode. The phrenic neurogram was amplified and monitored on an oscilloscope.

The arterial pressure was monitored continuously. Arterial blood gases were measured periodically. At predetermined intervals phrenic bursts (minimum of 10) were quantified for magnitude and frequency and minute phrenic nerve output calculated.

Arterial Chemoreceptors: Cell to System
Edited by R. O'Regan *et al*, Plenum Press, New York, 1994

Experimental design

Three groups of experiments (6 animals each) were performed.

Control hypoxia. In this group, mock CSF (0.1 ml.) was directly applied to the ventral surface of the medulla. Data were obtained during normoxia and 20 minutes of hypoxia (10% O_2).

Hypoxia and SP. Data were obtained during normoxia, followed by a 4 minute hypoxic challenge. Then, during normoxia SP 2 mM (0.1 ml.) was applied to the VMS. Five minutes later the animals were put on 10% O_2 for 20 minutes.

Hypoxia and SP/MK-801. In this group, the initial part of the experiment was similar to group 2. Then during normoxia MK-801 at 8 mM (0.1 ml.) was applied directly to the VMS. Ten minutes later SP was also applied to the VMS and then the animals were exposed to hypoxia.

RESULTS

Hypoxia and mock CSF: Phrenic nerve output increased by 60% in the first 2 minutes of hypoxia and then fell, but was 13% above baseline during the remaining 20 minutes of hypoxia. The same response occurred whether mock CSF was applied to the VMS or not.

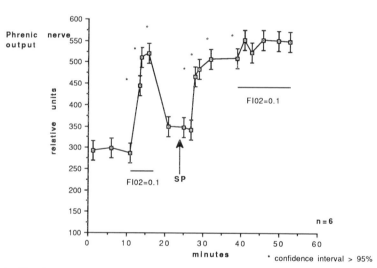

Figure 1. Phrenic nerve output in anesthetized, mechanically ventilated rats during hypoxia and after application of substance-P. Mean values + SEM.

Hypoxia and SP: Application of SP to the VMS increased phrenic nerve output during normoxia by 45%. Addition of hypoxia increased the output to 50% above baseline and there was no "roll-off".

Hypoxia and MK-801/SP: Application of NMDA antagonist, MK-801, to the VMS depressed phrenic nerve output by 90% and there was no response to hypoxia. Addition of SP during hypoxia did not overcome the depressive effect of MK-801.

282

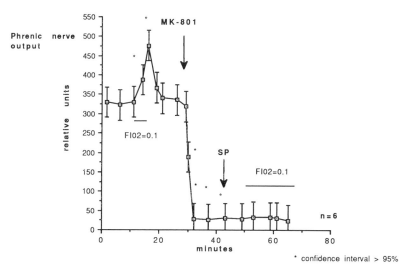

Figure 2. Phrenic nerve output in anesthetized, mechanically ventilated rats during hypoxia and after application of MK-801 and SP. Mean values + SEM.

DISCUSSION

The mammalian ventilatory response to acute sustained hypoxia is biphasic. There is an initial rise in ventilation and a subsequent fall in ventilation to a level above the pre-hypoxic value, the "roll off" effect (Bureau et al., 1984; Vizek et al., 1987). The mechanism(s) of this characteristic response is unclear. Glutamate and SP are excitatory CNS neurotransmitters and may play a major role in the initial hyperventilatory response to hypoxia. The findings of this study are that the initial increase in phrenic nerve output during acute sustained hypoxia is predominantly glutamatergic and that SP effects during normoxia and hypoxia are not present if glutamate receptors are blocked.

Substance-P is a known central respiratory stimulant. However, our findings suggest that SP effect during normoxia and hypoxia is through glutamatergic mechanisms.

Our prior work has shown that increased level of central glutamate, whether exogenous or endogenous, stimulates ventilation (Kazemi et al., 1989; Kazemi & Hoop, 1991). We have also shown that acute hypoxia increases glutamate turnover centrally. Interruption of the hypoxia sensing apparatus by carotid body denervation reduces the hyperventilatory response to hypoxia and decreases glutamate turnover centrally (Ang et al., 1992). This study corroborates our previous studies that blockade of brain stem NMDA receptors with MK-801, similarly abolishes the hyperventilatory response to acute hypoxia. These findings suggest an important role for glutamate in mediating the initial hyperventilatory response to acute hypoxia. We conclude that blockade of NMDA receptors on the ventral surface of the medulla with MK-801 decreases phrenic nerve output and prevents the initial rise in output in response to acute hypoxia. Application of SP to the VMS during normoxia and hypoxia does not overcome the glutamate blockade of phrenic nerve output. These findings suggest the presence of tonic glutamatergic input to basal ventilatory output. Facilitated glutamatergic transmission is important in the initial rapid rise in ventilation in response to acute hypoxia. The SP excitatory effect on ventilation during normoxia and hypoxia is probably mediated through glutamatergic mechanisms. The VMS is an important site for the action of excitatory neurochemicals in the hypoxic ventilatory response.

Ivan Soto-Arape was supported by the Will Rogers Memorial Fund.

REFERENCES

Ang, R.C., Hoop B., & Kazemi, H. (1992). Role of glutamate as the central neurotransmitter in the hypoxic ventilatory response. J.Appl. Physiol. 72:1480-1487.

Bureau, M.A., Zinman, R., Foulon, P., & Begin, R. (1984). Diphasic ventilatory response to hypoxia in the newborn lamb. J. Appl. Physil. 56: 84-90.

Dempsey, J.A., Olsen, E.B., & Skatrud, J.B. (1986). Hormones and neurochemicals in the regulation of breathing. In: Handbok of Physiology. The respiratory system. Control of breathing. Am. Physiol. Soc., Bethesda, MD, sect. 33, vol. II, chapt. 7, p.181-221.

Kangra, I., & Randic, M. (1990). Tachykinins and calcitonin gene related peptide enhance release the endogenous glutamate and aspartate from the rat spinal dorsal horn slice. J. Neurosci. 10:2026-2038.

Kawanno, H., & Chiba, T. (1984). Distribution of substance P immunoreactivity nerve terminals within the nucleus tractus solitarius of the rat. Neurosci. Lett. 45: 175-179.

Kazemi, H., Chiang, H. & Hoop, B. (1989). Role of medullary glutamate in the hypoxic ventilatory response. In: Chemoreceptors and Reflexes in Breathing, S. Lahiri., ed., New York: Oxford Univ. Press, p.233-242.

Kazemi, H., & Hoop, B. (1991). Glutamic acid and gamma-aminobutyric acid neurotransmitters in central control of breathing. J. Appl. Physiol. 70: 1-7.

Vizek, M., C.K. Pickett, & Weil, J.V. (1987). Biphasic ventilatory response of adult cats to sustained hypoxia has central origin. J. Appl. Physiol. 63: 1658-1664.

CAROTID CHEMORECEPTOR ACTIVITY AND HEART RATE RESPONSIVENESS TO HYPOXIA AFTER INHIBITION OF NITRIC OXIDE SYNTHASE

Andrzej Trzebski[1], Akio Sato[2], Yuko Sato[3] and Atsuko Suzuki[2]

[1]Department of Physiology, Medical Academy, Krakowskie Przedmiescie 26/28, 00-325 Warsaw, Poland; [2]Department of Autonomic Nervous System, Tokyo Metropolitan Institute of Gerontology, 35-2 Sakaecho, Itabashiku, Tokyo 173, Japan; [3]Division of Physiology, Tskuba College of Technology, Tsukubashi, Ibaragi 305, Japan

INTRODUCTION

Nitric oxide (NO), a free radical gas messenger in endothelial cells of blood vessels and in some central neurons (for references, Moncada et al., 1991) appears an interesting candidate to be considered in the mechanism of carotid body cells chemotransduction in view of its rapid inactivation by oxygen and by superoxides. Nitric oxide synthases (NOS) display close molecular homology with cytochrome P-450 reductase (Snyder, 1991). NOS molecule tightly bound with flavin adenine dinucleotide (FAD) transfers electrons successively between NADPH and flavins as a part of its catalytic activity (for references, Bredt et al., 1992). A similar molecular mechanism has been proposed as a molecular pathway of chemotransduction by Acker et al. (1992).

If generation of NO in carotid body plays a role in chemotransduction, a blockade of NOS should influence responsiveness of carotid chemoreceptor afferent activity to hypoxic stimuli. Furthermore, if endogenous NO modulates transmission in the pathway of the chemoreceptor-induced sympathetic cardiac reflex, NOS inhibition should affect the cardiac reflex response to hypoxia. The purpose of the present study was to check these possibilities.

METHODS

15 normotensive Wistar adults rats anaesthetized with urethane (0.9- 1.0 g/kg), paralyzed and artificially ventilated were used. Techniques of carotid sinus nerve dissection, recording and computing compound chemoreceptor afferent discharge, continuous recording of end-tidal O_2 and CO_2 concentration and other details of methods were presented elsewhere (Fukuda et al., 1987; Fukuda et al., 1989). In order to block NOS activity N-nitro-L-arginine methyl ester (L-NAME or L-NO_2-Arg) was used in a dose of 10 mg/kg.w. i.v. To reverse and overcome the blocking effect of L-NAME a 30 times greater dose of L-arginine was applied (300 mg/kg.w. i.v.). For statistical analysis the number of compound

spikes in the last 5s of hypoxic stimulation was counted in 2-3 control trials and several times in the 20-30 min period after L-NAME administration. After 30 min L-arginine was administered intravenously and hypoxic stimuli were repeated again. The gain of the reflex cardioacceleratory response to unloading of the arterial baroreceptors was estimated as the ratio of the peak response of heart rate acceleration (ΔHR) to the lowest value of arterial blood pressure during hypoxia. The gain of the reflex cardioinhibitory response was calculated as the ratio of the maximum reduction in heart rate (ΔHR) to the maximal increase in arterial blood pressure produced by hyperoxia or by L-NAME alone. Results were expressed as the mean ± S.E.M. Student's paired test was used to evaluate statistical significance.

RESULTS

Brief acute hypoxia at F_{ET} 6% O_2 produced a sharp and pronounced increase in mass activity of the peripheral end of the carotid sinus nerve (C.S.N., Fig. 1), a fall in the arterial blood pressure and an increase in the heart rate (Fig. 2).

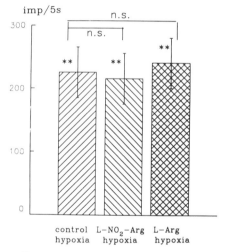

Figure 1. Lack of a significant effect of NOS inhibition on augmented carotid chemoreceptor discharge produced by F_{ET} 6% O_2 hypoxia. Vertical bars ± SEM. * P<0.05, ** P<0.01, *** P<0.001.

As the arterial blood pressure decreased during hypoxia, augmented C.S.N. afferent activity can not be accounted for baroreceptor activity. C.S.N. baroreceptor afferent activity does not significantly modify the primary carotid chemoreceptor response to hypoxia in rats (Fukuda et al. 1987, Fig 2). Following NOS blockade, the arterial blood pressure fall during hypoxia was significantly attenuated and the heart rate response enhanced (Fig. 2). Afferent chemoreceptor activity showed some variability, yet after all data were pooled, computed and expressed as respective means, no systematic and significant change in the chemoreceptor response to hypoxia could be found over the 20-30 min after L-NAME administration and after subsequent L-arginine administration (Fig. 1). In rats with aortic nerves cut hypoxia produced a cardioacceleration which was not significantly different from that observed before L-NAME administration. The gain of the baroreceptor cardiac reflex was significantly augmented after NOS inhibition: from 0.2 ± 0.05 to 0.9 ± 0.1 during hypoxic hypotension and from 0.52 ± 0.09 to 1.33 ± 0.21 during blood pressure rise. The

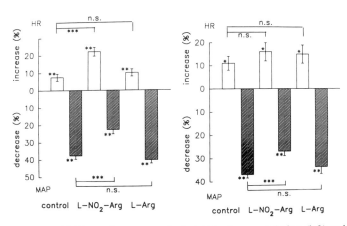

Figure 2. Effects of NOS inhibition on heart rate and arterial blood pressure before (left) and after bilateral aortic nerve section (right). Abbreviations as in Fig. 1.

cardioacceleratory effect of electrical stimulation of the sympathetic cardiac nerve was not influenced by L-NAME administration.

DISCUSSION AND CONCLUSIONS

Our data do not support the hypothesis that endogenous nitric oxide and/or nitric oxide synthesis within glomic or endothelial cells play a role in the mechanism of chemotransduction in the rat. L-NAME was used in a dose exceeding that which was used to prevent the peripheral vasodilator effect of hypoxia (Sun & Reis, 1992). However, some caution is needed. Adequate oxygen supply is required to sustain NOS - mediated NO production (Rengasamy & Johns, 1991) and even brief hypoxia may compromise NO synthesis. On the other hand, low tissue oxygen extends the half-life time and duration of effect of NO. Two opposite effects of hypoxia in the glomic cells might produce a null net effect, thus masking a real role for NO. A significant increase in cardioacceleratory response to hypoxia produced by NOS inhibition and reversed by L-arginine appears to be due to enhanced responsiveness of cardiac baroreceptor reflex. Bilateral section of aortic nerves, a major baroreceptor afferent input in rats (Sapru & Krieger, 1977; Fukuda et al., 1987), abolished the augmented increase in heart rate during hypoxia after NOS inhibition. Gain of the baroreceptor reflex heart rate response was significantly higher after NOS inhibition. The facilitatory effect of NO blockade upon the baroreceptor reflex can not be accounted for by altered responsiveness of the sympathetic effector side, as the heart rate response to electrical stimulation of the cardiac sympathetic nerve remained unchanged. The modulatory effect of endogenous NO upon the arterial baroreceptor cardioinhibitory reflex requires further research.

This study was supported by K.B.N. grant No 4 1728 91 01p/03

REFERENCES

Acker, H., Bolling, B, Delpiano, M.A., Dufau, E., Gorlach, A. & Holterman, H. (1992). The meaning of H_2O_2 generation in the carotid body cells for PO_2 generation. J. Auton. Nerv. Syst. 41:41-52.

Bredt, D.S., Hwang, P.H., Glatt, C., Loewenstein, C., Reed, R.R. & Snyder, S.H. (1991). Cloned and expressed nitric oxide synthase structurally resembles cytochrome P-reductase. Nature 352:714-718.

Bredt, D.S. & Snyder, S.H. (1992). Nitric oxide, a novel neuronal messenger. Neuron 8:3-11.

Fukuda, Y., Sato, A. & Trzebski, A. (1987). Carotid chemoreceptor discharge responses to hypoxia and hypercapnia in normotensive and spontaneously hypertensive rats. J. Auton. Nerv. Syst. 19:1-11.

Fukuda, Y., Sato, A., Suzuki, A. & Trzebski, A. (1989). Autonomic nerve and cardiovascular responses to changing blood oxygen and carbon dioxide levels in the rat. J. Auton. Nerv. Syst. 28:61-74.

Moncada, S., Palmer, R.M. & Higgs, E.A. (1991). Nitric oxide: physiology, pathophysiology, and pharmacology. Pharm. Rev. 43:109-142.

Rengasamy, A. & Johns, R.A. (1991). Characterization of endothelium-derived relaxing factor/nitric oxide synthase from bovine cerebellum and mechanism of modulation by high and low oxygen tensions. J. Pharmacol. Exp. Therap. 259:310-316.

Sapru, H.N. & Krieger, A.J. (1977). Carotid and aortic chemoreceptor function in the rat. J. Appl. Physiol. 42:344-348.

Sun, M.K. & Reis, D.J. (1992). Evidence that nitric oxide mediates the vasodepressor response to hypoxia in sino-denervated rats. Life Sciences 50:555-565.

EFFECTS OF ENDOTHELINS ON RESPIRATION AND ARTERIAL CHEMORECEPTOR ACTIVITY IN ANAESTHETISED RATS

Daniel S. McQueen[1], Michael R. Dashwood[2], Vanessa J. Cobb[1] and Charles G. Marr[1]

[1]Department of Pharmacology, University of Edinburgh Medical School, 1 George Square, Edinburgh, UK and [2]Department of Physiology, Royal Free Hospital School of Medicine, London, UK

INTRODUCTION

The endothelins (ETs) are a family of peptides (ET-1, ET-2, ET-3) that can be released from the endothelium by hypoxia. Two subtypes of ET receptor have been identified - ET_A and ET_B (see Haynes et al., 1993).

We have previously demonstrated ET-binding sites in the carotid body, carotid sinus, and nucleus of the tractus solitarius (NTS) in the cat (Spyer et al., 1991) and also provided some electrophysiological evidence suggesting that ETs can affect the activity of cat carotid body chemoreceptors (McQueen et al., 1991).

The present investigation was undertaken to determine whether ETs affect ventilation in anaesthetised rats and, if they do, whether carotid chemoreceptors are involved. We also undertook an autoradiographic study to establish if binding sites for ETs are present in the rat carotid body and NTS.

METHODS

Experiments were performed on adult male Wistar rats. Full details for the ventilatory and electrophysiological experiments on pentobarbitone - anaesthetised rats can be found in McQueen et al. (1989); details for autoradiography are provided in Spyer et al. (1991). The endothelin antagonist FR139317 was generously provided by the Fujisawa Pharmaceutical Company (Osaka, Japan).

RESULTS

Ventilation

ET-1 caused a dose-related transient increase in respiratory minute volume (RMV) when injected i.v. (0.1 - 3µg; 40pmoles - 1.2nmoles), as illustrated in Fig.1A. The increase in ventilation was due mainly to an increase in respiratory frequency. Cutting both carotid sinus nerves abolished the reflex increase in ventilation evoked by sodium cyanide (100 µg i.v.) and also abolished the increase in ventilation seen following ET-1 1µg (400 pmoles) (Fig.1B).

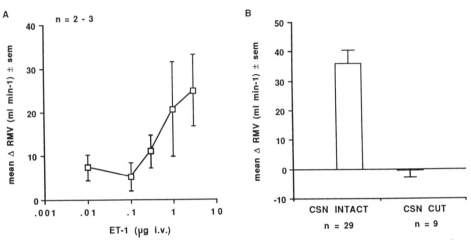

Figure 1. Effects of ET-1 on ventilation. **A** shows the dose-related increase in RMV. **B** Illustrates that the increase in RMV evoked by ET-1 (1µg) was abolished after cutting both carotid sinus nerves.

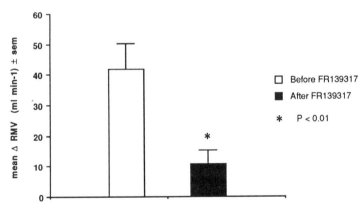

Figure 2. Ventilatory response to ET-1 (1µg i.v.) before and after injection of the ET_A antagonist FR139317 (1mg.kg^{-1} i.v.). Basal RMV was 115 ± 9 mls.min^{-1} before, and 113 ± 7 mls.min^{-1} after the antagonist, n = 5 before and after.

Mean blood pressure showed biphasic changes following ET-1, a fall in BP of about 40 mmHg being followed by a rise of about 25 mmHg. The increase in ventilation occurred during the 30 s period following injection of ET-1, i.e. during the hypotension. ET-3 (0.1 - 0.3µg) caused only hypotension and a slight increase in RMV. Ventilatory responses to hypoxia (10% oxygen in 90% nitrogen for 3 minutes) were not significantly different after ET-1 or ET-3 (1µg dose). FR139317 (ET_A antagonist, 1mg kg^{-1} i.v.) significantly reduced the increase in ventilation caused by ET-1 (Fig.2) and abolished the secondary hypertension; the antagonist had no significant effect on ventilatory responses to hypoxia nor to cyanide. Inhibition of nitric oxide synthase with L-NAME (10mg kg^{-1} i.v.) significantly reduced the primary hypotension caused by ET-1 (1µg i.v.), but did not significantly reduce the concurrent increase in RMV.

Neural Recording

Recordings of chemosensory activity from the peripheral end of the sectioned carotid sinus nerve showed a dose-related increase in discharge occurred at the same time as RMV increases had been observed following ET-1 (1 µg i.v.).

Autoradiography

The binding studies revealed that the rat carotid body and NTS contain ET-binding sites. Binding of radiolabelled ET-1 in the carotid body was displaceable by the ET_A antagonist FR139317, suggesting that ET_A receptors predominate there.

DISCUSSION

ET-1 causes a dose-related hyperventilation when injected i.v. in anaesthetised rats. This effect was abolished by cutting both carotid sinus nerves, suggesting that carotid body arterial chemoreceptors are involved: confirmation that ET-1 does cause chemoexcitation came from neural recordings of carotid sinus nerve activity. The autoradiographic study demonstrated that, as in the cat (Spyer et al., 1991), ET-binding sites are present in the rat carotid body and NTS, and the fact that radiolabelled ET-1 could be displaced by the ET_A antagonist FR139317 (see Haynes et al., 1993) is strong evidence that ETA receptors in the carotid body are responsible for chemoexcitation. This accords with the finding that ET-1 was much more potent than ET-3 (much weaker ET_A agonist) in causing hyperventilation.

Both ET-1 and ET-3 caused an initial hypotension when injected i.v.. It seemed unlikely that this hyperventilation could be secondary to ET-evoked vasodilatation, particularly since ET-3 had less effect on ventilation. However, since the hypotension is attributed to activation of the ET_B receptor which in turn leads to release of nitric oxide (Fozard & Part, 1992), we used the nitric oxide synthase inhibitor, L-NAME to reduce the hypotension and found that the hyperventilation associated with ET-1 was unaffected, or even increased in some experiments, following L-NAME. Thus, the chemoexcitation seen following these fairly high doses of ET-1 is not secondary to the hypotension and doesn't appear to involve nitric oxide.

Further studies are required to establish the physiological role of ET-1 and ET_A receptors in the carotid body, and to determine whether endothelins play a part in sensory transduction.

REFERENCES

Fozard, J.R. and Part, M.L. (1992). The role of nitric oxide in the regional vasodilator effects of endothelin-1 in the rat. Br. J. Pharmacol. 105:744-750.

Haynes, W.G., Davenport, A.P. and Webb, D.J. (1993). Endothelin: progress in pharmacology and physiology. Trends in Pharmacological Science, 14:225-228.

McQueen, D.S., Ritchie, I.M. and Birrell, G.J. (1989). Arterial chemoreceptor involvement in salicylate-induced hyperventilation in rats. Br. J. Pharmacol. 98:413-424.

McQueen, D.S., Dashwood, M.R. and Sykes, R.M. (1991). Effects of endothelin-1 on carotid baroreceptor and chemoreceptor activity in the anaesthetised cat. J. Physiol. (Lond.) 438:89P.

Spyer, K.M., McQueen, D.S., Dashwood, M.R., Sykes, R.M., Daly, M. de B. and Muddle, J.R. (1991). Localisation of [^{125}I]endothelin binding sites in the region of the carotid bifurcation and brainstem of the cat : possible baro- and chemoreceptor involvement. J. Cardiovascular Pharmacol. 17 (Suppl.7):S385-389.

CHANGES IN BLOOD GLUCOSE CONCENTRATION IN THE CAROTID BODY MODIFY BRAIN GLUCOSE RETENTION

Ramón Alvarez-Buylla,[1] and Elena Roces de Alvarez-Buylla[2]

[1]Centro Universitario de Investigaciones Biomédicas, Universidad de Colima, Colima, Col. México and [2]CINVESTAV, México D.F., México

INTRODUCTION

In a previous study we have shown that a decrease in baroreceptor output, elicited by carotid occlusion (Hering reflex), or chemoreceptor stimulation with small doses of cyanide (NaCN) increase arterial glucose levels and enhance glucose uptake by the brain (Alvarez-Buylla & R. de Alvarez-Buylla, 1988). This suggested the participation of the carotid sinus receptors in glucose homeostasis. In this paper we show that changes in blood glucose concentration in the carotid sinus influence the amount of glucose retained by the brain.

METHODS

Experiments were performed on 36 Wistar rats (300-350 g weight). Anesthesia was induced and maintained by intraperitoneal administration of sodium pentobarbital. Respiration and body temperature were artificially controlled. Two rats were used for each experiment. The common carotid artery was cannulated in rat B to temporarily perfuse the vascularly isolated carotid sinus of rat A through its common carotid artery. Blood was sent back to rat B from the cannulated lingual artery in rat A to the jugular vein in rat B. In order to ensure that homeostatic responses were triggered by changes in the blood reaching the right carotid sinus of rat A, both aortic nerves and the left carotid nerve were sectioned in rat A.

Rat B was injected (i.v., femoral vein) with either NaCN (20 μg/kg), glucose (300 mg/dl) or insulin (10 U/kg). Since the effects of NaCN are immediate and direct on the carotid body (Alvarez-Buylla & R. de Alvarez-Buylla, 1988), the carotid sinus of rat A was perfused while rat B received the injection of NaCN. For the experiments in which the perfusate glucose concentration was modified by injections of glucose or insulin, we waited 2 and 10 min, respectively, for glucose concentration in rat B to reach a maximum or minimum before starting the perfusion. The time of NaCN injection or when perfusion started was considered as t=0 (indicated as an arrow in the Figures). Blood samples in rat A were obtained as described before. At each sample time, 0.2 ml of blood from each catheter was collected, t=-4 min, t=-2 min and t=0 (basal values), and at t=2 min, t=4 min, t=8 min and t=16 min after stimulation. Plasma glucose concentration was measured by the glucose

Arterial Chemoreceptors: Cell to System
Edited by R. O'Regan *et al*, Plenum Press, New York, 1994

oxidase method. Glucose uptake by the brain was recorded in μmol/g/min by measuring blood flow and arterio-venous glucose difference across the brain (Hawkins et al., 1974).

RESULTS

When the carotid body of rat A was perfused with normal blood from rat B (4.8 - 6.7 mM glucose), no changes from basal values were detected on brain glucose retention, or on the circulation levels of glucose in rat A. In contrast, between 2 and 16 min after perfusing the carotid sinus of rat A with blood from rat B that received an injection of NaCN, glucose retention by the brain increased significantly. This response was maximal 4 minutes after stimulation, when glucose retention reached 0.28 ± 0.08 μmol/g/min compared to 0.13 ± 0.05 μmol/g/min at t=0 (p=0.0001). This result confirmed our earlier observation and demonstrates that the carotid sinus, perfused by blood from rat B, is functional.

Next we tested the effects of hyper-or hypoglycemia to the carotid sinus on the retention of glucose by the brain. Hyperglycemic blood (16.7 mM) after the injection of glucose into rat B, induced a 43 % ±4 reduction in brain glucose retention in rat A (t=0 vs t=4; p=0.004) (columns in Fig. 1). This effect lasted for at least 16 min (p=0.034) and was noticeable soon after the stimulus, but did not reach significance at the earliest time sampled (t=2) (p=0.056). This decrease in brain glucose retention was accompanied by a slight increase in the circulating levels of glucose in rat A.

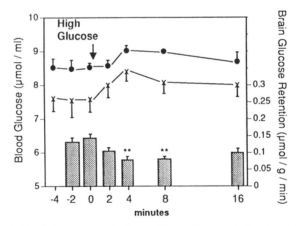

Figure 1. Changes in blood glucose concentration and brain glucose retention in rat A after perfusing its temporarily isolated carotid sinus with glucose-rich blood (300 mg/dl of glucose were injected into rat B, hyperglycemic blood 16.7 mM) (n=6). Solid circles: arterial glucose; crosses: venous glucose; columns: brain glucose retention. Mean±SEM, **P<0.01, *P<0.05.

In contrast, the perfusion of the isolated carotid sinus in rat A with hypoglycemic blood (2.7 mM), induced by insulin injection into rat B, had the opposite effect; brain glucose retention in rat A increased significantly from 0.13±0.03 μmol/g/min at t=0 to 0.23±0.06 μmol/g/min at t=4 (p<0.0073) (columns in Fig. 2). This effect was already significant at t=2 and lasted for at least 8 min. Hypoglycemic blood perfused to the carotid sinus, induced a noticeable hyperglycemia in arterial and venous blood of rat A.

DISCUSSION

Results showed an increase in glucose retention by the brain after perfusing the isolated carotid sinus with blood from an animal that had received i.v. NaCN. In a previous report, the denervation of the carotid sinus-body region abolished a similar reflex elicited by the direct infusion of NaCN to the carotid sinus, and led us to rule out the possibility that NaCN entering the general circulation had a direct effect on brain. The present experiments support this conclusion. Furthermore, we show that changes in blood glucose reaching only the carotid sinus affect the amount of glucose retained by the brain.

Since the carotid sinus is sensitive to several factors, including PO_2, PCO_2, pH and osmolarity, we decided to test its sensitivity to glucose, using an experimental system as close as possible to normal. However, the experiments perfusing the isolated carotid sinus with blood containing different concentrations of glucose, suggest, but do not demonstrate that the carotid sinus receptors are responsive to changes in blood glucose. Insulin or

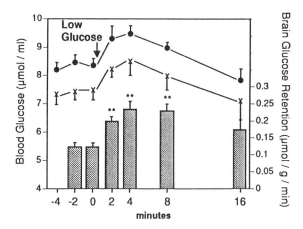

Figure 2. Changes in blood glucose concentration and brain glucose retention in rat A after perfusing its temporarily isolated carotid sinus with glucose-poor blood (insulin 10 U/kg was injected into rat B so that its blood was hypoglycemic-2.7 mM) (n=6). Symbols as in Figure 1.

glucose injections into rat B may affect an unknown factor that modifies carotid sinus activity, explaining the observed effects. Our experiments demonstrate that independent of the pathway by which glucose acts on the carotid sinus, the amount of glucose retained by the brain changes accordingly: high glucose perfused to the carotid sinus induces a decrease in brain glucose retention, and low glucose induces an increase in glucose retention by the brain. These results strengthen our previous conclusion that the carotid sinus receptors participate in glucose homeostasis. There are multiple pathways by which peripheral chemoreceptor inputs may influence central respiratory centers (Finley & Katz, 1992), and these pathways may also affect brain glucose regulation. Enkephalins, that seem to be involve in glucose regulation (Radosevich et al., 1989), and are present in higher concentration around the nucleus of the tractus solitarius (Watson & Barchas, 1979), could participate in humoral glucoregulation after carotid sinus receptor stimulation. Further work should explore if glucose acts directly on carotid sinus receptors and investigate the neural and humoral pathways that mediate these effects of glucose.

REFERENCES

Alvarez-Buylla, R. & R. de Alvarez-Buylla, E. (1988). Carotid sinus receptors participate in glucose homeostasis. Respir. Physiol. 72:347-360.

Finley, J. C. & Katz, D. M. (1992). The central organization of carotid body afferent projections to the brainstem of the rat. Brain res. 572:108-116.

Hawkins, R. A., Miller, A. L., Cremer, J. E. & Veech, R. L. (1974). Measurement of the rate of glucose utilization by rat brain in vivo. J. Neurochem. 23:917-923.

Radosevich, P. M., Lacy, D. B., Brown, L. L., Williams, P. E. & Abumrad, N. N. (1989). Central effects of β-endorphins on glucose homeostasis in conscious dog. Amer. J. Physiol. 256:E322-E330.

Watson, S. J. & Barchas, J. D. (1979). Anatomy of the endogenous peptides and related substances and the enkephalins, β-endorphin and ACTH, In "Mechanisms of Pain and Analgesic Compounds". R.F. Beer and E.G. Bassett, eds., Raven Press, New York pp. 227-238.

IS THE SECOND CAROTID BODY REDUNDANT?

Patricia A. Cragg[1] and Wilaiwan Khrisanapant[2]

[1]Department of Physiology, University of Otago, Dunedin, New Zealand;
[2]Department of Physiology, Khon Kaen University, Khon Kaen, Thailand

INTRODUCTION

The carotid bodies (CB) are the main detectors of arterial hypoxia. In the rat, bilateral denervation of these chemoreceptors abolishes most of the hypoxic stimulation of ventilation (Martin-Body et al., 1985; Khrisanapant & Cragg, 1988). The response that remains is attributed to the numerous but tiny carotid-body-like paraganglia found throughout the thorax and abdomen by McDonald & Blewett (1981). A simplistic approach is to expect that each of the inputs from the various chemoreceptors will act together in a purely additive manner. Alternatively there may be redundancy within the multiplicity of chemoafferent inputs.

Surprisingly few studies have examined the consequences on ventilation of denervating only one carotid body. Unilateral CB excision or nerve section has been reported to have no effect on the ventilatory responses to i.v. sodium cyanide or inhalation of 12% O_2 in the goat (Busch et al., 1983) whereas it causes modest reductions in the rat (Housley & Sinclair, 1988) and cat (Zapata et al., 1990). However our experience in the rat has been that failure to section adequately the nerve from one of the carotid bodies invariably resulted in a seemingly normal ventilatory response to hypoxia. This impression has now been formally examined.

METHODS

Anaesthesia in male Charles-Wistar rats (250-360 g body weight; n = 13) was induced with ether and after cannulation of the femoral vein was continued with i.v. pentobarbitone (initial dose: 30-40 mg/kg; maintenance dose: 12-16 mg/kg/h). Rectal temperature was maintained at 38°C with a thermostatically controlled heating pad and the trachea and femoral artery were cannulated. To measure ventilation, rats were placed supine in a plethysmograph with all cannulae exteriorized. Arterial blood pressure and end-tidal O_2 and CO_2 were also continuously monitored. Test gases (21, 16, 13, 10 and 8% O_2 in N_2 with no CO_2) were delivered sequentially in descending order, each for 2 min, and at a flow rate of ~1 litre/min past the tracheal opening.

All rats were tested before and immediately after a denervation procedure – thus each rat was its own control. CB denervation was achieved by sectioning the glossopharyngeal nerve, a procedure which took 15-20 min. Some of the rats which were sham denervated were subsequently tested after right or left CB denervation. Half of the rats which were unilaterally denervated were subsequently subjected to bilateral CB denervation. Data were grouped as follows: unilateral sham denervation (n = 4), left CB denervation (n = 7), right CB denervation (n = 6) and bilateral CB denervation (n = 7). Data are expressed as means ± S.E.M. and statistical significance was evaluated with paired t-tests.

RESULTS

In air, control rats (n = 13) breathed at a ventilation (V_E) of 52.5 ± 2.4 ml/100g/min, a tidal volume (V_T) of 0.574 ± 0.018 ml and a frequency (f) of 90.6 ± 2.5 /min; the mean arterial blood pressure was 134 ± 4 mmHg. Unilateral sham denervation (n = 4) did not modify the V_E response to hypoxia (for 8% O_2: control V_E 96.8 ± 8.2 ml/100g/min cf sham V_E 92.4 ± 10.3).

Left CB denervation (n = 7) had no effect on the V_E response to hypoxia except at 8% O_2 where the V_E was reduced from the control value of 92.6 ± 5.7 to 75.1 ± 6.4 ml/100g/min (P < 0.05). This reduction in the V_E response was entirely due to the frequency component (control f 133 ± 5.5 cf left CBD f 112 ± 8 /min; P < 0.05); the tidal volume was not affected (control V_T 0.697 ± 0.023 cf left CBD V_T 0.666 ± 0.016 ml/100g). In contrast, right CB denervation (n = 6) had no effect even at 8% O_2 (control V_E 91.9 ± 6.7 cf right CBD V_E 89.3 ± 3.1 ml/100g/min). When data for right and left CB denervation were pooled (n = 13) the reduction in V_E in 8% O_2 was no longer significant (Table 1).

Table 1. Effect of unilateral and bilateral CB denervation on V_E.

	21% O_2	16% O_2	13% O_2	10% O_2	8% O_2
Control	53 ± 2	69 ± 5	79 ± 1	87 ± 3	91 ± 6
Unilateral	56 ± 2	68 ± 3	81 ± 3	83 ± 3	83 ± 4
Bilateral	48 ± 2	58 ± 5	59 ± 4	63 ± 7	56 ± 10

Ventilation expressed as ml/min/100g b.w., mean ± SEM

As expected, bilateral CB denervation (n = 7) reduced V_E during air breathing and in response to all hypoxic gases, particularly 8% O_2 (P < 0.05; Table 1). The reductions in V_E were mainly due to a decrease in the frequency component (e.g. in 10% O_2, the control f and V_T were 131 ± 3 /min and 0.70 ± 0.04 ml/100g compared with a bilateral CBD f and V_T of 105 ± 5 /min and 0.61 ± 0.03 ml/100g).

DISCUSSION

Halving the CB input by means of a unilateral denervation did not halve the V_E response to hypoxia in rats. Denervation of the right CB appeared to be without effect whereas left CB denervation produced some reduction in the V_E response but only to severe hypoxia. Further experiments are required to substantiate this right/left difference. The conclusion from pooled data for unilateral CB denervation is that the input from one CB, in the presence of the other, appears to be completely redundant until severe hypoxia is encountered and even then the contribution is small.

A similar effect was found in adult rats treated neonatally with capsaicin (Cragg et al., 1992). Capsaicin halved both the number of axons in the carotid sinus nerves and the nerve activity at all levels of hypoxia but had little effect on V_E. As capsaicin-treatment produces a chronic rather than an acute denervation, central reorganisation of the remaining inputs may partly explain this V_E response.

Is there any evidence for chemoreceptor redundancy? Although Donoghue et al. (1985) found that subthreshold stimuli simultaneously applied to carotid and aortic chemoafferents acted on a single neuron in the nucleus tractus solitarius (NTS) in an additive manner, Eldridge et al. (1981) reported that simultaneous low-level electrical stimulation to right and left carotid sinus nerves caused only 70% of the predicted additive effect on phrenic nerve output. Data from Lipski et al. (1984) may offer another explanation. They showed that the carotid chemoreceptor input excites unilaterally not only the NTS but also the expiratory neurons of the Bötzinger complex, some of which in turn inhibit the inspiratory neurons of the contralateral NTS. Perhaps removal of one carotid body causes some disinhibition of the remaining contralateral input which partially masks the loss of the unilateral input.

REFERENCES

Busch, M.A., Bisgard, G.E., Mesina, J.E. & Forster, H.V. (1983). The effects of unilateral carotid body excision on ventilatory control in goats. Respir. Physiol. 54: 353-361.

Cragg, P.A., Kou, Y.R. & Prabhakar, N.R. (1992). Ventilatory and carotid chemoreceptor responses to hypoxia in neonatally capsaicin-treated rats. Fedn. Am. Soc. Exp. Biol. 6(4): A1172.

Donoghue, S., Felder, R.B., Gilbey, M.P., Jordan, D. & Spyer, K.M. (1985). Post-synaptic activity evoked in the nucleus tractus solitarius by carotid sinus and aortic nerve afferents in the cat. J. Physiol. (Lond.) 360: 261-273.

Eldridge, F.L., Gill-Kumar, P. & Millhorn, D.E. (1981). Input-output relationship of central neural circuits involved in respiration in cats. J. Physiol. (Lond.) 311: 81-95.

Housley, G.D. & Sinclair J.D. (1988). Localization by kainic acid lesions of neurones transmitting the carotid chemoreceptor stimulus for respiration in rat. J. Physiol. (Lond.) 406: 99-114.

Khrisanapant, W. & Cragg, P.A. (1988). Contribution of carotid body and vagal chemoreceptors to ventilatory sensitivity to normocapnic hypoxia in anaesthetized rats. Proc. Univ. Otago Med. Sch. 66: 55-56.

Lipski, J., Trzebski, A., Chodobska, J. & Kruk, P. (1984). Effects of carotid chemoreceptor excitation on medullary expiratory neurons in cats. Respir. Physiol. 57: 279-291.

McDonald, D.M. & Blewett, R.W. (1981). Location and size of carotid-body-like organs (paraganglia) revealed in rats by the permeability of blood vessels to Evans blue dye. J. Neurocytol. 10: 607-643.

Martin-Body, R.L., Robson, G.J. & Sinclair, J.D. (1985). Respiratory effects of sectioning the carotid sinus, glossopharyngeal and abdominal vagus nerves in the awake rat. J. Physiol. (Lond.) 361: 35-45.

Zapata, P., Larrain, C. & Eugenin, J. (1990). Restoration of chemoreflexes alter unilateral carotid deafferentation. In "Chemoreceptors and Chemoreceptor Reflexes". H. Acker, A. Trzebski & R.G. O'Regan, eds., Plenum Press, New York.

ACTIVITY OF CARDIAC VAGAL PREGANGLIONIC NEURONES DURING THE PULMONARY CHEMOREFLEX IN THE ANAESTHETIZED CAT.

James F.X. Jones, Yun Wang, and David Jordan.

Department of Physiology, Royal Free Hospital School of Medicine, Rowland Hill Street, London NW3 2PF

INTRODUCTION

The pulmonary chemoreflex is a primitive stereotyped response which occurs when phenylbiguanide (PBG) is injected into the pulmonary circulation. This is a chemical which activates receptors located near the pulmonary capillaries and supplied by small unmyelinated nerve fibres running in the vagus. The reflex response of the animal to this chemical flooding the pulmonary circulation is a cessation of breathing and a slowing of the heartbeat. With smaller doses of PBG there is little effect upon respiration although the cardiac effect is still obvious. This bradycardia is of interest because in the cat, it appears to unmodulated by central inspiratory activity (Daly, 1991). This is in marked contrast to the bradycardia of the carotid body chemoreflex which demonstrates such tight cardiorespiratory coupling. This result is still obtained after cardiac sympathetic denervation, indicating that cardiac vagal motoneurones are responsible. It has been postulated that these two reflexes utilize two different populations of cardiac vagal motoneurones, and that one population may not be coupled to the central respiratory network. There is some anatomical support for this two population hypothesis. When horseradish peroxidase is applied to the cardiac branch of the cat (Bennett et al., 1981; Jordan et al., 1986), labelled cells are seen in two very different locations. One group is found in the vicinity of the nucleus ambiguus in the ventral part of the medulla oblongata, and the other group is near the dorsal vagal motor nucleus. The experiments of McAllen & Spyer (1978) have clearly demonstrated that the ventral group play an important part in cardioinhibitory reflexes. This group of neurones exhibit strong respiratory related activity and have axons in the B-fibre range. The function of the dorsal group is unknown. The question arises then, how do these two populations behave during the pulmonary chemoreflex ?

METHODS

In sixteen cats anaesthetized with chloralose (50mg/kg) and urethane (0.5g/kg) i.p. the right cranial cardiac vagal branch was stimulated to evoke antidromic activity in the medulla, as described in detail previously (McAllen & Spyer, 1976; Gilbey et al., 1984). The right phrenic nerve was dissected, desheathed and placed on recording electrodes to provide an index of central inspiratory activity. A right atrial cannula was used to inject phenylbiguanide

(PBG) (7-30 µg/kg) into the pulmonary circulation. In order to expose the medulla, the occipital bone was opened and the dura over the cerebellum excised and reflected. Extracellular recordings of medullary neurones were made with single and multibarrel microelectrodes, in which one barrel was filled with DL-homocysteic acid (DLH), (0.2M, pH8.5). The location of antidromically evoked neurones was determined histologically following ionophoresis of pontamine sky blue into the responsive sites.

RESULTS

Cardiac vagal preganglionic neurones are concentrated just ventral to the two motor nuclei of the vagus, though none of the neurones are actually in these compact nuclei. The majority of the antidromically evoked responses were considered to arise from cell bodies rather than axons since many showed a fractionation of the spike into IS-SD components and had durations greater than 2 ms. Ionophoresis of DLH produced an increased firing and this is considered to affect cell bodies but not axons. The dorsal group of vagal preganglionic neurones (n=27) were located in the nucleus intercalatus and the ventral group (n=5) ventrolateral to the nucleus ambiguus. All the dorsal group neurones had axons which conducted in the C-fibre range (0.54-1.4 m/sec) and the ventral group neurones had B-fibre axons (4.2-9.3 m/sec). Nine cells of the C-fibre group exhibited spontaneous activity whereas the other eighteen were silent. Two cells showed long latency synaptic excitation (210-260ms) from the cardiac branch. In contrast, five cells had properties indicating that they received an inhibitory input from the cardiac branch. These included poor frequency following, IS-SD failure and inhibition of spontaneous discharge by cardiac branch stimulation. Two of the three spontaneously active neurones and none of the 8 silent neurones recorded during a PBG evoked bradycardia showed an increase in activity. One of the two spontaneously active neurones of the B-fibre group were excited during a PBG evoked bradycardia. There is a dramatic difference in the basal firing pattern of the B and C-fibre cardiac preganglionic neurones. Whereas the B-fibre group exhibit powerful respiratory modulation when spontaneously active, the C-fibre group discharge is of low frequency and unrelated to central respiration. The spontaneous activity of one cardiac C-fibre preganglionic neurone was recorded long enough to construct peristimulus time histograms triggered from the integrated phrenic nerve discharge, the ECG and the tracheal pressure. No obvious relation was found in the discharge pattern to any of these variables.

DISCUSSION

This study is an attempt to explain the oddity of the pulmonary chemoreflex. The finding that both groups of cardiac preganglionic neurones are excited during this reflex is perhaps not that surprising since in addition to bradycardia the pulmonary chemoreflex is associated with negative inotropy, negative dromotropy, and cholinergic coronary vasodilatation (Coleridge & Coleridge 1985). However, the fact that the dorsal C-fibre cardiac preganglionic neurones lack respiratory modulation suggests that potentially they could be involved in the powerful negative chronotropic response of the pulmonary chemoreflex. In this regard we have previously demonstrated that selective cardiac C-fibre efferent stimulation in a variety of species can slow the heart (Jones & Jordan 1993). Perhaps it is the combined firing pattern of the two populations of cardiac vagal preganglionic neurones descending on the final common pathway at the cardiac ganglion that determines the cardiac response.

This work was supported by the MRC and the Wellcome Trust.

REFERENCES

Bennett, J.A., Kidd, C., Latif, A.B., & McWilliam, P.N. (1981). A horseradish peroxidase study of vagal motoneurones with axons in cardiac and vagal branches of the cat and dog. Q. J. Exp. Physiol. 66: 145-154.

Coleridge, J.C.G. & Coleridge, H.M. (1984). Afferent vagal C-fibre innervation of the lungs and airways and its functional significance. Rev. Physiol. Biochem. Pharmacol. 99: 1-110.

Daly, M. de B. (1991). Some reflex cardioinhibitory responses in the cat and their modulation by central inspiratory neuronal activity. J. Physiol. (Lond.) 439: 559-577.

Gilbey, M.P., Jordan, D., Richter, D.W. & Spyer, K.M. (1984). Synaptic mechanisms involved in the inspiratory control of vagal cardio-inhibitory neurones in the cat. J. Physiol. (Lond.) 356: 65-78.

Jones, J.F.X. & Jordan, D. (1993). Evidence for a chronotropic response to cardiac vagal motor C-fibre stimulation in anaesthetized cats rats and rabbits. J. Physiol. (Lond.) 467: 148P.

Jordan, D., Spyer, K.M., Withington-Wray, D.J. & Wood, L.M. (1986). Histochemical and electrophysiological identification of cardiac and pulmonary vagal preganglionic neurones in the cat. J. Physiol. (Lond.) 372: 87P.

McAllen, R.M. & Spyer, K.M. (1976) The location of cardiac vagal preganglionic motoneurones in the medulla of the cat. J. Physiol. (Lond.) 258: 187-204.

McAllen, R.M. & Spyer, K.M. (1978) Two types of vagal preganglionic motoneurones projecting to the heart and lungs. J. Physiol. (Lond.) 282: 353-364.

TROPHIC REGULATION OF CAROTID BODY AFFERENT DEVELOPMENT

Torbjörn Hertzberg,[1,3] James C.W. Finley,[2] and David M. Katz[1,2]

[1]Department of Neurosciences, School of Medicine, Case Western Reserve University, Cleveland, OH, USA; [2]Department of Medicine, University Hospitals, Cleveland, OH, USA and [3]Department of Pediatrics, Karolinska Hospital, Stockholm, Sweden

INTRODUCTION

The ventilatory reflex response to hypoxia matures postnatally, from the biphasic pattern seen in the newborn to the more sustained hyperventilation typical of the adult (Eden & Hanson, 1987). Several mechanisms have been proposed to underlie this maturation, including an increase in chemoreceptor sensitivity and a decreased suprapontine inhibitory influence. However, the role of chemosensory afferent development in shaping the ventilatory response has been relatively unexplored. Primary afferent neurons in the glossopharyngeal petrosal ganglion (PG) convey chemosensory information from the carotid body to the brainstem. A large subset of carotid body afferents express dopaminergic traits including tyrosine hydroxylase (TH) and dopa decarboxylase, and 84% of these cells project to the carotid body via the sinus nerve (Katz et al., 1987). Moreover, TH immunoreactive (TH[+]) cells in the PG make synaptic contact with carotid body type I cells, further supporting a role in chemoreception (Finley et al., 1992; Katz, unpublished). Immunoreactivity for TH can therefore be used as a highly selective marker for carotid body afferents in the PG. The observation that the number of TH[+] neurons in the PG increases during the last trimester of gestation, following the onset of carotid body innervation, suggests that the carotid body may regulate maturation of these neurons (Katz & Erb 1990). This is consistent with the concept that development of innervating neurons requires interaction with target tissues. The present study demonstrates that glomectomy in newborn rats causes a marked loss of TH[+] neurons in the PG and that this loss can be attenuated by administration of brain-derived neurotrophic factor (BDNF). We conclude that postnatal development of chemosensory neurons is dependent on peripheral target innervation, and propose that target-derived influences are mediated by BDNF, or similar factors.

METHODS

Sprague-Dawley rats were used throughout the study. Newborns, <24 h old, and 3 week-old animals were anesthetized with ketamine (25 mg/kg) and xylazine (40 mg/kg) i.p., and the right carotid body was exposed through a ventral incision in the neck. Care was taken not to damage surrounding tissues, and major nerves and vessels were left intact. The carotid body was either removed or left undisturbed (sham), and after recovery, the newborn pups were returned to their mothers. Three weeks later, the animals were deeply anesthetized with ether and transcardially perfused with fixative. The PGs were dissected out and processed for immunocytochemical staining of TH and neurofilament proteins as previously described (Katz & Erb, 1990). Neurofilament staining was used to identify neurons that did not express TH. Since the overwhelming majority of TH^+ cells are located in the distal third of the ganglion, only cells in this area were considered (Finley et al., 1992). The number of TH^+ cells as well as total neuron counts were determined using fluorescence microscopy. The numbers of soma profiles were corrected for double counts by Abercrombie's formula, using nuclear size to calculate the correction factor (see Katz & Erb, 1990).

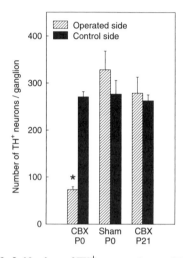 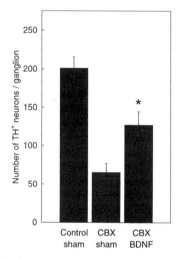

Figure 1. Left: Numbers of TH^+ neurons (mean±SEM) in the ipsi- and contralateral PG three weeks after glomectomy (CBX P0; n=4) or sham surgery (Sham P0; n=3) at birth, and 3 weeks after glomectomy at 3 weeks of age (CBX P21; n=3). There was a 73% reduction in TH^+ cells after ipsilateral glomectomy in the newborn (*p<0.05 vs. control side, t-test).
Right: Number of TH^+ neurons in the PG 3-4 days after glomectomy with (CBX BDNF; n=5) or without (CBX sham; n=4) BDNF replacement compared to sham operated controls with sham pledgets (Control sham; n=4). The loss of neurons following glomectomy was significantly attenuated by BDNF treatment (*p<0.05, t-test).

In a second set of experiments, one day-old pups were unilaterally glomectomized as described and a small Gelfoam pledget, soaked in either BDNF (2.3-4.6 µg) or vehicle, was placed adjacent to the PG. BDNF is a neurotrophin known to support survival of cranial and other sensory neurons in culture (Lindsay et al., 1985). Three to four days later the animals were perfused and the PGs were processed for immunocytochemical staining of TH and neurofilament proteins.

RESULTS

Unilateral glomectomy in the newborn animals resulted in a 73% loss of TH^+ neurons in the ipsilateral PG compared with the control side. This was accompanied by a decrease in the total number of neurons in the distal PG (763±125 ipsilateral vs. 1485±122 contralateral; mean±SEM; n=3, p<0.05 by t-test). In contrast, TH^+ cell numbers were unaffected by sham surgery. These findings indicate that in newborn rats, carotid body afferent cells in the PG are dependent on the carotid body for survival. No effect on afferent cell number was observed in animals glomectomized at 3 weeks of age, suggesting that the carotid body is required for trophic support only during a restricted period of development. BDNF treatment in glomectomized newborn pups was found to partially prevent the loss of TH^+ cells (Fig.), indicating that BDNF can substitute for target-derived influences at this stage.

CONCLUSION

We have found that carotid body afferent neurons in the newborn PG are dependent on peripheral target tissues for survival. This dependence appears to be confined to a critical period of development since glomectomy in adolescent rats failed to affect TH^+ cell number in the PG. Moreover, the loss of neurons seen after glomectomy in the newborn could be partly prevented by administration of BDNF. This is consistent with our finding that BDNF, but not other neurotrophins, supports survival of TH^+ neurons in the PG *in vitro* (Hertzberg et al., submitted). Our results highlight the fact that chemoafferent neurons exhibit marked plasticity at a time when chemoreflex function undergoes profound maturational changes. We hypothesize that extracellular cues, such as BDNF or similar molecules, play an essential role in the normal development and maturation of the carotid body afferent pathway.

This work was supported by PHS grant HL-42131 (DMK) and Wenner-Gren Foundation, Swedish Medical Research Council, Swedish Society of Medicine, Sällskapet Barnavård, the Crownprincess Lovisa's Foundation and the Swedish Parental Support Organization for SIDS (TH).

REFERENCES

Eden, G.J. & Hanson, M.A. (1987). Maturation of the respiratory response to acute hypoxia in the newborn rat. J. Physiol. 392:1-9.

Finley, J.C., Polak, J. & Katz, D.M. (1992). Transmitter diversity in carotid body afferent neurons: dopaminergic and peptidergic phenotypes. Neuroscience. 51:973-987.

Katz, D.M., Adler, J.E. & Black, I.B. (1987). Catecholaminergic primary sensory neurons: autonomic targets and mechanisms of transmitter regulation. Fed. Proc. 46:24-29.

Katz, D.M. & Erb, M.J. (1990). Developmental regulation of tyrosine hydroxylase expression in primary sensory neurons of the rat. Dev. Biol. 137:233-242.

Lindsay, R.M., Thoenen, H. & Barde, Y.A. (1985). Placode and neural crest-derived sensory neurons are responsive at early developmental stages to brain-derived neurotrophic factor. Dev. Biol. 112:319-328.

CAROTID BODY DOPAMINE RESPONSE TO ACUTE HYPOXIA IN DEVELOPING RABBITS

A. Bairam,[1,4] F. Marchal,[1] H. Basson,[1] J. M. Cottet-Emard,[2]
J.M. Pequignot,[2] J. M. Hascoet[3] and S. Lahiri

[1]Laboratoire de Physiologie, Faculté de Médecine ;[3]INSERM 272 Nancy;
[2]CNRS 1195 Lyon, France ; [4]Centre de Recherche HSFA Québec, Canada

INTRODUCTION

Dopamine (DA) is present at high concentration in the carotid body (CB) of different mammalian species, and may influence the functional properties of chemosensory cells, particularly their response to hypoxia. Long-term exposure to hypoxia produces a significant increase in DA synthesis and utilization; while short-term exposure to low PO_2 induces a decrease in carotid body DA content indicating an increased release from glomus cells. This release has been shown to be proportional to both the level of PO_2 and the carotid chemosensory activity (see for review Fidone et al. (1990)). In adult as in newborn animals in vivo and in vitro, studies have shown that dopamine may induce an inhibition and/or an excitation of carotid chemoreceptors activity (Fidone et al., 1990; Marchal et al., 1992; Zapata, 1975). The excitatory effect is predominant in young animals especially in hypoxia (Marchal et al., 1992). The variation in DA effect may be due to developmental changes in either chemoreceptor response to DA or in carotid body dopamine response to hypoxia. The aim of this study was to characterize the carotid body dopamine content and release in response to acute hypoxia in developing rabbits.

MATERIALS AND METHODS

Studies were carried out on carotid bodies (CB) of 70 rabbit pups aged respectively 1 day (n = 9), 5 days (n = 27), 15 days (n = 18), and 25 days (n = 16), and 1 group of adult rabbits ≥ 1 year (n = 11).

Animals were tracheotomized and artificially ventilated. The carotid bifurcation was dissected and carotid bodies were removed after 10-15 min of ventilation with 100 % O_2, and placed individually in vials containing 400 μl of HEPES (10 mM) + EDTA (0.029 mM), pH 7.40 (adjusted with 0.1 N NaOH). Then, they were immediately incubated in a closed-circuit circulated with either 100 % O_2 or 8 % O_2 in N_2 bubbling for one hour into the survival medium. At the end of the incubation period, each carotid body was placed in 300 μl and each survival medium in 40 μl perchloric acid (0.1 M) containing 400 μl of sodium bisulfate. Samples were immediately frozen on dry ice and stored at -80° C until dopamine measurement by HPLC (Pequignot et al., 1986).

Total DA was calculated as the sum of DA concentration in the CB (DAcb) and in surviving medium (DAm). The fraction of DA released was then calculated as : [DAm] x 100 / [total DA]. An ANOVA test was used for comparison. Results are expressed as mean ± SEM.

RESULTS

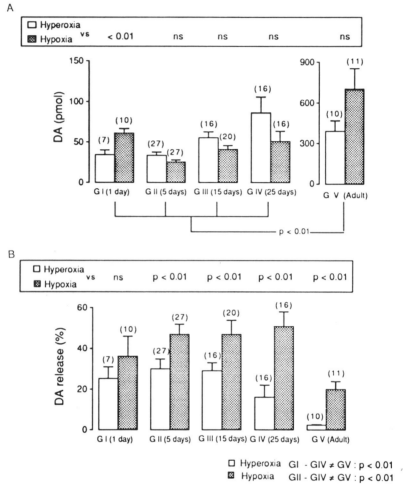

Figure 1. (A) Total DA and (B) fraction released in hyperoxia and hypoxia in developing and adult rabbits Numbers in brackets indicate number of samples. Note different scale for adult and pups in panel A.

Dopamine content (fig. 1A)

In hyperoxia, there was a significant increase of total DA with age (p < 0.01). A similar relationship was observed in hypoxia : total DA in the adult group was higher compared to younger groups (p < 0.01). However, total DA was not significantly different between hypoxia and hyperoxia in any age group except in 1 day old rabbits (61.14 ± 5.47 vs 35.2 ± 5.43 ; p < 0.01).

Dopamine release (fig. 1B)

The fraction of DA released in response to hypoxia was higher than in hyperoxia in all groups (p < 0.01) except in 1 day old rabbits. However, the fraction of DA released in hyperoxia (2.3 ± 0.4 %) and in hypoxia (20.5 ± 4.1 %) in adult was lower compared with all pup groups in hyperoxia (p < 0.01) and with rabbits aged ≥ 5 days in hypoxia (p < 0.01).

DISCUSSION

Hyperoxia was used as control, since prolonged hypoxia has been shown to stimulate carotid body glucose metabolism and cyclic AMP which in turn stimulate DA synthesis and release (Obeso et al., 1989; Perez-Garcia et al., 1991). The age-related increase in total dopamine may reflect the increase in carotid body mass rather than maturation of DA metabolism, since DA is expressed as content per CB. To study the dopamine response to hypoxia in different age groups, we have expressed DA secreted as per cent release from total DA, assuming that total DA at the onset and at the end of the incubation period was unchanged, i.e., no significant metabolism of DA had occurred. Although this may not be strictly true, the rate of DA metabolism over short periods of time - such as 20 or 60 minutes (Hanbauer & Hellstrom; Leitner, 1992) - is not different in hyperoxia and hypoxia, so that comparing the fraction of DA released in these two conditions may be interpreted as the change in the amount of DA secreted. The fact that total DA was not significantly increased by hypoxia, except in very early neonatal rabbits, is consistent with the lack of a significant increase in DA synthesis. In fact, when hypoxia has been shown to increase DA synthesis, the CB were exposed for 3 hours to hypoxia (Fidone et al., 1982). In newborns, although the number of studied CB was small, the higher DA content observed in hypoxia may express a higher sensitivity of DA metabolism to hypoxia.

Our results also indicate that pup carotid bodies respond to hypoxia by an increase in DA release that appears relatively larger than in adults. Biochemical evidence support the existence of presynaptic D2 dopamine receptors. If these receptors are autoreceptors, they may be activated by the release of endogenous dopamine to regulate further release (Parker & Cebeddu, 1985). In the carotid body, DA autoreceptor mechanisms may exist since both D2 mRNA and TH gene expression are present in the same type I cell (Czyzyk-Krzeska et al., 1992). In addition, DA released from nerve terminals in brain tissue is mainly removed from the synaptic cleft by an uptake mechanism (Iversen, 1975). Hence, it is possible that in developing animal, immature presynaptic DA autoreceptors and DA uptake sites explain the relatively larger amount of DA released by hypoxia than in adults. These data are also in keeping with an excitatory effect of DA on carotid chemosensory activity resulting from predominant postsynaptic receptor stimulation frequently observed in newborns.

The authors thank J. Beyrend, G. Colin, N. Bertin and C. Choné for skillful technical assistance and C. Creusat for the typing. This work was supported in part by a grant from La Fondation Pour la Recherche Médicale.

REFERENCES

Czyzyk-Krzeska, M.F., Lawson, E.E., & Millhorn, D.E. (1992) Expression of D2 dopamine receptor mRNA in the arterial chemoreceptor afferent pathway. J. Autonm. Nerv. Sys. 41:31-40.

Fidone, S.J., Gonzalez, C. & Yoshizaki, K. (1982) Effects of hypoxia on catecholamines synthesis in rabbit carotid body in vitro. J. Physiol. 333:81-91.

Fidone, S.J., Gonzalez, C., Obeso, A., Gomez-Nino, A. & Dinger, B. (1990) Biogenic amine and neuropeptide transmitters in carotid body chemostransmission: Experimental findings and perspectives In "Hypoxia: The adaptations." J.R. Sutton, G. Coates and J.E. Remmers, eds., Marcel Decker, Philadelphia.

Hanbauer, I. & Hellström, S. The regulation of dopamine and noradrenaline in the rat carotid body and its modification by denervation and by hypoxia. J. Physiol. 282:21-34.

Iversen, L.L. (1975) Uptake processes for biogenic amines. In "Handbook of psychopharmacology" L.L Iversen ., S.D. Iversen , S.H. Synder, eds., Plenum Press, New York.

Leitner, L.M. (1992) Dopamine metabolism in the rabbit carotid body in vitro : effect of hpoxia and hypercapnia. In : Neurobiology and Cell Physiology of Chemoreception, P.G. Data ., H. Acker and S. Lahiri, eds., Plenum Press New York,(In press)

Marchal, F., Bairam, A., Haouzi, P., Hascoet, J.M., Crance, J.P., Vert, P. & Lahiri, S. (1992) Dual responses of carotid chemosensory afferents to dopamine in the newborn kitten. Respir. Physiol. 90:173-183.

Obeso, A., Gonzalez, C., Dinger, B. & Fidone, S. (1989) Metabolic activation of carotid body glomus cells by hypoxia. J. Appl. Physiol. 67:484-487.

Parker, E.M. & Cebeddu, L.X. (1985) Evidence for autoreceptor modulation of endogenous dopamine release from rabbit caudate nucleus in vitro. J. Pharmacol. Exp. Ther. 233:492-500

Pérez-Garcia, M.T., Almaraz, L. & Gonzalez C. (1991) Cyclic AMP modulates differentially the release of dopamine induced by hypoxia and other stimuli and increases dopamine synthesis in the rabbit carotid body. J. Neurochem. 57:1992-2000.

Pequignot, J.M., Cottet-Emard, J.M., Dalmaz, Y., Dehaut De Sigy, M. & Peyrin L. (1986) Biochemical evidence for dopamine and norepinephrine stores outside the sympathetic nerves in rat carotid body. Brain Res. 367:238-243.

Zapata, P. (1975) Effects of dopamine on carotid chemoreceptors and baroreceptors in vitro. J. Physiol. 244:235-251.

ATTENUATION OF THE HYPOXIC VENTILATORY RESPONSE IN AWAKE RABBIT PUPS; POSSIBLE ROLE OF DOPAMINE

Denise Bee,[1] Caroline Wright,[1] David Pallot.[2]

[1]Department of Medicine and Pharmacology, University of Sheffield, Royal Hallamshire Hospital, Sheffield, UK and [2]Department of Human Anatomy, UAE University EL Ain, UAE

INTRODUCTION

A failure of some part of the respiratory control apparatus has been quoted as the underlying cause of sudden and unexplained death in infants (Busuttil, 1992). This could be due to either a prevailing immaturity of central mechanisms or an inability of the carotid body to detect hypoxia. The ventilatory response to hypoxia was found to be poor in a group of near miss sudden infant death syndrome (SIDS) infants (Hunt et al., 1981). Bolton (1990) also found that 2% of infants in a normal population also demonstrated an attenuated response to hypoxia, which he suggested may help to identify the individuals at risk. Investigations of the animal carotid body have shown that this organ resets its function after birth (Eden & Hanson, 1987) but within a few days the "adult" responses are achieved (Hertzberg et al., 1990). However, SIDS deaths have a peak incidence at around 3-4 months of age, which suggests that the period of risk is not associated with this early resetting of the hypoxic response. This led us to investigate the longitudinal development of the hypoxic ventilatory response (HVR) in rabbits from birth until weaning. In a study of 10 rabbit pups we have established that a severe attenuation of the HVR occurred around week 6 of life (Bee et al., 1993) which showed partial recovery at weaning. The current investigation is aimed at elucidating the role of the inhibitory amine, dopamine, in this attenuated HVR.

METHOD

Seven dwarf rabbit pups of either sex were used, their HVR's were tested each week from birth. Each pup was placed inside a body plethysmograph with the head protruding through a rubber collar. Pressure changes within the box were measured using a differential manometer (Furness Controls, UK) and recorded on a Lectromed hot pen recorder; the trace was calibrated for volume and a time scale allowed measurement of frequency. Cylinder gases of O_2 and N_2 were mixed and adjusted to concentrations of O_2 between 30 and 10% which was analysed by a Servomex O_2 analyser. The mixture was delivered to the pup by a loose face mask, O_2 was reduced in 1 minute steps from 30% to 21%, 15% and 10%O_2. The HVR was taken as the change in ventilation found between the 30% and 10%

measurements. Domperidone, a D_2 dopamine receptor antagonist (10ug/100g BW), or its vehicle (placebo) was injected in a small volume (0.03-0.05ml) via an ear vein and the HVR measured at least 5 minutes later. HVR's were measured before and after dopamine blockade. Differences in sensitivity to hypoxia were shown by means of Students paired t test; P<0.05 was considered significant.

RESULTS

7 rabbit pups showed an attenuated HVR at mean ($\pm$ SEM) of 5.9 ($\pm$ 0.47) weeks of age; dopamine blockade raised this to near pre-phenomenon levels.

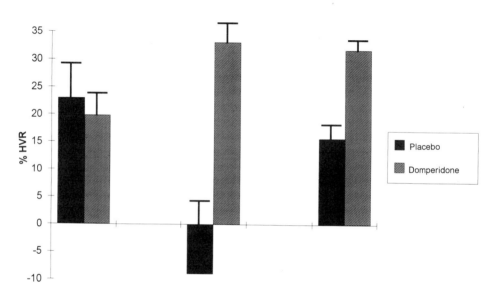

Figure 1. Effects of placebo and domperidone (10ug/100gBW) injection one week before, during and after minimum HVR. Values are mean $\pm$ s.e.m. HVR is expressed as the percentage increase in ventilation when F_IO_2 =0.10 compared with when F_IO_2 =0.30

One week prior to the maximum attenuation of HVR, domperidone treatment showed no significant effect on HVR when compared with placebo. However, at maximum attenuation domperidone injection significantly (p<0.05) increased HVR from -9.73% $\pm$ 9.7 (mean $\pm$ SEM) to 33.33% $\pm$ 5.5. One week post maximum attenuation, domperidone increased HVR from 15.5% $\pm$ 4.52 to 31.5% $\pm$ 4.85. The figure demonstrates domperidone has litttle effect on HVR until the peak attenuation occurs, one week after the peak attenuation domperidone still induces an increase in HVR but the increase is not as profound as that seen at minimum HVR.

DISCUSSION

The attenuation of the HVR is apparently a short lasting phenomenon that occurred in the current study at around 5-7 weeks of age. The age at which the attenuation occurs and its severity are variable. This may be due, in part, to the experimental protocol as measurements only took place once per week so the peak effect may have been missed. Domperidone treatment was shown to cause little effect before the period of attenuation but increased the HVR during this period. This suggested that dopamine acting through the D_2 receptor might be responsible for inhibiting the carotid body's response to hypoxia. A similar effect occurred in adult rats where chronic hypoxia caused attenuation of the HVR which was restored by dopamine blockade by domperidone (Wach et al., 1989).

We have shown that a developmental change in HVR in young rabbit pups occurs approximately two-thirds of the way to weaning and is a reasonably predictable event. The attenuation can be relieved by intravenous domperidone and may be due to increased production and release of dopamine or a change in D_2 receptor numbers and sensitivity, which requires further investigation.

We speculate that the peak incidence of SIDS at around 3-4 months of age might be associated with a loss of hypoxic sensitivity. This could be a developmental change, as indicated by our rabbit studies and constitutes a period of risk to the infant. In some babies if the changes are severe enough or complicated by respiratory infection or even sleep apnoea then death may be the result.

REFERENCES

Bee, D., Wright, C.E. & Pallot, D.J.(1993). Development of the hypoxic ventilatory response in awake rabbit pups. J. Physiol. (in press).

Bolton, D.P.G. (1990) The prevalence of immature respiratory control in a neonatal population. Aust. N. Z. Med. J. 103:89-92.

Busuttil, A.(1992). The SIDS phenomenon: an update. J. Clin. Pathol. 45:1-2.

Eden,G.J. & Hanson, M.A.(1987). Maturation of the respiratory response to acute hypoxia in the new-born rat. J. Physiol.(Lond.) 392:1-9.

Hunt, C.E., McCullock, K. & Brouillette, R.T.(1981). Diminished hypoxic ventilatory responses in near-miss sudden infant death syndrome. J. Appl. Physiol. 50:1313-1317.

Wach, R.A., Bee, D. & Barer, G.R. (1989). Dopamine and ventilatory effects of hypoxia and almitrine in chronically hypoxic rats. J. Appl. Physiol. 67:186-192.

D_2-DOPAMINE RECEPTOR mRNA IN THE CAROTID BODY AND PETROSAL GANGLIA IN THE DEVELOPING CAT

Estelle B. Gauda,[1] Machiko Shirahata,[2] and Robert S. Fitzgerald.[2]

[1]Department of Pediatrics and [2]Environmental Health Sciences; Johns Hopkins Medical Institutions, Baltimore, Maryland 21287-3200 USA

INTRODUCTION

Dopamine content is elevated in the carotid body of newborn rats and is associated with a blunted chemoreflex during the first few days of life (Hertzberg & Hellstrom, 1990). The purpose of this study was to establish the presence of mRNA coding for the D_2-dopamine receptor (D_2-R) in the carotid body and petrosal ganglia in the cat, and compare the levels of expression of D_2-R mRNA in these tissues at two stages during development. We hypothesized that D_2-R mRNA would be present in both the carotid body and petrosal ganglia. Because of the blunted chemoreflex observed at birth, we further hypothesized that there would be a greater expression of the mRNA coding for the D_2-R in the petrosal ganglia and less in the carotid body at birth than at 14 weeks postnatal age.

METHODS

Cats were anesthetized with ketamine (30 mg/kg) given intramuscularly. The caudate nucleus, carotid bodies and petrosal ganglia were harvested from 14 week (n=4) and 1 day old cats (n=2). Control tissues were obtained from adult rats. Caudate nuclei and liver tissue were used for positive and negative controls, respectively.

All tissues were frozen immediately on dry ice in RNAzol (Cinna/Biotecx). The frozen samples were homogenized and total cellular RNA was isolated by an acid-phenol extraction method. Glycogen was used as a carrier to facilitate precipitation of the nucleic acids in isopropanol. Slot blots were prepared by applying 8 and 4 microgram aliquots of denatured total RNA to a charged nitrocellulose membrane. In order to determine the specificity of the probes, Northern blots were also prepared. Twenty micrograms of total RNA obtained from rat and cat caudate nuclei and rat liver were electrophoresed through a 1.4% formaldehyde-agarose gel and transferred to a membrane. Full-length rat complementary DNA (cDNA) probes specific for the D_2-R and cyclophilin mRNAs were radiolabeled with [^{32}P]deoxycytidine triphosphate to specific activities of around 1-3 x 10^9 cpm/μg DNA using the random priming method. Slot and northern blots were prehybridized and hybridized in standard solutions at 42^0C, washed in solutions of increasing stringency and temperature, exposed to x-ray film and developed after 4-5 days. The blots were first probed with D_2-R cDNA, stripped and reprobed with cyclophilin cDNA. The amount of

D_2-R mRNA was quantitated by densitometry and normalized to the expression of cyclophilin mRNA, a housekeeping gene. Experiments presented were performed in duplicate.

RESULTS

Northern blot analysis of cat and rat tissue hybridized with rat cDNA showed a single band at the expected molecular weight for the D_2-R (2.5 kilobases) and cyclophilin (0.7 kilobases) mRNAs.

Slot blot autoradiograms showed that the D_2-R mRNA was easily detected in the carotid body and petrosal ganglia of cats at 14 weeks postnatal age (Table 1). However, the expression of the D_2-R mRNA was approximately 3 times greater in the petrosal ganglia than in the carotid body.

At birth, expression of the D_2-R mRNA in the carotid body was essentially undetectable with slot blot hybridization. However, it was easily detected and abundant in the petrosal ganglia. In comparison, expression of D_2-R mRNA is less in the carotid body and greater in the petrosal ganglia at birth than in adult cats.

Table 1. Relative Expression of D_2-R mRNA to Cyclophilin mRNA at birth and 14 weeks postnatal age.

	Carotid Body	Petrosal Ganglia
Birth	0.3	25
14 Weeks	3.0	17

DISCUSSION

In this study we have demonstrated that mRNA coding for D_2-R is present in the carotid body and petrosal ganglia in the adult cat. A new finding is that the expression of the D_2-R mRNA in these tissues changes during development. At birth, D_2-R mRNA was virtually undetected in the carotid body but was abundant in the petrosal ganglia. Using slot blot hybridization techniques, in the adult, D_2-R mRNA expression was easily detected in the carotid body and petrosal ganglia. These findings suggest that the effect of dopamine on chemoreceptor output may differ during development.

Dopamine content is elevated in the carotid body of the newborn rat and this is associated with a blunted chemoreflex at birth (Hertzberg et al., 1990). Several studies have shown that exogenous dopamine decreases ventilation and neural output from the carotid body. In addition, superfusion of cat carotid bodies with dopamine causes hyperpolarization of chemoreceptor afferent nerve endings (Sampson & Vidruk, 1977). Our findings suggest that if dopamine does inhibit neural output from the carotid body that the depressant effect of dopamine could be greater at birth.

We are unable to determine the exact localization of the mRNA for the D_2-R because tissue homogenates were used to obtain total RNA from the carotid body and petrosal ganglia. We suspect that detection of the transcript in the carotid body is due to D_2-R mRNA expression in the type I cell as suggested by in situ hybridization in the adult rat carotid body (Czyzyk-Krzeska et al., 1992). Not all cell bodies in the petrosal ganglia project fibers to the carotid body. However, Czyzyk-Krzeska et al., (1992) showed that Fluoro-Gold injected into the region of the carotid body labelled cells in the petrosal ganglia. These retrograde labelled cells also contained D_2-receptor mRNA transcripts. Thus, we believe that our data supports other studies that suggest D_2-Rs are on type 1 cells and on the carotid sinus nerve.

The carotid sinus nerve is the postsynaptic neuron of the chemoreflex pathway. The type I cell in the carotid body is the presynaptic neuron. Although the function of D_2-Rs on type 1 cells in the carotid body has not been described, much is known about D_2-Rs in the nigrostriatal dopamine system. In this system, release of dopamine is modulated by D_2-Rs which are autoreceptors on the presynaptic neuron. Binding of dopamine to the autoreceptor causes a decrease in synthesis and/or release of dopamine. If the D_2-Rs on the type 1 cell function as autoreceptors, binding of dopamine to these receptors could further decrease the release and synthesis of dopamine from the type I cells. The very low level of expression of D_2-R mRNA in the carotid body that we have described in the animals at birth could suggest that there is less autoreceptor regulation of dopamine synthesis and release from type 1 cells. This could result in more available dopamine to bind to the D_2-Rs on the postsynaptic neuron resulting in a decrease in neural output.

In conclusion, we have demonstrated D_2-R mRNA in the carotid body and petrosal ganglia which supports a role for presynaptic and postsynaptic effects of dopamine in the chemotransductive process. We have also shown that the D_2-receptor mRNA is virtually undetectable in the carotid body and abundant in the petrosal ganglia at birth. The blunted chemoreflex observed in newborns may be explained by a larger population of D_2-Rs on the carotid sinus nerve resulting in decrease neural output from the carotid body.

REFERENCES

Czyzky-Krzeska, M.F., Lawson, E.E., & Millhorn, D.E. (1992). Expression of D_2 dopamine receptor mRNA in the arterial chemoreceptor afferent pathway. J. Auton. Nerv. Syst. 41:31-40.

Hertzberg T., Hellstrom S., Langercrantz H., & Pequignot J. M. (1990). Development of the arterial chemoreflex and turnover of carotid body catecholamines in the newborn rat. J. Physiol. 425:211-225.

Sampson, S.R., & Vidruk E.H. (1977). Hyperpolarizing effects of dopamine on chemoreceptor nerve endings from cat and rabbit carotid bodies in vitro. J. Physiol. 268:211-221.

THE ROLE OF ENDOGENOUS DOPAMINE AS AN INHIBITORY NEUROMODULATOR IN NEONATAL AND ADULT CAROTID BODIES

Stuart M. Tomares[1], Owen S. Bamford[1], Laura M. Sterni[1], Robert S. Fitzgerald[2], and John L. Carroll[1]

[1]The Eudowood Division of Pediatric Respiratory Sciences, Department of Pediatrics, The Johns Hopkins School of Medicine, Baltimore, Maryland, U.S.A.; [2]Departments of Environmental Health Sciences, Physiology, and Medicine, The Johns Hopkins Medical Institutions, Baltimore, Maryland, U.S.A.

INTRODUCTION

The carotid chemoreceptors, the major sensors of arterial oxygen concentration in mammals, mediate ventilatory and arousal responses to hypoxia that are crucial for survival of the neonate. Carotid chemoreceptor denervation in newborn animals markedly increases mortality rate during postnatal development (Hofer, 1984; Bureau et al., 1985; Donnelly & Haddad, 1990). We and others have previously demonstrated that carotid chemoreceptor responses to hypoxia are weak in neonates and increase during postnatal development (Carroll et al., 1993; Marchal et al., 1992). Ventilatory responses to hypoxia are also weak in newborns and increase during postnatal maturation (Bonora & Gautier, 1987; Eden & Hanson, 1987). The mechanisms by which carotid chemoreceptor and ventilatory responses increase during postnatal development are not known.

Dopamine has been shown to be present in the carotid bodies of immature and adult animals although its role in chemotransduction is uncertain. Studies of dopaminergic mechanisms on the carotid chemoreceptors using exogenously administered dopamine have been difficult to interpret. Carotid body neural responses to exogenous dopamine are complex since it may act at multiple sites within the carotid body in addition to modulating carotid chemoreceptor blood flow. Most studies using dopamine receptor antagonists have suggested that endogenous dopamine operates via D-2 receptors and that its predominant effect on the carotid chemoreceptor response to hypoxia is inhibitory.

Dopamine content and turnover in newborn rat carotid bodies has been shown to be elevated at birth and to decline significantly during the first week of life (Hertzberg et al., 1992). It has therefore been proposed that the weak responses of the newborn may be due to inhibition by high levels of endogenous dopamine secretion just after birth (Hertzberg et al., 1992). In this study we test this hypothesis by measuring the effects of domperidone, a specific dopamine D-2 receptor antagonist, on the carotid sinus nerve (CSN) activity in neonatal versus adult cats.

METHODS

Cats of either sex were studied at two age groups; adults and neonates (4-7 days). Both age groups were anesthetized with sodium pentobarbital (40 mg/Kg intraperitoneally), paralyzed with pancuronium bromide (0.1-0.2 mg/Kg intravenously), and mechanically ventilated using a rate of 40-50 breaths/minute. Body temperature was maintained at $38\pm1°C$ using a controlled heating pad. Blood glucose was checked by dextrostick, and femoral arterial blood pressure was continuously monitored. Hematocrit was determined at the beginning and end of each experiment.

The carotid body was exposed surgically as previously described (Carroll et al., 1993). The carotid sinus nerve (CSN) was located and carefully separated from the glossopharyngeal nerve and sectioned. Ganglioglomerular nerves were sectioned. Baroreceptor activity was eliminated by thermal and mechanical disruption of baroreceptor nerve fibers on the carotid sinus. CSN activity was recorded by placing the CSN onto platinum-iridium electrodes under mineral oil. Blood gases were maintained equivalent throughout the protocol via metabolic or ventilatory manipulation.

Dopamine 10 mcg/Kg was infused intravenously over 1 minute and CSN activity was then recorded at four levels of isocapnic O_2 (P_aO_2 35-45, 55-65, 90-100, >300 mmHg), and four levels of isooxic CO_2 ($ETCO_2$ 3, 5.5, 8.2, 11 percent). Placebo solution 2 ml/Kg was given intravenously and CSN activity recorded. Domperidone (0.5 mg/ml) 1 mg/Kg (2 cc/Kg) was then administered via slow intravenous infusion. The subjects were given 10 minutes to stabilize after drug administration and the previous protocol was repeated in the same manner as above. Dopamine 10 mcg/Kg was given intravenously over 1 minute at the end of the protocol to demonstrate that the D-2 block was still in effect.

RESULTS

Preliminary results show that all subjects at both ages significantly increased CSN activity in response to hypoxia. Dopamine infusion before D-2 receptor blockade with domperidone caused a decrease in CSN activity at both ages. However the effects of domperidone differed between neonatal and adult cats. In the neonatal group, domperidone had no significant effect on CSN output during normoxia or hyperoxia. CSN activity was significantly increased by domperidone only during hypoxia. In contrast, in adult cats, CSN activity was significantly increased at all levels of oxygenation by domperidone. The pattern of domperidone effect on the carotid chemoreceptor response to CO_2 also differed between neonates and adults. Following administration of domperidone the slope of the carotid chemoreceptor neural response to CO_2 was increased only in neonates; in adults domperidone caused an upward shift in the CSN response to CO_2 without a significant change in slope. In both age groups, DA infusion at the end of the protocol resulted in either a small increase in CSN activity or no change at all (confirming that D-2 receptor blockade was still effective). Blood glucose and hematocrit remained within acceptable limits during experiments and domperidone did not significantly affect arterial blood pressure.

DISCUSSION

The results of this study suggest that the weak carotid chemoreceptor responses of neonates are not due to inhibitory action of endogenous dopamine. In normoxia and hyperoxia, D-2 receptor blockade resulted in a significant increase in CSN output in adults but not in the 4-7 day old cats. CSN activity was significantly higher following domperidone only during hypoxia in the neonatal group. Neonatal cats had low levels of CSN activity in normoxia/hyperoxia, which remained low after D-2 receptor blockade. If CSN activity was low due to endogenous dopamine acting as an inhibitory modulator on type-I cells, a significant increase in activity following D-2 receptor blockade would be anticipated. The lack of a rise in CSN activity following domperidone suggests that the low level of CSN output in the neonate (during normoxia and hyperoxia) was not due to inhibition by high levels of endogenous dopamine acting at an inhibitory receptor. The apparently minimal inhibitory action of dopamine in neonates compared to adults could be explained by low levels of resting dopamine release, absent or fewer dopamine D-2 inhibitory autoreceptors on type-1 cells (Gauda et al., 1991), or different function of D2 receptors in neonatal cats. The significant increase in CSN activity in adult subjects under the same conditions following D-2 blockade suggests that the inhibitory role of endogenous dopamine in the carotid chemoreceptors takes time to mature during postnatal development.

During stimulation by hypoxia the effect of D-2 blockade was to increase CSN activity in both neonates and adults in a similar manner. These results are consistent with the hypothesis that endogenous DA release parallels carotid chemoreceptor activity; its effects on CSN activity being mainly inhibitory. Hertzberg et. al. proposed that high levels of endogenous dopamine could inhibit carotid chemoreceptor function just after birth and account for the weak CSN activity of newborns. Although our results do not support that hypothesis, it should be noted that they found that carotid body dopamine turnover dropped markedly with in the first 12 hours of life in rats (Hertzberg et al., 1992). Since our subjects were 4-7 days old, it is possible that a significant inhibitory dopamine effect occurs earlier during the rapid chemoreceptor resetting phase and therefore would not be detected by our study. Species differences may also be important.

Dr. Carroll is a recipient of National Heart, Lung, Blood Institute Clinical Investigator Award HL-02543. Dr. Tomares is a recipient of a fellowship grant from the American Lung Association of Maryland.

REFERENCES

Bonora, M., & Gautier, H. (1987). Maturational changes in body temperature and ventilation during hypoxia in kittens. Respir. Physiol. 68:359-370.

Bureau, M.A., Lamarche, J., Foulon, P., & Dalle, D. (1985). Postnatal maturation of respiration in intact and carotid body-chemodenervated lambs. J. Appl. Physiol. 59:869-874.

Carroll, J.L., Bamford, O.S., & Fitzgerald, R.S. (1993). Postnatal maturation of carotid chemoreceptor responses to O_2 and CO_2 in the cat. J. Appl. Physiol. (in press).

Donnelly, D.F., & Haddad, G.G. (1990). Prolonged apnea and impaired survival in piglets after sinus and aortic nerve section. J. Appl. Physiol. 68:1048-1052.

Eden, G.J., & Hanson, M.A. (1987). Maturation of the respiratory response to acute hypoxia in the newborn rat. J. Physiol. (Lond). 392:1-9.

Gauda, E.B., Radin, A., Craig, R., & Fitzgerald, R.S. (1991). Effect of postnatal development on D2-dopamine receptor mRNA in the carotid body of kittens. FASEB. J. 5:A1120.

Hertzberg, T., Hellstrom, S., Holgert, H., Lagercrantz, H., & Pequignot, J.M. (1992). Ventilatory response to hyperoxia in newborn rats born in hypoxia - possible relationship to carotid body dopamine. J. Physiol. (Lond). 456:645-654.

Hofer, M.A. (1984). Lethal respiratory disturbance in neonatal rats after arterial chemoreceptor denervation. Life Sciences 34:489-496.

Marchal, F., Bairam, A., Haouzi, P., Crance, J.P., Di-Giulio, C., Vert, P., & Lahiri, S. (1992). Carotid chemoreceptor response to natural stimuli in the newborn kitten. Respir. Physiol. 87:183-193.

INTRACELLULAR CALCIUM RESPONSES TO HYPOXIA AND CYANIDE IN CULTURED TYPE I CELLS FROM NEWBORN AND ADULT RABBITS.

Laura M. Sterni,[1] Marshall H. Montrose[2], Owen S. Bamford[1], Stuart M. Tomares[1], and John L. Carroll[1]

[1]The Eudowood Division of Pediatric Respiratory Sciences, Department of Pediatrics, The Johns Hopkins School of Medicine, Baltimore, Maryland, U.S.A.; [2]Department of Gastroenterology, The Johns Hopkins School of Medicine, Baltimore, Maryland, U.S.A

INTRODUCTION

Carotid chemoreceptor responses to hypoxia and CO_2 are weak just after birth and take time to mature to adult levels (Kholwadwala & Donnelly, 1992; Marchal et al., 1992; Carroll et al., 1993). The mechanisms underlying changes in carotid chemoreceptor function during development are not known. Possible mechanisms include developmental changes in carotid body blood flow, increased synaptic density of sensory innervation on type-I cells, maturation of neurotransmitter or neuromodulator mechanisms, and increased sensitivity of the type-I cell's ability to respond to oxygen. The purpose of this study was to determine if carotid chemoreceptor development is due to increasing sensitivity of the type-I cell response to hypoxia.

An increase in intracellular calcium ($[Ca^{2+}]_i$) has been shown to be an important component of carotid chemoreceptor type-I cell responses to hypoxia and CO_2 (Biscoe et al., 1989; Biscoe & Duchen, 1990; Sato et al., 1991). As in other sensory systems, the rise in $[Ca^{2+}]_i$ is thought to be the stimulus for neurotransmitter release. Thus changes in $[Ca^{2+}]_i$ in response to a stimulus can be used as a marker of type-I cell sensitivity.

We hypothesized that developmental changes in the carotid chemoreceptor responses to hypoxia and CO_2 are due to maturational changes in the transduction mechanism of the type I cell (rather than changes in blood flow or innervation). It was postulated that immature carotid type I cells would be unable to generate a rise in $[Ca^{2+}]_i$ in response to hypoxia or cyanide as in adult cells. We tested this hypothesis by measuring the $[Ca^{2+}]_i$ response to hypoxia or CN^- in primary cultures of type-I cells from newborn vs. adult rabbits.

METHODS

Carotid chemoreceptor cells were isolated using methods based on those described by Nurse (Nurse, 1987; Stea & Nurse, 1989). Carotid bodies were removed from anesthetized animals and placed immediately in ice-cold buffered salt solution. Carotid bodies from 3-4 pups were pooled to provide enough tissue for culture. The cleaned bifurcations were incubated in trypsin (0.1%) and collagenase (0.1%) for 45 min at 37°. They were then triturated in 200µl of nutrient medium and 50µl aliquots transferred to coverslips pretreated with polylysine to promote cell adhesion. The coverslips were placed in 3 cm petri dishes and incubated at 37° in 5% CO_2/air. Nutrient medium (Ham F12 + 10% fetal bovine serum, Gibco) was added after 90 minutes and the cells fed at 48-hr intervals thereafter.

Type-I cells were studied after 3-4 days in culture and $[Ca^{2+}]_i$ responses were measured using Fura-2. Cells were incubated for 5 minutes at 37° with 2 M Fura-2/acetoxymethyl ester (Fura-2 AM, Molecular Probes). Coverslips with attached cells were mounted in a temperature-controlled sealed chamber at 35-37° with ports for perfusion. Cells treated as above but without Fura-2/AM were used to determine background values (autofluorescence and camera dark level), and background was subtracted from all fluorescence values. Dead cells were identified using propidium iodide and eliminated from the analysis. Type-I cells were identified by visual criteria (size, shape, characteristic appearance) and identity confirmed with the formaldehyde/glutaraldehyde method to induce catecholamine fluorescence. Cells were visualized in a Zeiss Axiovert microscope with a 50X Leitz objective, and cellular fluorescence measured using a 75W xenon lamp as excitation source and a Hamamatsu intensified CCD (model C2400-97) as light detector. Neutral density filters attenuated the excitation light to 20% of full power, and under these conditions photobleaching of Fura-2 was not detectable. Fura-2 fluorescent emission was measured at 420-570 nm in response to alternating excitation wavelengths of 350 ± 10 nm and 380 ± 10 nm. Values were simultaneously obtained from up to 20 cells in the field of view, and results from all cells averaged at each time point for presentation. When conditions were stable the cells were exposed to BSS equilibrated with 5% CO_2 in N_2, (with 0.1mM sodium dithionite added) for 3 min. The cells were allowed to recover in normoxic BSS between hypoxia exposures. After the anoxic challenge, the response to NaCN (1mM in BSS) was measured. Finally the cells were exposed to ionomycin (Research Biochemicals International) which renders the membrane permeable to Ca^{++}. This maximal rise in intracellular Ca^{++} was measured, to ensure that the responses to anoxia were within the dynamic range of our measuring system. A two-point calibration was performed by measuring the fluorescence ratios in two solutions of known Ca^{++} concentration.

RESULTS

Preliminary data from 32 type I cells from 2 adult rabbits and 40 type I cells from 8 1-2 day old rabbit pups shows that intracellular calcium increased in response to anoxia and cyanide in approximately 90% of cells studied. In most cells, responses to anoxia and cyanide were not sustained and the shapes of responses were heterogeneous. Peak $[Ca^{2+}]_i$ responses to hypoxia and cyanide did not differ significantly between cells from neonates and adults. The proportion of cells with minimal calcium responses tended to be larger in the neonatal group but distributions have not been compared statistically.

DISCUSSION

It is known from studies performed *in vivo* that carotid chemoreceptor function in neonates is weak compared to adults. However, results obtained to date do not demonstrate a difference in the magnitude of type-I cell peak $[Ca^{2+}]_i$ responses to anoxia in newborn versus adult rabbit carotid chemoreceptor type-I cells. There are several possible explanations for this discrepancy. It is possible that there is, in fact, no difference in $[Ca^{2+}]_i$ responses of neonatal versus adult type-I cells and that functional differences found *in vivo* are due to differences in carotid body blood flow, innervation, or some other factor. However, available evidence suggests that postnatal alterations in blood flow do not explain chemoreceptor resetting (Clarke et al., 1990) and the rapidity with which resetting occurs makes development of innervation an unlikely explanation. Alternatively, the type-I cell may be modulated *in vivo* by some factor that is missing in cell culture conditions. Other possibilities are that the coupling of $[Ca^{2+}]_i$ to neurosecretion is different in the newborn or that the difference between newborn and adult carotid chemoreceptors responses lies further down the chemotransduction cascade (after the intracellular calcium response).

We believe that the most likely explanation for our findings is resetting of carotid body type-I cells from newborn to adult levels of function during the 3-4 days in culture. Several investigators have reported that the carotid chemoreceptors are unresponsive just after birth and increase function over the next few days (Biscoe & Purves, 1967; Blanco et al., 1984). The main trigger for postnatal resetting of the chemoreceptors is believed to be the increase in arterial oxygen tension at birth (Eden & Hanson, 1987; Blanco et al., 1988). Our cells in culture were kept in room air + 5% CO_2. Under these conditions the PO_2 would be > 100 mmHg, which is likely higher than it would be during the same time period *in vivo*. Therefore, if oxygen is the trigger for a chemoreceptor resetting process that requires several days, it is possible that our cells had already reset to adult levels by the time they were studied. Studies of freshly dissociated type-I cells and cells grown under hypoxic conditions are currently underway.

Dr. Carroll is a recipient of National Heart, Lung, Blood Institute Clinical Investigator Award HL-02543.

REFERENCES

Biscoe, T.J., & Duchen, M.R. (1990). Responses of type I cells dissociated from the rabbit carotid body to hypoxia. J. Physiol. (Lond). 428:39-59.

Biscoe, T.J., & Purves, M.J. (1967). Carotid body chemoreceptor activity in the new-born lamb. J. Physiol. (Lond). 190:443-454.

Biscoe, T.J., Duchen, M.R., Eisner, D.A., O'Neill, S.C., & Valdeolmillos, M. (1989). Measurements of intracellular Ca^{2+} in dissociated type I cells of the rabbit carotid body. J. Physiol. (Lond). 416:421-434.

Blanco, C.E., Dawes, G.S., Hanson, M.A., & McCooke, H.B. (1984). The response to hypoxia of arterial chemoreceptors in fetal sheep and new-born lambs. J. Physiol. (Lond). 351:25-37.

Blanco, C.E., Hanson, M.A., & McCooke, H.B. (1988). Effects on carotid chemoreceptor resetting of pulmonary ventilation in the fetal lamb in utero. J. Dev. Physiol. 10:167-174.

Carroll, J.L., Bamford, O.S., & Fitzgerald, R.S. (1993). Postnatal maturation of carotid chemoreceptor responses to O_2 and CO_2 in the cat. J. Appl. Physiol. (in press)

Clarke, J.A., de-Burgh-Daly, M., & Ead, H.W. (1990). Comparison of the size of the vascular compartment of the carotid body of the fetal, neonatal and adult cat. Acta. Anat. (Basel). 138:166-174.

Eden, G.J., & Hanson, M.A. (1987). Effects of chronic hypoxia from birth on the ventilatory response to acute hypoxia in the newborn rat. J. Physiol. (Lond). 392:11-19.

Kholwadwala, D., & Donnelly, D.F. (1992). Maturation of carotid chemoreceptor sensitivity to hypoxia: in vitro studies in the newborn rat. J. Physiol. (Lond). 453:461-473.

Marchal, F., Bairam, A., Haouzi, P., Crance, J.P., Di-Giulio, C., Vert, P., & Lahiri, S. (1992). Carotid chemoreceptor response to natural stimuli in the newborn kitten. Respir. Physiol. 87:183-193.

Nurse, C.A. (1987). Localization of acetylcholinesterase in dissociated cell cultures of the carotid body of the rat. Cell. Tissue. Res. 250:21-27.

Sato, M., Ikeda, K., Yoshizaki, K., & Koyano, H. (1991). Response of cytosolic calcium to anoxia and cyanide in cultured glomus cells of newborn rabbit carotid body. Brain. Res. 551:327-330.

Stea, A., & Nurse, C.A. (1989). Chloride channels in cultured glomus cells of the rat carotid body. Am. J. Physiol. 257:C174-C181.

EFFECTS OF ACETAZOLAMIDE ON THE TIME COURSE OF THE CO_2 RESPONSE OF CAROTID BODY IN THE NEWBORN KITTEN

B. Hannhart [1], A. Bairam [2], F. Marchal [2]

[1]INSERM-U 14 , and [2]Laboratoire de Physiologie, Université de Nancy, Vandoeuvre-lès-Nancy, France

INTRODUCTION

In adult cats, peripheral chemoreceptors respond to a step increase in PCO_2 by a rise in activity to a maximum and then adapt to a lower steady level within one minute. It has been shown that the transient peak response is entirely dependent on the catalyzed CO_2 hydration and disappears after carbonic anhydrase inhibition (Black et al., 1971). In newborn kittens, the dynamics of response of peripheral chemoreceptors are different from that observed in adult cats (Marchal et al., 1992). It is known that neither the chemosensory activity (Hanson, 1986) nor the carbonic anhydrase activity (Maren, 1967) is mature at birth. However, the dynamics of the hypercapnic response of the peripheral chemoreceptors in newborns remains unknown.

The present experiments were performed to investigate the role of catalyzed CO_2 hydration on the time course of the CO_2 response of the peripheral chemoreceptor over the first days of life. For this aim, the activity of the carotid body during hypercapnic stimulation was analyzed before and after inhibition of carbonic anhydrase by acetazolamide in newborn kittens.

MATERIALS AND METHODS

Eleven newborn kittens aged 0.5 to 25 days, were anesthetized with sodium thiopental (60 mg/kg, i.p.), artificially ventilated and paralysed with pancuronium bromide (0.5 mg/kg, i.v.). A catheter was placed in the femoral artery to measure blood pressure (Statham P23 ID) and to sample blood for arterial blood gases analysis (Ciba Corning 238). Core temperature was maintained at 38°C with a heating pad. The respiratory gases, F_IO_2 (Beckman OM11) and $F_{ET}CO_2$ (Instrument Laboratory, IL200), were continuously monitored.

One carotid sinus nerve was prepared for recording the whole nerve activity. The nerve was cut near the petrosal ganglion, carefully isolated from surrounding tissue and desheathed. Baroreceptor discharge was eliminated by crushing the carotid sinus until audible cardiosynchronous activity was abolished. Carotid body neural output was determined from the sinus nerve activity (SNA) recorded by platinum electrodes. The amplified signal was filtered and quantitated by the amplitude variance analysis method

Arterial Chemoreceptors: Cell to System
Edited by R. O'Regan *et al*, Plenum Press, New York, 1994

previously described (Hannhart et al., 1990). SNA signal, arterial blood pressure and respiratory gases were digitized and fed into a microcomputer (MacIntosh SE).

The dynamics of the peripheral chemosensory response to CO_2 was analyzed during a step change in F_ICO_2 (0.08), while a steady hypoxic background (F_IO_2 = 0.08) was maintained to enlarge the CO_2 response. Because absolute value of the amplitude variance is affected by resistance of the electrode-nerve contact, the SNA values were normalized in all animals by setting the hypoxic response (F_IO_2 decrease from 1.00 to 0.08) to one and expressing SNA relative to the individual hypoxic response (%hypox). To determine the potential role of the carbonic acid hydration, the time course of the CO_2 response of the peripheral chemoreceptor was studied before and 45 min after injection of 50 mg/kg i.v. acetazolamide (Diamox), a carbonic anhydrase inhibitor

RESULTS

Control

A representative recording obtained in a 1-day-old kitten is presented in the Fig. 1. While F_IO_2 was decreased to 0.08, a clear increase in SNA was observed and was arbitrarily set to one. Maintaining the steady hypoxia, CO_2 was abruptly added to the inspired gas. In all but 2 kittens, a prompt increase in the peripheral chemoreceptor activity by 50±7 %hypox was observed within the first 14±1 (± SEM) sec, followed by a more or less complete adaptation towards the initial hypoxic level within the subsequent 17±1 sec (Fig.1, left panel).

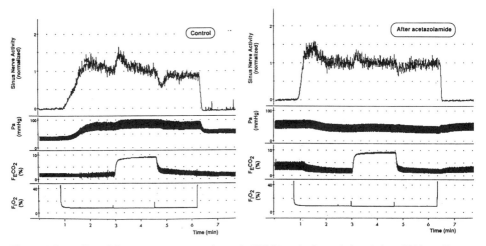

Figure 1. Recording of the response to a step change in FICO2 under hypoxia in a 1-day-old kitten. From top to bottom: Sinus nerve activity, systemic arterial pressure (Pa), F_ECO2 and F_IO2. Left panel = control; Right panel = after acetazolamide.

The younger the kittens, the more complete the adaptation. Therefore, as shown in Fig.2 (left panel), the late steady-state component of the CO_2 response is weak at birth compared with the hypoxic response and seems to develop during the first three weeks of life. On the contrary, the early transient peak response exists soon after birth and its magnitude seems to be independent of the age.

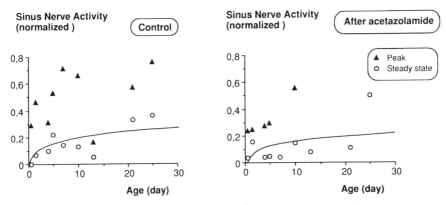

Figure 2. Effect of ageing on the two components of the CO2 response of the peripheral chemoreceptors. Left panel = control; Right panel = after acetazolamide.

After acetazolamide

After acetazolamide, acidosis developed in blood; arterial pH changing from 7.3 ± 0.04 to 7.06 ± 0.05. The basal activity of the sinus nerve, the amplitude of hypoxic responsiveness and the steady level of the CO_2 response were not significantly modified. On the contrary, the transient peak response disappeared, as in adults, in 4 out of the 5 older kittens (>1 wk old). As shown in the right panels of Fig.1 and 2, in the younger kittens under carbonic anhydrase inhibition, the early transient peak response still persisted although slightly decreased by $27\pm20\%$ and delayed (19 ± 3 sec, NS).

DISCUSSION

These results demonstrate that the chemosensitivity of the carotid body to CO_2 is already developed at birth, although modest relatively to the hypoxic response. Under hypoxia, the steady-state response to CO_2 of peripheral chemoreceptor is weak and progressively developed with ageing. This maturation of the peripheral CO_2 sensitivity could correspond to the maturation and the resetting of chemoreceptor responsiveness to hypoxia previously described in the lamb (Hanson, 1986).

The early transient peak CO_2 response of the peripheral chemoreceptor exists soon after birth. Such a transient response is usually observed in adult animals (Schwieler, 1968; Black et al., 1971, Lahiri and al., 1984). and corresponds to the rapid admission of CO_2 to the interior of the sensitive cells. However, since the rapid peak response was suppressed by inhibition of the carbonic anhydrase (Black et al., 1971; Gray, 1971), the molecular CO_2 appears to be inert on the chemosensory mechanism (Travis, 1971). Thus, the catalyzed hydration of CO_2 into H^+ ions is necessary to initiate the chemosensitive reaction and, as suggested by the acidic theory, the carotid chemoreceptors would respond to local pH changes (Torrance, 1976). The subsequent adaptation in the response depends on the slower proton buffering and extrusion via cellular ion exchangers.

Contrary to what is observed in adult animals, the initial peak discharge was only partially affected by carbonic anhydrase inhibition during the first week of life in kittens. It is unlikely that the reason is an incomplete inhibition of the enzyme by acetazolamide in the newborn. Indeed, the effective inhibition is reflected by the clear acidotic pH appearing in all kittens, at least in the blood. Therefore, at birth, the catalyzed CO_2 hydration does not seem to be the major factor that regulated the dynamics of the CO_2 response of the peripheral chemoreceptor. Other mechanisms have to be sought. They could also explain the early peak response to hypoxia often observed in newborn animals (Marchal et al., 1990). Such relatively large transient responses of the carotid chemoreceptors to natural stimuli could play a key role in the generation of unstable ventilatory control in neonates.

REFERENCES

Black, A.M.S., McCloskey, D.I. & Torrance, R.W. (1971). The responses of carotid body chemoreceptors in the cat to sudden changes of hypercapnic and hypoxic stimuli. Respir.Physiol. 13:36-49.

Gray, B.A. (1971). On the speed of the carotid chemoreceptor response in relation to the kinetics of CO_2 hydration. Respir.Physiol. 11:235-246.

Hannhart, B., Pickett, C.K. & Moore, L.G. (1990). Effects of estrogen and progesterone on carotid body neural output responsiveness to hypoxia. J.Appl.Physiol. 68:909-1916.

Hanson, M.A. (1986). Peripheral chemoreceptor function before and after birth. In "Respiratory control and lung development in the fetus and newborn." B.M. Johnson & P.D. Gluckman, ed, Ithaca, Perinatology Pres., New York, pp. 311-330.

Lahiri, S., Mulligan, E. & Mokashi, A. (1982). Adaptive response of carotid body chemoreceptors to CO_2. Brain Res. 234:137-147.

Marchal, F., Bairam, A., Haouzi, P., Crance, J.P., DiGiulio, C., Vert, P. & Lahiri, S. (1992). Carotid chemoreceptor response to natural stimuli in the newborn kitten. Respir.Physiol. 87:183-193.

Maren, T.H. (1967). Carbonic anhydrase; chemistry, physiology and inhibition. Physiol.Rev. 47:595-781.

Schwieler, G.H. (1968). Respiratory regulation during postnatal development in cats and rabbits and some of its morphological substrate. Acta Physiol Scand.Suppl. 304:1-123.

Torrance, R.W. (1976). A new version of the acid receptor hypothesis of carotid chemoreceptors. In: "Morphology and mechanisms of arterial chemoreceptors." A.S. Paintal, ed. Vallabhbhai Patel Chest Inst.Univ., Dehli, pp. 131-137.

Travis, D.M. (1971). Molecular CO_2 is inert on carotid chemoreceptor: demonstration by inhibition of carbonic anhydrase. J.Pharmacol.Exp.Ther. 178:529-540.

CARDIOVASCULAR RESPONSES TO HYPOXIA IN DEVELOPING SWINE

Phyllis M. Gootman and Norman Gootman

Department of Physiology, State University of New York-Health Science Center at Brooklyn, 450 Clarkson Avenue, Brooklyn, New York, USA

INTRODUCTION

Hypoxia, severe enough to lead to acidosis, is a common stress in the perinatal period. There have been some studies of cardiovascular (CV) responses to hypoxia in fetal and adult swine (Harris & Cummings, 1973), our animal model of human development (Gootman, 1991). We next decided to examine the effects of moderate and severe hypoxia at three different postnatal ages selected because of their maturational differences in reflex responsiveness (Gootman, 1991).

METHODS

Swine aged 2-4 days (n = 21), 2 weeks (n = 20) and 2 months (n = 24) were anesthetized with age-adjusted doses of sodium pentobarbital, paralyzed with C-10 and ventilated at constant rate and volume with a Palmer respirator to prevent ventilatory responses. Hydration and body temperature were maintained. Aortic pressure (AoP), heart rate (HR) and blood flows through the renal, superior mesenteric (intestinal) and femoral arteries were registered, and vascular resistances calculated by our standard methods (Buckley, 1986; Gootman, 1991). End-tidal CO_2 was continuously monitored (Sensormedic LB2 Infrared Analyzer). Arterial blood gas composition and pH, total hemoglobin concentration and O_2 saturation (% sat Hb), and total blood lactate concentration were determined by standard methods (Gootman, 1991). Each age group of swine was used for 3 different protocols: normoxia (N), moderate hypoxia (MH) or severe hypoxia (SH). Hypoxia was produced by decreasing the F_IO_2 to attain an arterial PO_2 of 50-65 torr for MH and 25-40 torr for SH. Arterial blood and CV parameters were measured at the end of a control period and at 20 min. after MH or SH was achieved. Normoxia was maintained and observations made at comparable times in the age-matched animals on protocol N. During the control period, AoP was lower and resistances higher in the youngest animals. Therefore changes in CV function during each protocol were expressed as % of baseline value in each animal. Observations at 20 min after MH or SH were cross-compared with age-matched N by ANOVA.

RESULTS

Hypoxia was achieved rapidly and sustained during the 20 min observation period. The % sat Hb decreased during both MH and SH and C_aO_2 decreased during SH, but significantly less in the youngest animals. Arterial PCO_2 remained virtually unchanged, but total blood lactate increased and arterial pH decreased during SH. Fig.1 shows the absence of HR change and the smaller AoP change during MH in the youngest animals. Tachycardia was seen in all animals. Significant changes in blood flows were seen only during SH (see Fig. 1). Fig. 2 shows the mean changes in renal, intestinal and femoral vascular R after 20 min of MH or SH.

DISCUSSION

The age-related pattern of pressor responses to the single stress of low P_aO_2 during MH was also characteristic of maturation of the baroreceptor reflex (Gootman, 1991). The

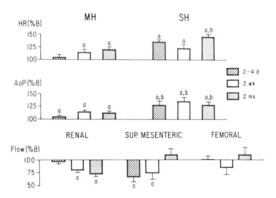

Figure 1. Changes in heart rate (upper panel) and mean aortic pressure (middle panel) during MH (left) and SH (right), and regional blood flows (lower panel) during SH, in 3 age groups of swine. Bars = group mean values; verticals = SEM; a = significantly different from age-matched N group (p<0.05) ; b = significant difference between responses to MH and SH (p< 0.05).

absence of reflex bradycardia to MH or SH in postnatal swine, as in fetal swine (Harris & Cummings, 1973), is further evidence for delayed maturation of the cardiac component of the baroreceptor reflex in swine (Gootman, 1991).

The multiple stress of low P_aO_2 and acidosis during SH reflected a switch from aerobic to anaerobic metabolism. It was accompanied by age-related changes in renal, intestinal and femoral resistances. All 3 vasculatures constricted in animals younger than one month of age, while autoregulatory intestinal and vasodilatory femoral mechanisms apparently minimized vasoconstriction in these regions in the oldest animals. The renal and intestinal vasoconstriction produced in animals young enough to be considered neonates (2-4 days old) could be hazardous for organ function.

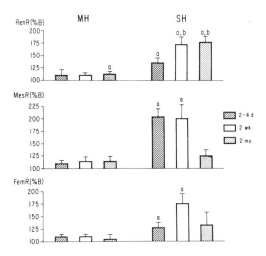

Figure 2. Changes in renal (upper), intestinal (middle) and femoral (lower) vascular resistances during MH (left) and SH (right) in 3 age groups of swine. Bars = group mean values; verticals= SEM; a= significantly different from age-matched N group (p<0.05); b = significant difference between responses to MH and SH (p <0.05).

Major elements in the postnatal development of CV responses to hypoxia stress include asynchronous maturation of components of the ANS (Buckley, 1986; Gootman, 1991). However it must also be noted that, in young swine, hypoxia depresses carotid chemoreceptor discharge, medullary vasomotor center responses to electrical stimulation, and spontaneous cervical sympathetic efferent discharge (Gootman, 1991).

This study was supported by USPHS NIH grants HL 20964 and HD-28931. The authors would like to acknowledge the invaluable help of Dr. N.M. Buckley with the preparation of the manuscript.

REFERENCES

Harris, W.H. & Cummings, J.N. (1973). Maternal and fetal responses to varying levels of oxygen intake in swine. J. Appl. Physiol. 34:584-589.

Gootman, P.M. (1991). Developmental aspects of reflex control of the circulation. In "Reflex Control of the Circulation". I.H. Zucker & J.P. Gilmore, eds. CRC Press, Boca Raton, Florida.

Buckley, N.M (1986). Regulation of regional vascular beds by the developing autonomic nervous system. In "Developmental Neurobiology of the Autonomic Nervous System". P.M. Gootman, ed. Humana Press, Clifton, New Jersey.

FETAL REFLEXES IN CHRONIC HYPOXAEMIA

Laura Bennet, Takanori Watanabe, John Spencer and Mark A. Hanson

Department of Obstetrics and Gynaecology
University College London Medical School
86-96 Chenies Mews
London WC1E 6HX

INTRODUCTION

Currently our physiological and clinical understanding of how the fetus responds to hypoxaemia or asphyxia is primarily based on observations of the effects of single acute episodes of these insults. We know very little about how the fetus responds and adapts to chronic hypoxaemia or asphyxia, yet it is becoming increasingly evident that the developing fetus is more likely to face either such continuous compromise or repeated acute insults. It is evident from a number of studies that what happens during fetal life has important consequences after birth. This observation raises several fundamental questions about how the fetus adapts to its abnormal intrauterine environment, how it is able to respond to further challenges and how these fetal adaptations affect postnatal life.

EXPERIMENTAL MODELS

Studies with a range of techniques have demonstrated that the sheep fetus is capable of adapting to 24-48 hours of hypoxaemia and that after this time fetal behaviour does not differ from that of control animals despite continued compromise (see Bocking, 1993, for review). However it is clear from these preliminary studies that even by 24 hours there are persistent hormonal and cardiovascular changes (Bocking et al, 1989; Kitanaka et al, 1989) and Hooper et al. (1991) found significant reduction in DNA synthesis in the fetal lung, skeletal muscle and thymus gland after 24 hours of hypoxaemia.

To date, however, chronic hypoxaemia has still only been induced for a relatively acute period of time; 24-48 hours. We have developed a method of prolonged reduction of uterine artery blood flow and present preliminary evaluations of the fetal responses to 2 weeks of hypoxaemia and the response of these chronically hypoxaemic fetuses to an additional superimposed episode of hypoxaemia. We examined two levels of hypoxaemia. In group 1 the fetal P_aO_2 was reduced to 11-13 mmHg and in group 2 the fetal P_aO_2 reduced to 15-17 mmHg.

In group 1 we found that the majority of fetuses did not survive severe hypoxaemia for more than 24-72 hours. While P_aO_2 remained constant, they became progressively acidotic. In those fetuses which did survive, HR fell initially and slowly returned to normal over

Arterial Chemoreceptors: Cell to System
Edited by R. O'Regan *et al*, Plenum Press, New York, 1994

several hours, as did femoral blood flow. BP rose initially and then returned to normal. Fetal breathing movements (FBM) ceased initially but returned 7-18 hours after the start of occlusion. These FBM were often initially continuous for some hours or occurred episodically in both high and low voltage electrocortical (ECoG) state. There was also a loss of ECoG signal power and of differentiation of activity during the first 3-15 hours. In those fetuses which died unexpectedly after 5 or 6 days the best predictor of imminent fetal death were these types of changes in ECoG activity. These changes were observed 6-18 hours before death, at a time where there were no other apparent changes in behaviour. In one fetus we conducted the acute hypoxaemic challenge after 8 days of occlusion. This fetus was primarily tachycardic during and post hypoxaemia.

In group 2, fetuses became transiently bradycardic then tachycardic for 5-8 hours. BP rose initially and remained elevated for 3-4 hours. Both HR and BP then returned to normal

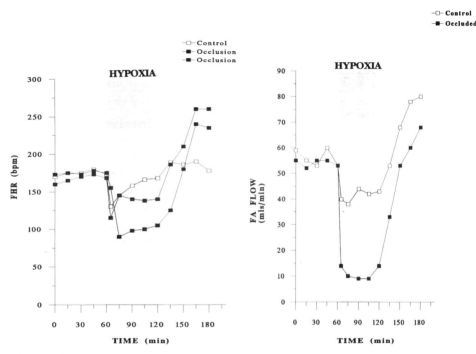

Figure 1. The effect of acute isocapnic hypoxia on fetal heart rate (FHR, left panel) and femoral artery (FA) blood flow (right panel) after two weeks of moderate chronic hypoxaemia in the late gestation fetal sheep.

and remained so throughout the occlusion period. FBM returned after 7-12 hours. Again these fetuses displayed FBM during both high and low voltage ECoG activity. Fetuses which became acidotic during the initial occlusion period also displayed a loss of ECoG differentiation and signal power and even those which did not showed a 2-4 hour period of reduced ECoG activity. The acute hypoxia protocol was conducted on two fetuses from this group (Fig. 1, left panel). Both fetuses remained bradycardic during hypoxia. Moreover, at the cessation of the acute hypoxaemia, there was a pronounced tachycardia. In one fetus we recorded femoral artery blood flow. During occlusion blood flow was slightly lower than control and in hypoxaemia it fell to very low levels compared to controls (Fig 1, right panel). This suggests that the hypoxic fetal chemoreflex response which redistributes blood flow away from the periphery is not blunted, but rather is increased. In conjunction with the effects on heart rate, it appears that the cholinergic and adrenergic efferent limbs of the reflex are enhanced.

CONCLUSIONS

Our preliminary findings suggest that although the fetus is capable of adapting to hypoxaemia (if acidemia does not develop), its cardiovascular responses to further episodes of hypoxaemia are altered. This alteration takes the form of an apparently <u>enhanced</u> peripheral chemoreflex response. Similar conclusions are drawn from studies on a species genetically adapted to chronic hypoxaemia (the llama, see Giussani et al in this volume). The mechanisms underlying this change in peripheral chemoreflex sensitivity are unknown.

Supported by Birthright, AFRC and The Wellcome Trust.

REFERENCES

Bocking, A.D., White, S.E., Gagnon, R. & Hansford, H. (1989) Effect of prolonged hypoxemia on fetal heart rate accelerations and decelerations in sheep. Am.J. Obst. Gynaecol. 161: 722-7.

Bocking, A.D. (1993) Effects of chronic hypoxaemia on circulatory control, In "Fetus and Neonate Physiology and Clinical Applications.", Volume 1, The Circulation," M.A. Hanson, J.A.D. Spencer, C.H. Rodeck, eds., Cambridge University Press, Cambridge.

Hooper, S.B., Bocking, A.D., White, S.E., Challis, J.R.G. & Han, V.K.M. (1991) Changes in lung liquid dynamics induced by prolonged hypoxaemia. Am.J.Physiol. 261: R508-R514.

Kitanaka, T., Alonso, J.G., Gilbert, R.D., Benjamin, L.S., Clemons, G.K. & Longo, L.D. (1989) Fetal responses to long-term hypoxemia in sheep. Am. J. Physiol. 256: R1348-R1354.

IS THE RAPID AND INTENSE PERIPHERAL VASOCONSTRICTION OCCURRING DURING ACUTE HYPOXAEMIA IN THE LLAMA FETUS AN ARTERIAL CHEMOREFLEX ?

Dino A. Giussani[3], Raquel A. Riquelme[2], Mark A. Hanson[3] and Aníbal J. Llanos[1]

[1]Departamento de Medicina Experimental, Campus Oriente, Facultad de Medicina, Universidad de Chile; [2]Departamento de Bioquímica y Biología Molecular, Ciencias Químicas Farmacéuticas, Universidad de Chile and [3]Department of Obstetrics and Gynaecology, University College London, London, WC1E 6HX, United Kingdom

INTRODUCTION

In lowland species the fetus responds to acute isocapnic hypoxaemia with an initial bradycardia, an increase in arterial blood pressure and a redistribution of the combined ventricular output (CVO) favouring the cerebral, myocardial and adrenal circulations and including a peripheral vasoconstriction (Boddy et al., 1974; Cohn et al., 1974; Giussani et al., 1993). This vasoconstriction is initiated by a carotid chemoreflex (Giussani et al., 1993) and maintained via increased plasma concentrations of vasoconstrictor hormones such as catecholamines (Jones & Wei, 1985), arginine vasopressin (Rurak, 1983) and angiotensin II (Broughton-Pipkin et al., 1974) and is modulated by endogenous opioids (Espinoza et al., 1989).

In contrast to lowland species the fetal llama, a species adapted to the chronic hypoxia of high altitude, responds to acute hypoxaemia without an increase in cerebral blood flow but it shows a more pronounced peripheral vasoconstriction (Riquelme et al., 1992). The mechanism mediating the enhanced peripheral vasoconstriction is unknown.

We have now monitored femoral blood continuously, in addition to measuring organ blood flow via radio-labelled microspheres during acute hypoxaemia, in 0.6-0.7 gestation llama fetuses to 1) examine whether the peripheral vasoconstriction is present earlier in gestation, and 2) to determine its rate of onset.

METHODS

Seven fetal llamas were chronically instrumented at 0.6-0.7 of gestation (fetal weights were 2384±317 g; mean±S.E.M, n=7; term is 7000-8000 g; see Fowler, 1989) under general anaesthesia (1% halothane in 50/50 O_2 and N_2O). Catheters were inserted in the ascending and descending aorta, inferior vena cava and the amniotic cavity. In addition, Transonic flow transducers (Transonics Inc., Ithaca, NY, USA) were implanted around a carotid and a femoral artery (Giussani et al., 1993). All catheters were filled with heparinized saline (1000 I.U.ml^{-1}), plugged with a copper wire and exteriorized with the flow transducer leads through a maternal flank. On the fourth post-operative day, fetal hypoxaemia was induced for one hour by reducing the maternal inspired PO_2. Arterial, venous and amniotic pressures and carotid and femoral blood flows were monitored continuously during the experimental protocol. Cardiac output and its distribution were measured with radiolabelled microspheres (^{57}Co, ^{113}Sn, ^{46}Sc; New England Nuclear, Boston, MA; see Heymann et al., 1977) after 45 minutes of control (normoxia) and 15 and 45 minutes after the onset of hypoxaemia.

Values are expressed as the mean±S.E.M. The Student's t test for paired data was used to compare values for a variable in control normoxia and hypoxaemia.

RESULTS

During hypoxaemia there was an increase in perfusion (arterial-venous) pressure ($P<0.05$; 37.7±3.3 vs 46.9±5.1 mmHg; 60 minutes of control normoxia vs. maximal increase during hypoxaemia), and a transient bradycardia, after which heart rate levels returned to, or to above, control values (Table 1). In addition, there was an increase in myocardial and adrenal blood flows, a pronounced fall in peripheral blood flow but no sustained increase in cerebral blood flow during the hypoxaemic episode (Table 1). Whilst there was no change in carotid vascular resistance (perfusion pressure/ carotid blood flow) during hypoxaemia, there was a large increase in femoral vascular resistance, occurring within 5 minutes of the onset of hypoxaemia ($P=0.01$; Fig. 1). The maximal increase in femoral vascular resistance during hypoxaemia in the llama fetus was 5 times greater than that observed for the sheep fetus (Giussani et al., 1993, 1994) (Fig. 1).

Table 1. Blood gases and cardiovascular data in 0.6-0.7 gestation fetal llamas after 45 minutes of normoxia and after 5, 15 and 45 minutes of isocapnic hypoxaemia.

	NORMOXIA		HYPOXAEMIA	
Time (min)	0	5	15	45
pHa	7.33±0.01		7.25±0.03 [a]	7.21±0.03 [a]
Pa,CO2 (mmHg)	41.1±1.7		44.1±3.2 [b]	45.1±4.0 [b]
Pa,O2 (mmHg)	24.0±1.5		13.8±0.5	14.7±1.3
Perfusion pressure (mmHg)	36.0±2.4	36.7±5.8	42.9±4.8	39.7±4.5
Fetal heart rate (bpm)	117.3±7.1	93.2±3.0 [a]	116.3±14.1	117.0±12.9
Organ blood flows (mls/min.100g)				
Brain	54.3±6.7		107.8±24.5	69.0±13.0
Heart	133.8±25.2		500.5±97.4 [a]	345.5±139.71
Adrenals	411.3±62.6		799.7±124.8 [a]	849.4±90.6 [b]
Carcass	8.6±0.7		3.7±0.9 [b]	3.2±0.7 [b]
Kidney	160.9±22.4		77.0±27.1 [b]	53.2±25.1 [b]
Liver	2.8±0.5		0.8±0.2 [b]	1.0±0.2 [a]

Values given are mean ± S.E.M. Significant differences, normoxia vs. hypoxaemia (Paired t test): a:$P<0.05$, b:$P<0.01$

DISCUSSION

One adaptive response to the chronic hypoxia of life at high altitude in the adult llama is a shift in its oxygen dissociation curve to a position similar to that of the fetal llama

(Meschia et al., 1960). This shift increases the O_2 affinity of adult haemoglobin at lower O_2 partial pressures and increases the O_2 content but it also necessitates a lower PO_2 in the tissues, including the placenta, for unbinding the O_2 carried. In addition, the fetal llama will be exposed to hypoxaemia if its mother is resident at high altitude.

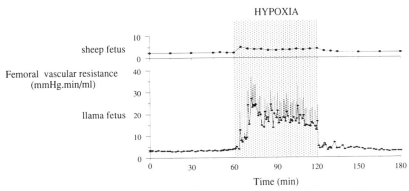

Figure 1. Comparison of changes in femoral vascular resistance during acute hypoxaemia between fetal llamas and fetal sheep. The increase in femoral resistance at the onset of hypoxaemia in fetal sheep is itself significant (from 1.3±0.1 to 3.8±0.8 mmHg.min/ml, control at 60 min vs. 5 minutes of hypoxaemia; paired t test, P<0.01) but that of llama fetuses is 5 times greater.

Teleologically, it is therefore reasonable for the llama fetus to have strong protective cardiovascular responses to acute hypoxaemia, ensuring a powerful redistribution of the CVO to the vital organs.

By analogy with fetal sheep, the speed of the initial femoral vasoconstriction in the llama fetus suggests it to be chemoreflex in nature. Furthermore, since the magnitude of the femoral vasoconstriction in the 0.6-0.7 gestation llama fetus is much greater than that observed in the sheep fetus in the late gestation, the chemoreflex response develops relatively early in the former. Alternatively, it may be that the fetal llama responses to hypoxaemia are much greater than those of fetal sheep due to an early maturation of strong endocrine responses. Further work is needed in order to discriminate between these possibilities.

D.A.G. was supported by an Astor Foundation fellowship and The Royal Society. Work funded in Chile by Fondecyt (grant N°1931033) and in the UK by The Wellcome Trust.

REFERENCES

Boddy, K., Dawes, G.S., Fisher, R., Pinter, S. & Robinson, J.S. (1974). Foetal respiratory movements, electrocortical and cardiovascular responses to hypoxemia and hypercapnia in sheep. J. Physiol. 243:599-618.

Broughton-Pipkin, F., Kirkpatrick, S.M.L., Lumbers, E.R. & Mott, J.C. (1974). Factors influencing plasma renin and angiotensin II in the conscious pregnant ewe and its foetus. J. Physiol. 243:619-637.

Cohn, E.H., Sacks, E.J., Heymann, M.A. & Rudolph, A.M. (1974). Cardiovascular responses to hypoxemia and acidemia in fetal lambs. Am. J. Obs. Gyn. 120:817-824.

Espinoza, M., Riquelme, R., Germain, A.M., Tevah, J., Parer, J.T. & Llanos, A.J. (1989). Role of endogenous opioids in the cardiovascular response to asphyxia in fetal sheep. Am. J. Physiol. 256, R1063-R1068.

Fowler, M.E. (1989). "Medicine and surgery of South American camelids: llama, alpaca, vicuña, guanaco." Ames, Iowa State University Press, pp 126-127.

Giussani, D.A., Spencer, J.A.D., Moore, P.J., Bennet, L. & Hanson, M.A. (1993). Afferent and efferent components of the cardiovascular reflex responses to acute hypoxia in term fetal sheep. J. Physiol. 461:431-449.

Giussani, D.A., Riquelme, R.A., Gaete, C.R., Moraga, F.A., Sanhueza, E.M., Hanson, M.A. & Llanos, J.A. (1994). Rapid, intense peripheral vasoconstriction in the llama fetus in utero during acute hypoxaemia at 0.6-0.7 of gestation (abstract). J. Physiol. in press.

Heymann, M.A., Payne, B.D., Hoffman, J.I.E. & Rudolph, A.M. (1977). Blood flow measurements with radionuclide-labelled particles. Prog. Cardiovasc. Dis. 20:55-79.

Jones, C. T. & Wei, G. (1985). Adrenal-medullary activity and cardiovascular control in the fetal sheep. In: "Fetal heart rate monitoring", W. Kunzel, ed., Springer-Verlag, Berlin:

Riquelme, R.A., Gaete, C.R., Garay, F., Carrasco, J., Espinoza, M., Cabello, G., Serón-Ferré, M., Parer, J.P. & Llanos, A.J. (1992). Lack of response of brain and adrenal blood flow to hypoxaemia in the fetal llama. Pediatric Res. 32:737.

Rurak, D.W. (1978). Plasma vasopressin levels during hypoxaemia and the cardiovascular effects of exogenous vasopressin in foetal and adult sheep. J. Physiol. 277:341-357.

Meschia, G., Prystowsky, H., Hellegers, A., Huckabee, W., Metcalfe, J. & Barron, D. (1960). Observations on the oxygen supply to the fetal llama. Q. J. Exp. Physiol. 45:284-291.

IS THE VENTILATORY DECLINE SEEN IN NEWBORNS DURING HYPOXAEMIA CENTRALLY MEDIATED?

Gareth L. Ackland, Peter J. Moore & Mark A. Hanson

Departments of Obstetrics & Gynaecology and Physiology,
University College London Medical School
86-96 Chenies Mews
London WC1E 6HX

INTRODUCTION

Breathing pattern in the newborn is often irregular and may be periodic or apnoeic, particularly during REM sleep. Clearly mild levels of hypoxaemia will be regularly experienced by many babies until respiratory control matures. A fall in P_aO_2 becomes even more significant when the newborn's respiratory response to acute, mild hypoxaemia is considered. This response is apparently paradoxical, with a brisk initial increase in ventilation (phase 1), being followed shortly afterwards by a decline to, or to below, pre-hypoxaemic levels (phase 2). Whilst phase 1 is attributed to peripheral chemoreceptor stimulation, the mechanism(s) underlying phase 2 have remained controversial. There is increasing evidence that the brainstem may cause the ventilatory decline in the newborn (Moore et al., 1991) whilst there is maintenance of increased afferent chemoreceptor drive throughout this phase (Blanco et al., 1984). If an inhibitory central mechanism is activated during mild hypoxaemia and acts to reduce ventilation, the central processing of afferent chemoreceptor discharge should be modulated. Therefore, we hypothesised that a carotid chemoreceptor-mediated reflex affecting breathing should be altered during hypoxaemia in young rabbits. We also anticipated that other non chemoreceptor-mediated effects on breathing would not be affected.

METHODS

New Zealand white rabbits (18-31 days) were sedated (ketamine, 25mg/kg i.m.) and anaesthetized (induction: 2-2.5% halothane in air; maintenance: urethane 1.2-1.6g/kg i.v.). Catheters were placed in a femoral artery and vein, depth of anaesthesia being monitored from arterial blood pressure and ECG. The animals were paralysed (gallamine triethiodide), vagotomized and artificially ventilated to maintain arterial pH and blood gases within normal physiological ranges. In addition body temperature was controlled. Three protocols were conducted in separate animals which involved the following additional preparation.

Arterial Chemoreceptors: Cell to System
Edited by R. O'Regan *et al*, Plenum Press, New York, 1994

Protocol A: Multifibre carotid chemoreceptor activity was recorded, and a catheter placed in the left external carotid artery for transient stimulation of carotid chemoreceptor fibres, using a bolus of 0.1-0.3ml CO_2-equilibrated saline.

Protocol B: Phrenic nerve activity was recorded, and catheters placed in each external carotid artery for retrograde, transient stimulation of the carotid chemoreceptors, again using bolus CO_2-saline injections.

Protocol C: The sciatic nerve was electrically stimulated (Isostim 2000) with silver bipolar electrodes and phrenic nerve activity was recorded.

RESULTS

Protocol A: Transient chemical stimulation of the carotid body (using CO_2-equilibrated saline) during both normoxaemia and isocapnic hypoxaemia, produced a

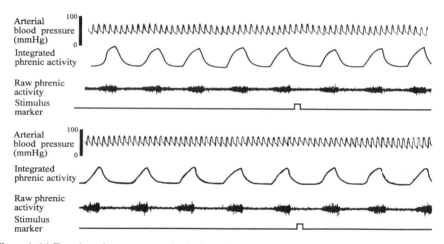

Figure 1. (a) Transient chemoreceptor stimulation, with intracarotid injection of a bolus of CO_2-saturated saline, delivered in early expiration during normoxaemia, prolongs that expiration. **(b)** After 8 minutes of hypoxaemia, the same stimulus fails to prolong expiration.

similarly marked and transient increase in multifibre carotid chemoreceptor discharge (206± 62% and 183±49% increase over baseline discharge respectively), with no sign of chemoreceptor adaptation to hypoxaemia.

Protocol B: Under normoxic conditions, transient stimulation of the carotid chemoreceptors using CO_2-equilibrated saline produced marked effects on central respiratory output, as recorded from the phrenic nerve (Black & Torrance, 1971; Eldridge, 1976). For analysis, the breath in which the transient chemoreceptor stimulation was delivered was compared to the preceding five breaths, in terms of breath duration and peak phrenic activity. Transient stimuli delivered during the start of an expiration (see Figure 1(a) below) significantly prolonged the duration of that breath, without any effect on other respiratory variables [1.40±0.06s (control) vs. 1.65±0.09s (stimulation breath) mean ± S.E.M.; P<0.01; Wilcoxon T test].

However, during isocapnic hypoxaemia (P_aO_2 40±3mmHg) there was no significant effect of this transient chemical stimulation on phrenic activity (Figure 1(b)) (at 7th minute of hypoxaemia - control 1.55±0.12s vs. stimulation 1.57±0.10s respectively, mean ± S.E.M.). Thus during hypoxaemia of around 40mmHg, transient chemoreceptor stimulation failed to produce significant changes in central respiratory output, even though the CO_2-saline bolus could produce a substantial increase in chemoreceptor discharge throughout the hypoxaemic period (Protocol A). However, in apnoea, transient chemoreceptor stimulation produced an immediate burst of phrenic activity.

Protocol C: The threshold required to increase central respiratory output by electrical stimulation of the sciatic nerve (frequency 20 or 100Hz; 0.4ms pulse width; 0.3-3mA current) was determined under normoxaemic conditions (Figure 2(a)) and after 5 min of isocapnic hypoxaemia (P_aO_2 38±3mmHg). Stimulation during isocapnic hypoxaemia, using the threshold parameters determined during normoxia, again caused a similar or even greater increase in respiratory output (Figure 2(b)).

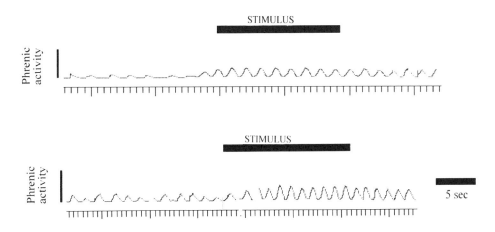

Figure 2. (a) Effect of stimulating sciatic nerve afferents on phrenic nerve discharge in normoxaemia. **(b)** Threshold parameters required to elicit phrenic response in normoxaemia produce a similar response after 5 minutes of hypoxaemia.

DISCUSSION

These results show that hypoxaemia inhibits the chemoreceptor-mediated transient reflex effect on central respiratory output, and supports the idea that the effect of peripheral chemoreceptor activity is modulated during hypoxaemia by a centrally activated mechanism (Schramm & Grunstein, 1987) which may involve the rostral pons (Moore et al., 1991). However, during severe hypoxaemia, that produces apnoea, chemoreceptor stimulation produces a burst of phrenic activity. Here, any inhibitory mechanisms initiated by hypoxaemia may be metabolically/pharmacologically inhibited by low brain tissue PO_2. This illustrates the fine balance that exists between the effects of peripheral chemoreceptor activity being gated out at milder P_aO_2 levels and the respiratory depression which occurs during severe hypoxaemia. Mild hypoxaemia does not seem to produce a generalised inhibition of afferent inputs, since threshold sciatic nerve stimulation under normoxaemic conditions still produces similar changes in central respiratory output during hypoxaemia.

This work is supported by The Wellcome Trust.

REFERENCES

Black, A.M.S & Torrance, R.W. (1971) Respiratory oscillations in chemoreceptor discharge in the control of breathing. Respir. Physiol. 13: 221-237

Blanco, C.E., Hanson, M.A., Johnson, P. & Rigatto, H. (1984) Breathing patterns of kittens during hypoxia J. Appl. Physiol. 56(1):12-17

Eldridge, F.L. (1976) Expiratory effects of brief carotid sinus nerve and carotid body stimuli. Respir. Physiol. 26:395-410

Moore, P.J., Parkes, M.J., Noble, R. & Hanson, M.A. (1991) Reversible blockade of the secondary fall of ventilation during hypoxia in anaesthetised newborn sheep by focal cooling of the brain stem. J. Physiol. 438:242P

Schramm,C.M., Grunstein, M.M. (1987) Respiratory influence of peripheral chemoreceptor stimulation in maturing rabbits. J. Appl. Physiol. 63:1671-1680

POSTMORTEM CHANGES IN THE HUMAN CAROTID BODY

M. Seker,[1] D.J. Pallot,[1] J-O Habeck,[2] and A. Abramovici[3]

[1]Department of Human Anatomy, University of the U.A.E.; [2]Department of Pathology, Municipal Hospital, Chemnitz, Germany; [3]Department of Pathology, Sackler School of Medicine, Tel Aviv, Israel

INTRODUCTION

Heath and his colleagues have described three varieties of Type I cells based upon differences in nuclear morphology (Heath et al., 1970); this is at odds with the situation in experimental animals. Pallot et al. (1992) examined rat carotid bodies fixed at various times after death of the animal. Their data showed that, with increasing delay in fixation of the carotid body, first Type I cells with dark nuclei became apparent and with further delay cells with pyknotic nuclei appeared. Here we correlate the percentage occurrence of clear, dark and pyknotic nucleated cells in the human carotid body with the delay between death of the patient and fixation of the tissue.

METHODS

A total of 75 carotid bodies were fixed in Zamboni's fluid at postmortem of and after routine processing sections were stained with H&E. Sections separated by a minimum gap of 250μm were examined and random fields using a x40 objective used to classify the Type I cells as either clear, dark or pyknotic.

RESULTS

Fig 1 shows a photomicrograph of carotid body tissue which had been fixed 3.5 hours after death of the patient. The three varieties of Type I cell, clear, dark and pyknotic are clearly seen.

All of the cases were ascribed to one of three groups on the basis of the time between death and fixation of the carotid body. The percentage occurrence of the three varieties of type I cells are illustrated in Fig 2. It can be seen that, with increasing delay, the number of clear cells decreased whilst the number of pyknotic cells increased. We also removed two carotid bodies and divided them into two parts; the first was fixed on removal whilst the second was stored at 4°C for 18 hours before fixation. After storage the number of pyknotic cells increased and the number of clear cells decreased (see Fig 2 D1,D2 & E1,E2).

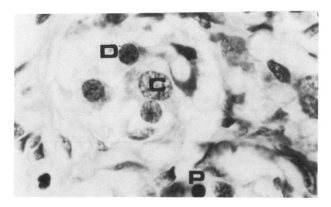

Figure 1. Photomicrograph of the human carotid body showing clear (C), dark (D) and pyknotic (P) cells.

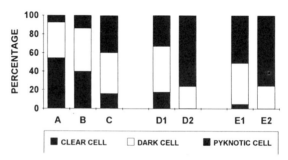

Figure 2. Distribution histograms of the percentage occurrence of the three cell varieties in the human carotid body at various times after death. A = 2-7, B = 7-15, C = >15 hours. D & E show similar data for two carotid bodies divided into two parts and fixed at 14 & 32 hours (D1, D2) and 21 & 38 hours (E1, E2) after death .

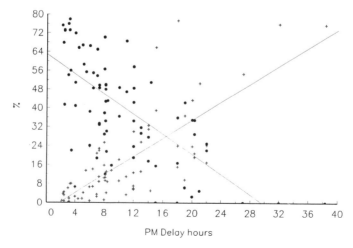

Figure 3. Plot of the percentage number of clear (dots) and pyknotic (crosses) cells against time.

Fig 3 illustrates a plot of the percentage occurrence of clear cells and pyknotic cells as a function of time together with the line of best fit. The linear correlation coefficient for clear cells against time was -0.77 (p>0.001) whilst for pyknotic cells it was 0.71 (p>0.001).

All of the above data indicate that there is a relationship between the number of the different varieties of Type I cells and the time that elapses between death and fixation of the tissue.

DISCUSSION

Like Heath and his colleagues we found three varieties of Type I cells in the human carotid body obtained postmortem (Heath et al., 1970); these were similar to those reported in the rat carotid body (Pallot et al., 1992). In essence the clear Type I cells possessed a lightly eosinophilic cytoplasm and pale nuclei with dispersed chromatin. In dark cells there was increased eosinophilia and a condensation of the nuclear chromatin. Pyknotic cells had only a small rim of cytoplasm around a dense nucleus. In both the rat and human carotid bodies there were increases in the number of pyknotic cells and decreases in the number of clear cells with increasing delay between death and fixation of the tissue. The evidence from the experiments on the rat carotid body (Pallot et al., 1992.) indicate that the dark and pyknotic variants of Type I cells represent postmortem changes, for when fixed very rapidly the carotid body consisted exclusively of clear Type I cells; delay resulted in the appearance of dark cells and then pyknotic cells. Our data show a reduction in the number of clear Type I cells and an increase in the number of pyknotic cells with increasing fixation delay.

REFERENCES

Heath, D., Edwards, C. & Harris, P. (1970). Postmortem size & structure of the human carotid body. Thorax 25: 129-140.

Heath, D., Khan, Q. & Smith, P. (1990). Histopathology of the carotid bodies in neonates and infants. Histopath. 17: 511-520.

Pallot, D.J., Seker, M. & Abramovici A. (1992) . Postmortem changes in the rat carotid body: possible implications for human histopathology. Virchows Archiv A. Pathol. Anat. 420:31-35.

EFFECTS OF VARIOUS DISEASES UPON THE STRUCTURE OF THE HUMAN CAROTID BODY

M. Seker,[1] D.J. Pallot,[1] J-O Habeck,[2] and A. Abramovici.[3]

[1]Department of Human Anatomy, University of the U.A.E.; [2]Department of Pathology, Municipal Hospital, Chemnitz, Germany; [3]Department of Pathology, Sackler School of Medicine, Tel Aviv, Israel

INTRODUCTION

It is well documented that the carotid body responds to a number of abnormal physiological stimuli such as chronic hypoxaemia and hypertension (Heath & Smith, 1992; Pallot, 1987). In both of these conditions there is an increase in the size of the carotid body and, in experimental animals, there is evidence that this increased size is brought about by a combination of hypertrophy and hyperplasia (Bee et al., 1986); in the human evidence of hyperplasia has not been obtained.

In this study we have examined human carotid bodies obtained at routine necropsy and examined three aspects of the carotid body structure, cell cluster size, lobule size and the amount of connective tissue within the lobules.

METHODS

Carotid bodies were removed at routine necropsy, fixed in Zambonis fluid, processed for embedding in paraffin wax, serially sectioned at 5um and stained with H&E. Sections separated by a minimum distance of 250um were then examined as below. The cases were divided into the following categories; chronic hypoxia, essential hypertension, diabetes mellitus, sepsis and non thoracic carcinoma; in addition there were a group of patients who lacked and evidence of these conditions in neither their medical history nor postmortem results, these were used as controls and referred to as unrelated cases.

Single sections were viewed with a x10 objective and the area of carotid body tissue, the outline of each lobule and the outline of all of the cell clusters within the field drawn using a camera lucida; the areas of these drawings was determined using a Videoplan. By simple subtraction the area occupied by connective tissue was calculated from the field area minus the lobule plus cell cluster area. A cumulative mean technique was used to ascertain that a sufficient sample had been analysed.

RESULTS

Table 1 illustrates all of the data relating area of the lobules, cell clusters and connective tissue. From this table it may be seen that hypoxia and hypertension result in an increase in size of all three parameters; what is surprising however is that sepsis and diabetes mellitus both increase the area of lobules. Diabetes mellitus also increases the amount of connective tissue, an effect not seen in patients with sepsis.

Table 1. The area of lobules and cell clusters and the area of connective tissue within our various cases. All data are means and standard deviations. * not significantly different from unrelated, ** p<0.05 as compared to unrelated (t test)

DISEASE	NUMBER	LOBULE AREA	CELL CLUSTER AREA	CONN. TISSUE AREA
UNRELATED	8	0.094 ± 0.023	0.0392 ± 0.010	0.0547 ± 0.013
COPD	13	0.165 ± 0.062**	0.0644 ± 0.022**	0.1000 ± 0.042**
HYPERTENSION	25	0.133 ± 0.031**	0.0470 ± 0.011**	0.0859 ± 0.023**
D. MELLITUS	19	0.121 ± 0.042**	0.0417 ± 0.013*	0.0793 ± 0.032**
CARCINOMA	13	0.106 ± 0.035*	0.0413 ± 0.014*	0.0649 ± 0.026*
SEPSIS	7	0.143 ± 0.075**	0.0565 ± 0.028*	0.0859 ± 0.052*

We divided the chronic hypoxia cases into those with pneumonia and chronic hypoxia due to chronic obstructive pulmonary disease (COPD) and those who lacked the infection; the data showed little difference in the two situations.

We also calculated the area fraction of each lobule occupied cell clusters and connective tissue (see Table 2). The table shows how there is no change in the area fractions of the carotid body lobule occupied by cell clusters and connective tissue in cases of COPD, carcinoma and sepsis, but that the area fractions of the lobule occupied cells in both hypertension and diabetes is decreased whilst there is an increase in the area occupied by connective tissue.

Table 2. Area fraction of lobules occupied by connective tissue and cell clusters in our various cases plus standard deviations. * not significantly different from unrelated, ** p<0.05 when compared to unrelated (t test)

DISEASE	NUMBER	LOBULE AREA	CELL CLUSTER AREA FRACTION	CONN. TISSUE AREA FRACTION
UNRELATED	8	0.094 ± 0.023	41.8 ± 4.1	58.2 ± 4.2
COPD	13	0.165 ± 0.062**	39.9 ± 5.6*	60.1 ± 5.6*
HYPERTENSION	25	0.133 ± 0.031**	35.7 ± 5.5**	64.3 ± 5.5**
D. MELLITUS	19	0.121 ± 0.042**	35.1 ± 6.1**	64.9 ± 6.1**
CARCINOMA	13	0.106 ± 0.035*	39.3 ± 9.5*	60.7 ± 9.5*
SEPSIS	7	0.143 ± 0.075**	40.8 ± 11.1*	59.1 ± 11.1*

DISCUSSION

Our data show, as previously reported, that chronic hypoxia and hypertension result in hypertrophy of the lobules and cell clusters of the human carotid body (see review by Heath & Smith; 1992); in addition to this there is an increase in the amount of connective tissue within the lobule. The new data relates to diabetes mellitus which also increases the lobule area and amount of connective tissue; cell cluster size is also increased in diabetes mellitus. Interestingly the area fraction of each lobule occupied by cell clusters and connective tissue remain unchanged indicating that the hypertrophy and/or hyperplasia occurs uniformly in both elements in the case of COPD whilst in diabetes and hypertension there is a reduction in the proportion of the lobule occupied by cell clusters and a consequent increase in the area of connective tissue. We have no data at the moment to address the issue of hypertrophy versus hyperplasia; counts are in progress to determine the numbers of cells in normal and hypoxaemic carotid body lobules.

MS is grateful to the University of the U.A.E. and the University of Selcuk, Turkey for support.

REFERENCES

Bee, D., Pallot, D.J. & Barer, G.R. (1986) Division of Type I and endothelial cell nuclei in the hypoxic rat carotid body. Acta Anat. 126: 226-230.

Heath, D. & Smith, P. (1992) "Disease of the Human Carotid Body ", Springer Verlag, Berlin, Heidelberg, New York, London.

Pallot, D.J. (1987) The mammalian carotid body. Adv. Anat. Embryol. & Cell Biol. 102: 1-91.

MODIFICATION OF THE RABBIT CAROTID BODY TYPE I CELL MITOCHONDRIA BY HIGH ALTITUDE EXPOSURE AND THE EFFECTS OF DRACOCEPHALUM HETEROPHYLLUM

Xue Dahai[1], Yang Fengxiang[2], and Denise Bee[1]

[1]Department of Experimental Medicine, Medical School, University of Sheffield, UK, and [2]Department of Histology and Embryology, Qinghai Medical School, Xining, China

INTRODUCTION

The carotid body is the principal peripheral chemoreceptor. It is sensitive to hypoxaemia and hypercapnia, and controls ventilation through neural reflex mechanisms. De Castro (1926) pioneered research into carotid body sensitivity to hypoxia, and since then there have been many studies investigating the activity of the carotid body in response to alterations of oxygen concentration in the blood. Morphometric analyses of the carotid body have been conducted by Laidler et al. (1975a,b); Pallot et al. (1986a,b) and others. These studies mainly concentrated on the changes in the volume of structures but few studies give a detailed description of membranes and surfaces. We have made a novel stereological investigation into the effects of high altitude hypoxia with morphometric studies of the mitochondria of rabbit carotid bodies exposed to sustained hypoxia (30 days at high altitude) and the effects of the herb *Dracocephalum heterophyllum Benth*.

METHODS

Eleven male Japan White rabbits born and reared at the altitude of 2200 meters, (weights 1.6-2.4kg), were randomly divided into 3 groups: (1) Control (n=4): these animals remained at a low altitude (2200m) where the bifurcations were dissected. (2) High-Altitude Group (HA) (n=4): these animals were moved to an altitude of 3416m where they remained for 30 days before the carotid bifurcations were dissected. (3) *D. heterophyllum* Treated Group (AM) (n=3): these animals were moved to 3416m where they remained for 30 days before the bifurcations were dissected. These animals were provided with food mixed with a crude powder of the herb *D. heterophyllum* (4g/day).

The animals were anaesthetised with sodium barbiturate (40mg/kg, i.p.) and killed by chest opening. A cannula was inserted into the aorta through the left ventricle. Blood was flushed out with 0.9% sodium chloride for 2 minutes, followed by fixation with 100ml 2% glutaraldehyde in 0.02M phosphate buffer sucrose (pH 7.4). The carotid bifurcations were

Arterial Chemoreceptors: Cell to System
Edited by R. O'Regan *et al*, Plenum Press, New York, 1994

dissected out and stored in 2.5% glutaraldehyde at 4°C overnight. The carotid bodies were dissected out, re-fixed in osmium tetroxide and embedded in Epon 812.

After location of the carotid body with the use of semithin sections, 60nm ultrasections were made and double stained with uranium acetate and lead nitrate. 25 to 40 micrographs were taken from each group at 20,000× magnification. Gundersen's quadric grid and point counting were applied to determine the volume density (Vv), average volume (V), numerical density (Nv), surface/volume ratio of the outer membrane (SVR), and surface/volume ratio of the cristae (SVRc) of the Type-I cell mitochondria. Statistical analyses were performed by Student's t-test.

RESULTS

After 30 days at high altitude (HA Group), the Vv of mitochondria of the rabbit type-I cells increased from 17.20±1.14% (mean ± SEM) to 21.63±1.54% (P<0.01). This increase

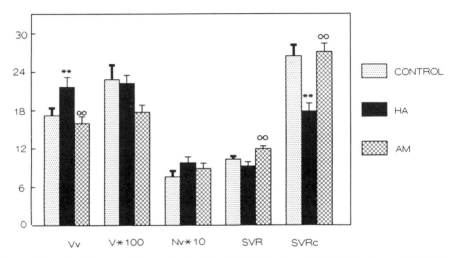

Figure 1. Hypoxic rabbit carotid body mitochondria. CONTROL: low altitude (2200m) group, HA: high altitude (3416m) group, AM: high altitude and *D. heterophyllum* treated group, Vv: volume density (%), V: average volume (μm^3), Nv: numerical density ($\mu m^2/\mu m^3$), SVR: surface volume ratio ($\mu m^2/\mu m^3$), SVRc: surface volume ratio of the cristae ($\mu m^2/\mu m^3$) **: Control vs other groups, P<0.01; oo: HA vs AM, P<0.01.

was probably due to a tendency for the number of mitochondria to increase (Nv increased from 0.756±0.091•μm^{-3} to 0.976±0.091•μm^{-3}, NS) but there was no change in the average volume. SVR showed a tendency to reduce, suggesting dilation of the mitochondria. SVRc significantly (P<0.01) decreased from 26.46±1.70$\mu m^2/\mu m^3$ (control) to 17.80± 1.28$\mu m^2/\mu m^3$ (HA).

After 30 days treatment with *D. heterophyllum* at high altitude, the Vv of the mitochondria (15.69±1.05%) was not significantly different from control values and showed a significant reduction (P<0.01) when compared to HA. Both volume and number tended to decrease with drug treatment. The SVR was significantly higher (P<0.01) than the untreated hypoxic group (11.93±0.46$\mu m^2/\mu m^3$ vs. 9.23±0.66$\mu m^2/\mu m^3$). This together with the reduction in V suggests inhibition of mitochondrial dilation. SVRc was significantly reduced (P<0.01) at high altitude but *D. heterophyllum* prevented this decrease, the SVRc was not significantly different from the control level (SVRc=27.12±1.30$\mu m^2/\mu m^3$, P<0.01 vs. HA, NS vs. control). (Figure 1).

DISCUSSION

After sustained hypoxia the volume density of mitochondria increased showing compensatory hyperplasia as there is a tendency for an increase in the number of mitochondria but the average volume was unaltered. The cristae, however, were severely injured, showing maladaptation to hypoxic exposure. In rats, the same length of hypoxia exposure (from 397 meters to 3416 meters) caused deterioration of the mitochondria, including the injury of the cristae and the dilation of the mitochondria. Shorter exposure (7 days), on the other hand, caused compensatory hyperplasia (Xue et al., 1993). The less severe effects found in rabbits may be due to the less dramatic change of altitude (from 2200 meters to 3416 meters). The large blood supply of the carotid body does not seem to be able to prevent the cells from being damaged (MacDonald, 1989).

Current work (Acker et al., 1989) suggests that the chemoreceptive mechanism may be related to the enzymes and the components of the respiratory chain. It is especially noticeable that the cytochrome a/a_3 on the mitochondrial cristae of the type-I cells has a very low affinity for O_2 and this might be the O_2 sensitive trigger. A more recent study has suggested that cytochrome b may also play an important role in O_2 sensitivity (Acker et al., 1992). The attenuation of O_2 sensitivity after prolonged hypoxia may be related to the injury of the mitochondrial cristae.

The morphometric analysis of the hypoxic rabbit carotid body with the administration of *D. heterophyllum* showed that the herb had a marked protective effect on the mitochondria. The volume density of the mitochondria remained at the control level. A more detailed analysis established that *D. heterophyllum* prevented the mitochondria from dilating (SVR was significantly larger than that of the HA Group) and also prevented the destruction of the cristae.

Compared to other anti-hypoxic herbs and drugs, the investigations of *D. heterophyllum* are very limited. It has been reported that the herb has the effect of inhibiting the rise of catecholamines in the hypoxic cardiac muscle and brain (Peng, 1971-1977) and reducing the depletion of tissue cAMP. It lowers the oxygen consumption of hypoxic rats, and this effect is much greater than most of the other anti-hypoxic herbs and microbiological products (Peng, 1971-1977). Investigations on the ultrastructure of rabbit lungs found that *D. heterophyllum* was able to reduce the lamina bodies in the type II epithelia of the alveoli, which increase after hypoxic exposure. Our results and these observations suggest that *D. heterophyllum* may have a beneficial protective effect on the cellular and subcellular structures when exposed to hypoxia. Previous studies have shown that the toxicity of the herb is slight (He, 1971-1977). *D. heterophyllum* may therefore have potentially selective properties for the treatment of hypoxia but further studies are required to investigate its effective components, mechanisms of action and clinical applications.

REFERENCES

Acker, H., Delpiano, M.A & Pietruschka (1989) Possible mechanisms of oxygen sensing in the carotid body. In "Chemoreceptors and reflexes in breathing-cellular and molecular aspects" S. Lahiri et al., eds. New York. pp 121-132

Acker, H., Bolling, B., Delpiano, M.A., Dufau, E., Gorlach, A. & Holtermann, G. (1992) The meaning of H_2O_2 generation in carotid body cells for PO_2 chemoreception. J. Autonom. Nerv. Syst. 41:41-51

De Castro, F. (1926) Sur la structure et l'innervation de la glande intercarotidienne (glomus caroticum) de l'homme et de mammiferes, et sur un nouveau systeme d'innervation autonome du nerf glossopharyngien. Etudes anatomique et experimentale. Trab. Lab. Invest. Biol. Univ. Madrid 24:356-432

He, Y.H. (1971-1977) The toxicology study of D. heterophyllum. In "A Collection of Army Researches of Medicine: Volume II", China, pp 183-185

Laidler, P. & Kay, J.M. (1975a) The effect of chronic hypoxia on the number and nuclear diameter of type I cells in the carotid bodies of rats. Am J Path 79:311-320

Laidler, P. & Kay, J.M. (1975b) A quantitative morphological study of the carotid bodies of rats living at a simulated altitude of 4300 metres. J Path 117:183-191

MacDonald, D. M. (1989) Route for blood flow through the rat carotid body. In "Chemoreceptors and reflexes in breathing-cellular and molecular aspects" S. Lahiri et al., eds. New York. pp 5-12

Pallot, D.J. & Blakeman, N. (1986a) Quantitative ultrastructural studies of cat carotid body. III: The type I cells. Acta Anat. 124:35-41

Pallot, D.J. & Blakeman, N. (1986b) Quantitative ultrastructural studies of rat carotid body type I cells. Acta Anat. 126:187-192

Peng, H.F. (1971-1977) The effects of anti-hypoxia drugs to the catecholamines and cAMP in the hypoxic rat heart and brain. In "A Collection of Army Researches of Medicine: Volume III", China, pp 1-8

Xue, D.H., Yang, F.X. & Bee, D. (1993) Modification of the rat carotid body type I cell mitochondria by high altitude exposure. J. Physiol. (In press).

BREATHING FREQUENCY AND TIDAL VOLUME ARE INDEPENDENTLY CONTROLLED IN GARTER SNAKES: THE ROLE OF CO_2-RISE TIME

Robert A. Furilla

Department of Physiology, University of Puerto Rico, School of Medicine
San Juan, PR 00936-5067

INTRODUCTION

Oscillations in pH and PCO_2 resulting from tidal breathing have been noted in mammals for many years (Nims & Marshall, 1938; Band et al., 1969), and there is some evidence that they play a role in ventilatory control (Cross et al., 1982). These oscillations are particularly prominent in some reptiles because of their large tidal volumes and intermittent breathing patterns. The rate of rise of intrapulmonary PCO_2 after each breath is an index of the metabolic rate, and Furilla (1991) showed a strong correlation between this rate of rise and ventilation in garter snakes.

The purpose of this study is to determine the influence of tonic and phasic airway CO_2 on breathing frequency and tidal volume in snakes. Because snakes have a tubular lung, they can be unidirectionally ventilated, virtually eliminating dead space. In this study, the animal can control its mean plasma pH because a gas mixer arranged as a servo-feedback system delivers CO_2 to the unidirectionally ventilated lung.

METHODS

Snakes were restrained and unidirectionally ventilated according to the procedures in Furilla (1991). A gas mixer connected to a personal computer delivered gas containing CO_2 to the lung. The output of a pneumotachograph placed downstream from the animal was also connected to the computer. When the computer sensed the beginning of inspiration, CO_2 was removed from the airstream, thus simulating the situation during natural breathing. At the end of inspiration, CO_2 was made to rise according to the formula $a\text{-}be^{-rt}$, where a & b set the limits, t is time in seconds, and r is a variable that can be set from the computer keyboard to adjust CO_2-rise time. In this way, the animal can control when and how often it receives fresh air, but the investigator determines the speed and the amplitude of the rising CO_2. One group of animals had the vagus nerves cut. In another set of experiments the gas mixer was replaced with a solenoid valve that could be switched between air containing no CO_2, and air containing CO_2. During inspiration, CO_2 could either be removed or clamped high. The animal, therefore, may or may not be able to adjust its arterial pH, depending on the computer's setting.

RESULTS

Breathing frequency was highly correlated with the rate of rise of CO_2. Over a 128-fold span of CO_2-rise times, breathing frequency varied by 22-fold, but tidal volume varied by only 1.5-fold (Fig. 1). However, tidal volume increased by 1.5-fold if the peak amplitude of CO_2 was doubled. Bilateral vagotomy virtually eliminated the breathing frequency response to the rate of rise of CO_2. After vagotomy, breathing frequency was 0.3 to 0.5 min^{-1} over the entire range of CO_2-rise times, and tidal volume approximately doubled with no change in the sensitivity to the rate of rise of CO_2

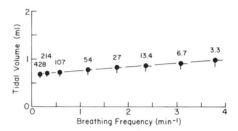

Figure 1. The numbers above the points represent the time in seconds to reach 5% CO_2. The circles are means and the horizontal and vertical lines represent 1 SE. Errors smaller than the symbols are not shown.

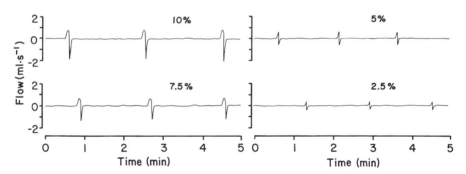

Figure 2. Sample traces showing tidal flow at 4 tonic levels of airway CO_2. When airway CO_2 was zero, breathing ceased. Expiration is shown by a positive flow.

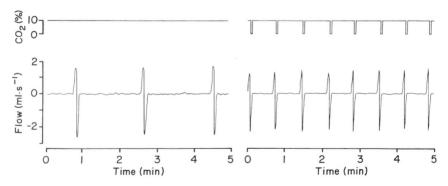

Figure 3. Sample traces showing tidal flow and airway CO_2 for tonic and phasic stimuli. The left trace was recorded when airway CO_2 was high even during inspiration. In the right trace, CO_2 fell during inspiration. Expiration is shown by a positive flow.

362

When airway CO_2 was held high even during inspiration, tidal volume was correlated with the level of CO_2 in the airstream, but breathing frequency was virtually the same regardless of the level of airway CO_2 (Fig. 2). If CO_2 was allowed to fall on inspiration, however, breathing frequency increased, and tidal volume decreased (Fig. 3). After bilateral vagotomy, breathing frequency and tidal volume were similar to those shown in Figure 2 (upper left trace, high tidal volume & low breathing frequency).

DISCUSSION

In 1991, Furilla et al. demonstrated arterial isocapnia in snakes whose venous PCO_2 was elevated using the skin as a gas exchanger. In addition, end expired PCO_2 did not change during venous CO_2 loading. In the absence of venous chemoreceptors and significant alterations in arterial pH and blood gas levels, the central respiratory controller must be responding to another stimulus. Yamamoto and Edwards (1960) suggested a link between oscillating PCO_2 and ventilation, and in 1982, Cross et al. showed a correlation between the level of venous PCO_2 and the first derivative of the falling arterial pH in cats. They also showed a relationship between the rate of fall of arterial pH and ventilation, suggesting a mechanism whereby animals adjust ventilation to changes in metabolic rate.

In addition to arterial chemoreceptors, birds and reptiles have receptors in the lung that are sensitive to airway PCO_2. These intrapulmonary chemoreceptors (IPCs) are in a good location to monitor CO_2 flux from the blood to lung air. In fact, snakes are able to adjust ventilation to the rate at which CO_2 rises in the lung (Furilla, 1991), which may account for the arterial isocapnia seen in snakes during venous CO_2 loading. The fact that pulmonary vagotomy virtually eliminates the response to the rate of change of airway CO_2 implicates IPCs and suggests that either the output of IPCs depends on the first derivative of the stimulus, or that the central controller is acting as a differentiator.

The data from this study indicate that the two components of ventilation (volume & frequency) are adjusted independently. Because breathing frequency remains unchanged at all tonic levels of airway CO_2, mean intrapulmonary or arterial PCO_2 appears to have no influence on the central rhythm generator; whereas, tidal volume is greatly affected by tonic levels of PCO_2. On the other hand, tidal volume is little affected by the rate at which PCO_2 changes, but breathing frequency is closely correlated with the rate of rise of CO_2. It is difficult to relate these findings directly to the control of breathing during activities such as exercise because non-chemical peripheral and central stimuli can influence ventilation as well. However, PCO_2 dynamics likely aid in the regulation of blood chemistry during exercise in a way that non-chemical stimuli can not.

I thank Dr. M. H. Bernstein of New Mexico State Univ. without whose help this study would not have been possible. This work was supported by NSF Grant BSR-8806604 to M. H. B. and NIH-RCMI grant RR-03051 to the Univ. of Puerto Rico.

REFERENCES

Band, D. M., Cameron, I. R. & Semple, S. J. G. (1969). Oscillations in arterial pH with breathing in the cat. J. Appl. Physiol. 26: 261-267.

Cross, B. A., Davey, A., Guz, A., Katona, P. G., MacLean, M., Murphy, K., Semple, S. J. G. & Stidwell, R. (1982). The pH oscillations in arterial blood during exercise; a potential signal for the ventilatory response in the dog. J. Physiol. (Lond.) 329: 57-73.

Furilla, R. A. (1991). The rate of rise of intrapulmonary CO_2 drives breathing frequency in garter snakes. J. Appl. Physiol. 71: 2304-2308.

Furilla, R. A., Coates, E. L. & Bartlett, D., Jr. (1991). The influence of venous CO_2 on ventilation in garter snakes. Respir. Physiol. 83: 46-60.

Nims, L. F. & Marshall, C. (1938). Blood pH in vivo. I. Changes due to respiration. Yale J. Biol. Med. 10: 561-564.

Yamamoto, W. S. & Edwards, M. W., Jr. (1960). Homeostasis of carbon dioxide during intravenous infusion of carbon dioxide. J. Appl. Physiol. 15: 807-818.

EFFECTS OF CHRONIC HYPOXIA ON RAT CAROTID BODY AND TOAD CAROTID LABYRINTH GLOMUS CELLS

Frank L. Powell,[1] Tatsumi Kusakabe,[2,3] and Mark H. Ellisman[2]

[1]Department of Medicine and [2]San Diego Microscopy and Imaging Resource, Department of Neurosciences, University of California, San Diego, La Jolla, California, USA; [3]Department of Anatomy, Yokohama City University School of Medicine, Yokohama 236, Japan

INTRODUCTION

Chronic hypoxia causes enlargement and ultrastructural changes of mammalian carotid body glomus cells. Recently, we reported several ultrastructural features in glomus cells from chronically hypoxic rats that were typical of amphibian carotid labyrinth glomus cells, including incomplete covering of glomus cells by support cells, long thin cytoplasmic projections in the intervascular stroma, and intimate contacts between glomus cells and pericytes, endothelial cells, plasma cells, fibrocytes and other glomus cells (Kusakabe et al., 1993). We also observed large vesicles (400-800 nm dia.) with eccentric dense cores in hypoxic, but not normoxic, rats. To determine if these changes represent a generalized vertebrate glomus cell response to hypoxia, we made a comparative study of glomus cell ultrastructure from normoxic and chronically hypoxic amphibians and mammals.

METHODS & RESULTS

Rats (Sprague-Dawley) and toads (*Bufo marinus*) were exposed to (1) normobaric or hypobaric hypoxia (PO_2 = 80 Torr) or (2) normoxia in ambient air for 4-12 wks. Their carotid bodies and labyrinths were perfusion fixed and studied with transmission electron microscopy as described previously (Kusakabe et al., 1993; Kusakabe, 1992).

Figure 1 compares the ultrastructure of glomus cells from chronically hypoxic rats and toads. As we previously observed, chronic hypoxia induced ultrastructural changes in rat glomus cells so they resembled amphibian glomus cells. In contrast, chronic hypoxia caused no striking changes in toad glomus cells. Both normoxic and hypoxic toads showed glomus cells having extensive direct contact with intervascular stroma and other glomus cells, and two types of dense cored vesicles (80-100 and 100-180 nm).

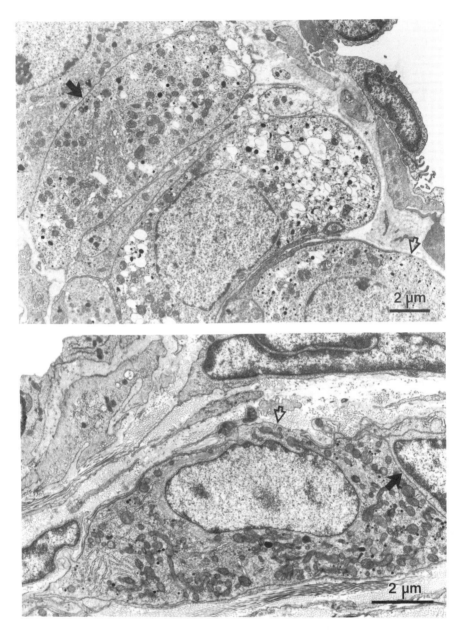

Figure 1. Electron micrographs of glomus cells from chronically hypoxic rat carotid body (upper) and chronically hypoxic toad carotid labyrinth (lower) showing large areas of glomus cells in direct contact with each other (filled arrows) and the intervascular stroma (open arrows). Large spaces in rat glomus cells are dilated eccentric dense core vesicles (cf. Kusakabe et al., 1993).

DISCUSSION

Chronic hypoxia in toads did not cause ultrastructure changes in carotid labyrinth glomus cells like it did in carotid body glomus cells. We hypothesize that this is because P_aO_2 is already relatively low in normoxic toads, so toads exhibit a glomus cell morphology that is typical of chronically hypoxic vertebrates. Arterial PO_2 is only 50 Torr in awake toads breathing room air (West et al., 1987), i.e. more similar to that in hypoxic than in normoxic rats (Kusakabe et al., 1993). Both the carotid body and labyrinth can sense P_aO_2 changes (Ishii et al., 1966), so it is reasonable that vertebrate glomus cells may share other O_2-sensitive processes too. Recent studies show the hypertrophic response of rat glomus cells to chronic hypoxia can be induced in culture (Mills & Nurse, 1993). Culturing toad glomus cells at normoxic mammalian P_aO_2 levels, and looking for more mammalian-like ultrastructure characteristics, could provide a test of this hypothesis.

We thank E. Parker and L. Hempleman for their technical assistance. This work was supported by grants from the NIH grants P41-04050 and HL-17731.

REFERENCES

Ishii, K., Honda, K. & Ishii, K. (1966). The function of the carotid labyrinth in the toad. Tohoku J. Exp. Med. 88: 103-116.

Kusakabe, T. (1992). Intimate apposition of the glomus and smooth muscle cells (g-s connection) in the carotid labyrinth of juvenile bullfrogs. Anat. Embryol. 185: 39-44.

Kusakabe, T., Powell, F.L. & Ellisman, M.H. (1993). Ultrastructure of the glomus cells in the carotid body of chronically hypoxic rats: with a special reference to the similarity of the amphibian glomus cells. Anat. Rec. 237:

Mills, L. & Nurse, C. (1993). Chronic hypoxia *in vitro* increases volume of dissociated carotid body chemoreceptors. NeuroReport 4: 619-622.

West, N.H., Topor, Z.L. & Van Vliet, B.N. (1987). Hypoxemic threshold for lung ventilation in the toad. Respir. Physiol. 70: 377-390.

THE STIMULUS MODALITY OF THE HYPOXIC VENTILATORY RESPONSE IN RODENTS

Rhonda J. Garland, Richard Kinkead, and William K. Milsom

Department of Zoology, University of British Columbia,
6270 University Blvd., Vancouver, British Columbia, Canada

INTRODUCTION

Exposure to reduced ambient O_2 concentrations decreases both arterial oxygen content (C_aO_2) and partial pressure (P_aO_2). In many species the P_aO_2 at which ventilation begins to increase is correlated with the P_aO_2 of the inflection point on the oxygen equilibrium curve (OEC) where C_aO_2 begins to significantly decrease. Although suggestive of chemoreceptors responsive to changes in C_aO_2, most authors have concluded that this correlation is a consequence of natural selection acting on the P_aO_2 threshold of the hypoxic ventilatory response (HVR) in a manner which optimally protects arterial oxygen saturation (Van Nice et al, 1980; Boggs & Birchard, 1983; Birchard & Tenney, 1986). In species that experience natural fluctuations in P_{50}, however, the relationship between the threshold of the HVR and the inflection point of the OEC is retained (Glass et al, 1983; McArthur & Milsom, 1991). It has been suggested that for animals that undergo wide fluctuations in body temperature and exhibit a left-shifted OEC accompanied by an intraspecific decrease in P_{50}, C_aO_2 would be a better indicator of the oxygen status of the blood than would P_aO_2 (Wood, 1984).

Based on these observations, the present study was undertaken to examine the comparative ventilatory responses to concurrent decreases in P_aO_2 and C_aO_2 as well as to decreases in C_aO_2 alone, of rodent species which do (golden-mantled ground squirrels) and do not (rats) hibernate.

METHODS

The experiments were performed on sodium pentobarbitol anesthetized Wistar rats and golden-mantled ground squirrels. The trachea, both femoral arteries and one femoral vein were cannulated. Tidal volume (V_T) and breathing frequency (f) were monitored by attaching a small pneumotachograph onto the tracheotomy tube. Arterial blood gases (P_aO_2 and P_aCO_2) and pH were monitored continuously by connecting one arterial cannula in series with the venous cannula *via* O_2, CO_2 and pH microelectrodes. The second arterial cannula was connected to a pressure transducer to monitor arterial blood pressure. Arterial oxygen content was measured on 20µl blood samples using a Tucker chamber. Body temperature was monitored and maintained at 37°C. For each species, the animals were divided into two groups. The first group was made progressively hypoxic by decreasing the fraction of

Arterial Chemoreceptors: Cell to System
Edited by R. O'Regan *et al*, Plenum Press, New York, 1994

inspired O_2 in the air through the addition of N_2 (hypoxic hypoxia). In the second group hypoxia was induced through the addition of carbon monoxide to the air (CO-hypoxia). In both groups the animals were maintained isocapnic by the addition or removal of CO_2 from the gas mixture. Animals exposed to CO-hypoxia were maintained isoxic through alterations of the N_2 concentration in the gas mixture. The level of hypoxia was increased until C_aO_2 decreased to 50% of the original measurement.

RESULTS

Hypoxic hypoxia, which reduced both P_aO_2 and C_aO_2, produced a brisk ventilatory response in both species. Minute ventilation (V_E) increased by 10-fold in the squirrels but only 6-fold in the rats. When expressed as a function of C_aO_2, the ventilatory response curves for hypoxic hypoxia were linear for both species over the experimental range (Fig. 1A). During exposure to CO, the P_aO_2 did not deviate significantly from the normoxic level and similar drops in C_aO_2 were produced in both species. The effects of lowering C_aO_2, independent of P_aO_2, on the ventilation of squirrels and rats are presented in Fig. 1B. Again, the squirrels underwent a proportionately greater increase in V_E (5-fold) than did the rats (3-fold). In both species, pH, P_aCO_2 hematocrit and blood pressure were maintained relatively constant throughout both experimental series.

The slopes of the least squares linear regression lines describing the ventilatory responses to hypoxic hypoxia were significantly different between species, while those describing the ventilatory responses to CO-hypoxia were not. There were no intraspecific differences between the slopes describing the relationship between V_E and C_aO_2 for the two forms of hypoxia. In both species, changing C_aO_2 alone could only produce 60% of the ventilatory response that occurred when both P_aO_2 and C_aO_2 were altered together.

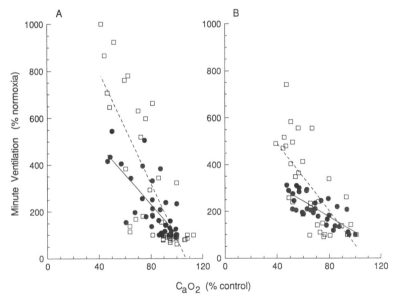

Figure 1. Relationship between C_aO_2 and minute ventilation, expressed as % change from normoxic values, during graded hypoxic hypoxia (A) and graded carbon monoxide hypoxia (B) (Rats= ●; Squirrels= □). Least squares linear regression lines are drawn for the rat (——) and for the squirrel (- - - -).

DISCUSSION

The present study indicates that rodents possess chemoreceptors capable of responding to changes in C_aO_2. Reductions in C_aO_2 alone can elicit 60% of the HVR produced when P_aO_2 and C_aO_2 are reduced concomitantly. This ability was not exclusive to the heterotherms. That both heterothermic and nonheterothermic rodents respond to changes in C_aO_2 alone suggests that either the carotid bodies in these animals are sensitive to changes in C_aO_2 or that O_2 chemoreceptors other than the carotid bodies sensitive to changes in C_aO_2 produce a significant HVR in rodents. The retention of a brisk HVR in carotid body denervated ground squirrels (Webb & Milsom, 1990) supports the latter conclusion.

REFERENCES

Birchard, G. F. & Tenney, S. M. (1986). The hypoxic ventilatory response of rats with increased blood oxygen affinity. Respir. Physiol. 66:225-233.

Boggs, D. F. & Birchard, G. F. (1983). Relationship between hemoglobin O_2 affinity and the ventilatory response to hypoxia in the rhea and pheasant. J. Exp. Biol. 102:347-352.

Glass, M. L., Boutilier, R. G. & Heisler, N. (1983). Ventilatory control of arterial PO_2 in the turtle Chrysemys picta bellii: effects of temperature and hypoxia. J. Comp. Physiol. 151:145-153.

McArthur, M. D. & Milsom, W. K. (1991). Ventilation and respiratory sensitivity associated with hibernation in Columbian (Spermophilus columbianus) and golden-mantled (Spermophilus lateralis) ground squirrels. Physiol. Zool. 64(4):921-939.

Van Nice, P., Black, C. P. & Tenney, S. M. (1980). A comparative study of ventilatory responses to hypoxia with reference to hemoglobin O_2-affinity in llama, cat, rat, duck and goose. Comp. Biochem. Physiol. 59(6):1955-1960.

Wood, S. C. (1984). Cardiovascular shunts and oxygen transport in lower vertebrates. Am. J. Physiol. 247:R3-R14.

Webb, C. L. & Milsom, W. K. (1990). Carotid body contribution to hypoxic ventilatory responses in euthermic and hibernating ground squirrels. In "Arterial Chemoreception." C. Eyzaguirre, S. J. Fidone, R. S. Fitzgerald, S. Lahiri & D. M. McDonald, eds., Springer-Verlag, New York.

HISTOCHEMICAL DEMONSTRATION OF CARBONIC ANHYDRASE IN THE LARYNX

Z.H. Wang[1], Ronan G. O'Regan[1], and James J. Giles[2]

[1]Department of Human Anatomy and Physiology, and [2]Electron Microscopy Unit, University College, Earlsfort Terrace, Dublin 2, Ireland

INTRODUCTION

It has been repeatedly demonstrated by recordings from the superior laryngeal nerve afferent fibres that airway CO_2 modifies laryngeal mechanoreceptor activity (Boushey et al., 1974; Bradford et al., 1990). This effect occurs rapidly following the onset of CO_2 exposure to the larynx. In a recent study using the isolated, perfused larynx, airway PCO_2 modified laryngeal mechanoreceptor activity independent of the pH of the media perfusing the larynx (O'Regan et al., 1993). These results indicate that carbonic anhydrase (CA), the enzyme which catalyses the reversible reaction of CO_2 hydration, is involved in mediating the laryngeal CO_2 chemoreception.

The purpose of this study was to determine histochemically whether CA was present in the larynx.

METHODS

The larynx of adult cats and rats and also trachea of rats were studied. The superior laryngeal nerves (SLNs) and recurrent laryngeal nerves (RLNs) of both species were also examined. As a positive control tissue for CA, rat kidney was used. Tissue fixation was performed by intracardial perfusion of phosphate buffered 2.5% glutaraldehyde (pH 7.4) for 10 minutes followed by tissue immersion in the same fixative for 3-6 hours. Cryosections of 15 m were cut from tissue quick frozen in liquid nitrogen. Histochemical staining was performed according to Hansson's cobalt-phosphate method (Hansson, 1967). For control staining, the CA inhibitor acetazolamide was included in the incubation medium (10^{-6}-10^{-5}M).

RESULTS

Rat kidney stained positively and the staining pattern was consistent with results reported by others (Lonnerholm et al., 1971). In the distal convoluted tubules, the staining was restricted to the basal parts of the cells. The proximal convoluted tubules were stained evenly. In contrast, the glomeruli were unreactive except for red blood cells within the capillaries.

In the larynx of both cats and rats, surface epithelial cells stained positively at all levels (Fig. 1. A-C). Nerve branches and terminals along the surface epithelium also gave a positive reaction. Overall, the intensity of CA reactivity at different levels of the cat larynx was not very dissimilar and staining was readily obtained within a 10 minute incubation time. In many parts of the rat larynx, however, staining was weaker or less readily obtained. A slightly longer incubation time may be needed. In other parts of the rat larynx, such as the epithelium that covers the medial aspect of the arytenoid cartilage, the subglottic area and the cricoid cartilage level, staining activity was stronger and similar to that found in the cat (Fig. 1C). In contrast, the rat tracheal surface epithelial cells were unreactive apart from very few scattered cells which were considered to be goblet cells in view of their shape and distribution (Fig. 1D).

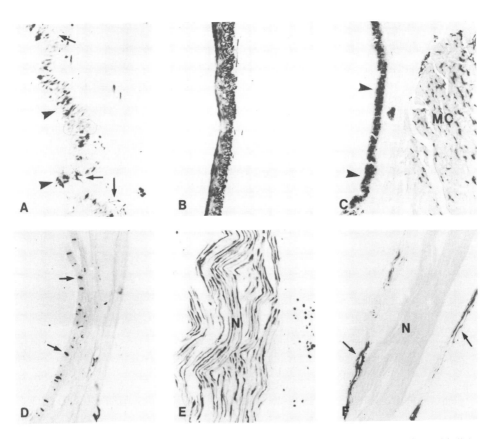

Figure 1. **A**. A section cut through the top of the cat arytenoid cartilage showing stained surface epithelial cells (arrow heads) and nerve terminals (arrows). ×80. **B**. Intensively stained surface squamous epithelium of the cat glottis. ×40. **C**. Darkly stained surface columnar epithelium (arrows) at cricoid level of the rat larynx. Capillaries in the skeletal muscle (MC) also stained positively. ×40. **D**. A section of the rat middle trachea showing stained goblet cells (arrows) ×40. **E**. Darkly stained cat superior laryngeal nerve (N). ×40. **F**. Unstained nerve fibres (N) in cat recurrent laryngeal nerve contrasts with the stained nerve sheath (arrows) ×40.

A strong reaction was observed in the SLNs with almost all the nerve fibres stained in the cat (Fig. 1E) while a lower proportion (40-70%) of fibres stained in the rat. In contrast, most of the fibres in the RLNs in both cats and rats were unreactive (Fig. 1F).

The staining of the above surface epithelia and nerve fibres was consistently blocked by 10^{-6}M acetazolamide which shows the specificity of the method and that the CA present in the larynx was highly sensitive to inhibition.

DISCUSSION

CA exists wherever the speed of CO_2 and H^+ ion inter-conversion is important. The essential role of CA in the prompt CO_2 chemoreception of the carotid body is proven by the delayed, reduced response to CO_2 after inhibition with sulfonamides as reported elsewhere (Travis, 1971; Iturriaga et al., 1991). The histochemical confirmation of the presence of CA in the larynx (but not in the trachea) is in support of the hypothesis that this enzyme is involved in mediating the laryngeal CO_2 chemoreception as well. The location of the enzyme in the surface epithelial cells and in the intra- or sub-epithelial nerve endings coincide with the suggested superficial location of the laryngeal CO_2 receptors (Boushey et al., 1974). The close relationship between the stained sensory nerve endings and the surface epithelial cells may indicate that the enzyme in these locations are jointly involved in CO_2 chemoreception although ordinary somatic sensory nerves are also reported to be CA positive (Riley & Lang, 1984).

In the ever growing family of the CA isozymes, CA I, CA II, and CA III are still the major cytoplasmic forms. Membrane-associated isozyme, CA IV, has also been detected in a wide range of tissues (Wistrand, 1984). It is not possible to specify the form of isozyme(s) in the present study though CA III is unlikely to be involved as this isozyme is resistant to acetazolamide inhibition. Immunohistochemical techniques are required to determine the type of isozyme(s) and the pattern of distribution.

Supported by The Health Research Board, R3261.

REFERENCES

Boushey, H.A., Richardson, P.S., Widdicombe, J.G. & Wise, J.C.M. (1974). The response of laryngeal afferent fibres to mechanical and chemical stimuli. J. Physiol. (Lond.) 240:153-175.

Bradford, A., Nolan, P., McKeogh, D., Bannon, C. & O'Regan, R.G. (1990). The responses of superior laryngeal nerve afferent fibres to laryngeal airway CO_2 concentration in the anaesthetized cat. Exp. Physiol. 75:267-270.

Hansson, H.P.J. (1967). Histochemical demonstration of carbonic anhydrase activity. Histochem. 11:112-128.

Iturriaga, R., Lahiri, S. & Mokashi, A. (1991). Carbonic anhydrase and chemoreception in the cat carotid body. Am. J. Physiol. 261:C565-573.

Lonnerholm, G. (1971). Histochemical demonstration of carbonic anhydrase activity in the rat kidney. Acta Physiol. Scand. 81:433-439.

O'Regan, R.G., Wang, Z.H., Nolan, P. & Bradford, A. (1993). Airway PCO_2 modifies laryngeal mechanoreceptors independent of the pH of the media perfusing the isolated larynx in the anaesthetised cat. Proc. XXXII IUPS Congress, Glasgow, 1993, 183.3/P.

Riley, D.A.& Lang, D.H. (1984). Carbonic anhydrase activity of human peripheral nerves: A possible histochemical aid to nerve repair. J. Hand Surg. 9A(1):112-120.

Travis, D. M. (1971). Molecular CO_2 is inert on carotid chemoreceptor: demonstration by inhibition of carbonic anhydrase. J. Pharmacol. Exp. Ther. 178:529-540.

Wistrand, P.J. (1984) Properties of membrane-bound carbonic anhydrase. Ann. N.Y. Acad. Sci. 429:195-206.

EFFECTS OF INTRALARYNGEAL CO_2 AND H^+ ON LARYNGEAL RECEPTOR ACTIVITY IN THE PERFUSED LARYNX IN CATS

Z.H. Wang[1], Aidan Bradford[2] and Ronan G. O'Regan[1]

[1]Department of Human Anatomy and Physiology, University College, Earlsfort Terrace, Dublin 2, Ireland. [2]Department of Physiology, Royal College of Surgeons in Ireland, Dublin 2, Ireland

INTRODUCTION

Intralaryngeal CO_2 alters discharges of superior laryngeal nerve (SLN) afferent fibres (Boushey et al., 1974; Bradford et al., 1990) and reflexly enhances the activity of upper airway dilating muscles (Nolan et al., 1990; Bartlett et al., 1992a), decreases ventilation (Boushey et al., 1974; Nolan et al., 1990) and phrenic nerve activity (Bartlett et al., 1992a). These reflex effects are abolished by SLN section. The above results suggest that laryngeal CO_2 receptors may play an important role in maintaining upper airway patency. To elucidate mechanisms of CO_2-induced effects on laryngeal mechanoreceptors, an in situ, isolated, perfused larynx has been developed. Part of this study has been briefly reported elsewhere (O'Regan et al., 1993).

METHODS

Experiments were performed on 16 cats anaesthetized with pentobarbitone sodium (induction, 42-48 mg kg^{-1} i.p.; maintenance, 6-12 mg i.v. hourly), paralysed (pancuronium 0.8 mg i.v. as required) and artificially ventilated through a low cervical tracheostomy. The larynx was isolated and perfused by means of an inflow cannula inserted cranially via a tracheostomy with its tip just below the cricoid cartilage and an outflow cannula passed through the mouth with its tip at the epiglottis and fixed in place by a tie encircling the hypopharynx. Physiological solutions at 37°C were perfused through the larynx (15-20 ml min^{-1}). An acapnic solution equilibrated with air with a pH value of 7.4 served as control solution. Hypercapnic solutions equilibrated with 9% CO_2 in air had pH values of either 6.8 (solution A) or 7.4 (solution B). The effects of an acidic acapnic solution with pH 6.8 (solution D) were also tested. Following periods of perfusion (2-5 min), waves of pressure oscillating 5-10 cmH$_2$O around zero with a frequency of 30 cycles min^{-1} were applied to the larynx through a side arm of the outflow cannula. Laryngeal pressure was continuously monitored through a catheter inserted into the larynx via a side arm of the inflow cannula. Single SLN afferent fibre activity was recorded using conventional techniques.

Afferent fibres were classified into 'quiescent' or 'tonic' depending on their discharge frequency while the larynx was perfused with control solution at zero pressure. The fibres were further categorized according to their responses to pressure. Cold receptors increased their discharge in response to a reduction in temperature of the perfusing control solution.

Each trial consisted of successive perfusions with control solution, test solution A or B or D and control solution again. The differences in mean discharge frequency between control periods and periods of test solutions were analysed with two-tailed Student's t tests. When both solutions A and B were tested on the same fibre, the changes in mean fibre discharge caused by either hypercapnic solution over control were calculated. For all the fibres that had trials with both solutions A and B, the mean differences in excitation or inhibition between the two solutions were compared with paired t test ($p<0.05$ being considered statistically significant).

RESULTS

A total of 42 SLN sensory fibres were modified by intralaryngeal CO_2 with either acidic or neutral pH. Among the 23 quiescent units responsive to negative pressure, 18 were

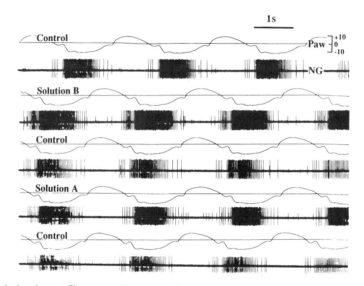

Figure 1. A quiescent fibre responding to negative pressure was excited by both acidic and neutral hypercapnic solutions. Paw: laryngeal airway pressure (cmH_2O); NG: neurogram.

excited and 5 inhibited. Among the 5 quiescent fibres responsive to positive pressure, 3 were excited and the rest inhibited. All of the 11 tonic fibres (9 responding to negative pressure and 3 to positive pressure) were inhibited by CO_2. Also recorded were 3 quiescent fibres with no consistent response to pressure all of which were excited by CO_2 with one fibre being confirmed as a cold receptor. (All above results $p<0.05$).

A total of 18 fibres were subjected to both hypercapnic solutions. The responses of each fibre to the hypercapnic solutions with either acidic or neutral pH were similar in general in both direction and magnitude. An example is shown in figure 1. Quantitatively, with all the fibres tested with both solutions A and B, the mean changes in fibre discharge caused by solutions A and B show no significant difference.

On the other hand, the acidic acapnic solution (solution D) had little or no effect on 12 fibers which were either excited or inhibited by CO_2.

DISCUSSION

It has been repeatedly shown that intralaryngeal CO_2 alters laryngeal mechanoreceptor activity in the artificially ventilated larynx (Anderson et al., 1990; Bradford et al., 1990; Bartlett et al., 1992b). The present study shows that intralaryngeal CO_2 has similar effects on the saline perfused larynx. It is generally believed that molecular CO_2 is inert and peripheral arterial CO_2 chemoreception is mediated by H^+/HCO_3^- (Iturriaga et al., 1991). The fact that our results showed similar effects with either acidic or neutral hypercapnic solutions and no effect with the acidic acapnic solution on CO_2 sensitive receptors suggests that laryngeal CO_2 chemoreception occurs intracellularly. Presumably H^+ can not enter the cells as rapidly as CO_2 in order to generate a rapid change in intracellular H^+ ion concentration. There is evidence that carbonic anhydrase, the enzyme that speeds up CO_2 and H^+ inter-conversion, is involved in carotid body CO_2 chemoreception (Black et al., 1971; Iturriaga et al., 1991). This enzyme has also been shown to exist in the surface epithelial cells and sensory nerve terminals of the larynx (Wang et al., 1993) which coincides with the suggested superficial location of CO_2 sensitive laryngeal receptors. However, whether carbonic anhydrase is involved in mediating laryngeal CO_2 chemoreception remains to be investigated.

This work was supported by The Health Research Board, R3261.

REFERENCES

Anderson, J.W., Sant'Ambrogio, F.B., Orani, G.P., Sant'Ambrogio, G. & Mathew, O.P. (1990). Carbon dioxide-responsive laryngeal receptors in the dog. Respir. Physiol. 82:217-226.

Bartlett, D.Jr., Knuth, S.L. & Gdovin, M.J. (1992a). Influences of intralaryngeal CO_2 on respiratory activities of motor nerves to accessory muscles. Respir. Physiol. 90:289-297.

Bartlett, D.Jr. & Knuth, S.L. (1992b). Responses of laryngeal receptors to intralaryngeal CO_2 in the cat. J. Physiol. (Lond) 475:187-193.

Black, A.M.S., McCloskey, D.I. & Torrance, R.W. (1971). The responses of carotid body chemoreceptors in the cat to sudden changes of hypercapnic and hypoxic stimuli. Respir. Physiol. 13:36-49.

Boushey, H.A., Richardson, P.S., Widdicombe, J.G. & Wise, J.C.M. (1974). The response of laryngeal afferent fibres to mechanical and chemical stimuli. J. Physiol. (Lond.) 240:153-175.

Bradford, A., Nolan, P., McKeogh, D., Bannon, C. & O'Regan, R.G. (1990). The responses of superior laryngeal nerve afferent fibres to laryngeal airway CO_2 concentration in the anaesthetized cat. Exp. Physiol. 75:267-270.

Iturriaga, R., Lahiri, S. & Mokashi, A. (1991). Carbonic anhydrase and chemoreception in the cat carotid body. Am. J. Physiol. 261:C565-573.

Nolan, P., Bradford, A., O'Regan, R.G. & McKeogh, D. (1990). The effects of changes in laryngeal airway CO_2 concentration on genioglossus muscle activity in the anaesthetized cat. Exp. Physiol. 75:271-274.

O'Regan, R.G., Wang, Z.H., Nolan, P. & Bradford, A. (1993). Airway PCO_2 modifies laryngeal mechanoreceptors independent of the pH of the media perfusing the isolated larynx in the anaesthetised cat. Proc. XXXII IUPS Congress, Glasgow, 1993, 183.3/P.

Wang, Z.H., O'Regan, R.G., & Giles, J.J. (1993). Histochemical demonstration of carbonic anhydrase in the larynx. This volume.

THE EFFECTS OF AIRWAY CO_2 ON LARYNGEAL PRESSURE, 'DRIVE' AND COLD RECEPTORS IN SPONTANEOUSLY BREATHING CATS

Aidan Bradford,[1] Donogh McKeogh,[2] Ronan G. O'Regan,[2] and Philip Nolan[2]

[1]Department of Physiology, Royal College of Surgeons in Ireland, St. Stephen's Green, Dublin 2, Ireland; [2]Department of Human Anatomy and Physiology, University College, Earlsfort Terrace, Dublin 2, Ireland

INTRODUCTION

We have previously demonstrated that the activity of superior laryngeal nerve afferents is affected when CO_2 is applied continuously to the laryngeal lumen using an isolated, artificially ventilated upper airway (UA) preparation in anaesthetized, paralysed cats (Bradford, et al., 1990a).

However, in this preparation, neuromuscular blockade precluded the study of the effects of CO_2 on 'drive' receptors, i.e. laryngeal receptors sensitive to contraction of intrinsic laryngeal muscles and/or laryngeal movements. Furthermore, laryngeal ventilation, although mimicking physiological conditions, was not identical to pulmonary ventilation. The present study uses a servo-respirator to ventilate the isolated larynx by matching spontaneous tracheal airflow in timing, waveform and magnitude in anaesthetized, spontaneously breathing cats in order to study the effects of CO_2 on laryngeal receptors including 'drive' receptors.

METHODS

Five adult cats were anaesthetized (induction: alphaxalone 0.9% w/v and alphadalone acetate 0.3% w/v, 1.5 ml/kg i.m.; maintenance: pentobarbitone sodium 20 mg i.v. initially and 6-12 mg i.v. as required) and breathed room air spontaneously through a cannula inserted into a low-cervical tracheostomy. A second cannula was inserted through a high-cervical tracheostomy and directed rostrally to lie at the level of the cricoid cartilage. A third cannula was inserted through the mouth to lie at the level of the epiglottis. The mouth and nose were sealed except for the opening of the oral cannula. The UA was ventilated using a servo-respirator which matched spontaneous tracheal airflow (measured using a pneumotachograph attached to the low-cervical tracheostomy cannula) in timing, waveform and magnitude (see McKeogh et al., 1991). UA airflow, pressure and CO_2 concentration were recorded. Laryngeal receptor activity was recorded from easily identifiable single units of the superior laryngeal nerve and receptors were classified as previously described (Bradford et al., 1990). Units which retained a respiratory modulation when UA ventilation was stopped were identified as 'drive' receptors. Activity was recorded in response to increasing UA CO_2 concentrations from 0 to 5 and 9% (balance 21% O_2 in N_2).

RESULTS

We identified 5 quiescent negative pressure receptors, 4 cold receptors, 4 'expiratory drive' receptors, 3 quiescent positive pressure receptors, 2 tonic negative pressure receptors and 2 tonic positive pressure receptors. Five and/or 9% CO_2 significantly excited all quiescent negative pressure, cold and 'expiratory drive' (see Fig.1) receptors and inhibited all quiescent positive pressure and tonic negative pressure receptors and 1 out of 2 tonic positive pressure receptors ($p < 0.05$, Student's t-test).

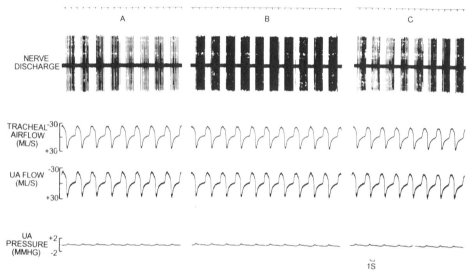

Figure 1. The activity of an 'expiratory drive' receptor (nerve discharge) before (A). during (B) and after (C) the application of 9% CO_2 continuously to the UA.

DISCUSSION

These results show that in spontaneously breathing cats, laryngeal receptors are sensitive to physiological concentrations of CO_2 in the laryngeal lumen when UA airflows, pressures, temperatures and humidities closely resemble those of a normal respiratory cycle. These effects were qualitatively similar to those previously described for paralysed, artificially ventilated cats (Bradford et al., 1990a,b). In the only other study on the effects of CO_2 on 'drive' receptors, Anderson et al. (1990) described an inhibitory effect in dogs of blowing 10% CO_2 continuously over the larynx in an expiratory direction on receptors which had an inspiratory modulation and which were inhibited by UA occlusion (which we interpret to be 'inspiratory drive' receptors).

The functional significance of these opposing effects of CO_2 on inspiratory 'drive' receptors (inhibition in the Anderson et al. (1990) study) and expiratory 'drive' receptors (excitation in the present study) is unclear. We have previously demonstrated that intralaryngeal CO_2 inhibits breathing and excites the genioglossus muscle in spontaneously breathing cats through a superior laryngeal nerve-mediated reflex (Nolan et al., 1990). These findings have been recently corroborated (Bartlett et al., 1992). We proposed that a build up of CO_2 in the larynx may contribute to the reflex activation of UA muscles caused by UA occlusion, a reflex believed to be important in preserving UA patency (Mathew et. al., 1982). We suggested that CO_2 would act by exciting and inhibiting quiescent negative and positive pressure receptors respectively. However, many 'drive' receptors are also pressure sensitive (Mathew et al., 1988) and therefore, their responses to CO_2 may participate in reflexly regulating UA patency.

Supported by the Health Research Board (Ireland) and the Wellcome Trust.

REFERENCES

Anderson, J.W., Sant'Ambrogio, F.B., Orani, G.P., Sant'Ambrogio, G & Mathew, O. P. (1990). Carbon dioxide-responsive laryngeal receptors in the dog. Respir. Physiol. 82, 217-226.

Bartlett Jr., D., Knuth, S.L & Leiter J. C. (1992). Alteration of ventilatory activity by intralaryngeal CO_2 in the cat. J. Physiol. 457, 177-185.

Bradford, A., Nolan, P., McKeogh, D., Bannon, C. & O'Regan, R.G. (1990a). The responses of superior laryngeal nerve afferent fibres to laryngeal airway CO_2 concentration in the anaesthetized cat. Exp. Physiol. 75, 267-270.

Bradford, A., Bannon, C., Nolan , P. & O'Regan R. G. (1990b). A study of the effects of airway carbon dioxide (P_{aw} CO_2) on superior laryngeal nerve afferents using an isolated, artificially ventilated closed laryngeal preparation in the anaesthetized cat. In "Chemoreceptors and Chemoreceptor Reflexes". H. Acker et al., ed. Plenum Press, New York.

Mathew, O.P., Abu-Osba, Y,.K. & Thach, B.T. (1982). Influence of upper airway pressure changes on genioglossus muscle respiratory activity. J. Appl. Physiol. 52, 438-444.

Mathew, O.P., Sant'Ambrogio, F.B. & Sant'Ambrogio, G. (1988). Laryngeal paralysis on receptor and reflex responses to negative pressure in the upper airway. Respir. Physiol. 74, 25-34.

McKeogh, D., Nolan, P., O'Regan, R.G. & Bradford, A. (1991). Artificial ventilation of the isolated larynx in the anaesthetized cat using a servo-controlled pump. J. Physiol. 446, 396P.

Nolan, P., Bradford, A., O'Regan, R.G. & McKeogh, D. (1990). The effects of changes in laryngeal airway CO_2 concentration on genioglossus muscle activity in the anaesthetized cat. Exp. Physiol. 75, 271-274.

LARYNGEAL RECEPTORS ARE SENSITIVE TO EXPIRATORY CONCENTRATIONS OF CO_2

Aidan Bradford,[1] Ronan G. O'Regan,[2] Philip Nolan,[2] and
Donogh McKeogh[2]

[1]Department of Physiology, Royal College of Surgeons in Ireland,
St. Stephen's Green, Dublin 2, Ireland; [2]Department of Human Anatomy and
Physiology, University College, Earlsfort Terrace, Dublin 2, Ireland

INTRODUCTION

It is well established that upper airway (UA) luminal CO_2 modulates the activity of laryngeal receptors (Boushey et al., 1974; Bradford et al., 1990a; Anderson et al., 1990). However, in all of these studies, the CO_2 was presented continuously to the larynx whereas, during normal breathing, CO_2 fluctuates between 0% and end-tidal concentrations during inspiration and expiration respectively. The purpose of the present investigation is to determine if laryngeal receptors are sensitive to such fluctuations in CO_2 using an isolated, artificially ventilated laryngeal preparation in anaesthetized, paralysed cats.

METHODS

Experiments were performed on 8 anaesthetized (pentobarbitone sodium, induction 42-48 mg/kg i.p.; maintenance 12 mg i.v. hourly), paralysed (pancuronium 0.8 mg i.v. as required) cats artificially ventilated through a low cervical tracheostomy. A cannula was inserted through a high cervical tracheostomy and directed rostrally to the level of the cricoid cartilage. Another cannula was inserted through the mouth to the level of the epiglottis. The mouth and nose were sealed around this cannula. The isolated larynx was artificially ventilated as described previously (Bradford et al., 1990b) so that laryngeal pressures, temperatures, airflows and humidities were similar to those of a normal respiratory cycle. Laryngeal pressure, airflow, temperature and CO_2 concentration were continuously recorded. Laryngeal receptor activity was recorded from easily identifiable single units of the superior laryngeal nerve and receptors were classified as described previously (Bradford et al., 1990b). Laryngeal CO_2 concentration was increased from 0 to 5 and 9% (balance 21% O_2 in N_2) during both inspiration and expiration and during expiration only.

RESULTS

Applying 5 and/or 9% CO_2, both continuously and during expiration only, significantly excited (p < 0.05, Student's t-test) quiescent negative pressure receptors (9 out of 12 receptors studied), fibres with no response to occlusion (2 out of 2) and the one cold receptor studied (see Fig. 1). The remaining 3 quiescent negative pressure receptors were unaffected. On the other hand, quiescent positive pressure receptors (4 out of 6) and tonic positive pressure receptors (3 out of 5) were significantly inhibited. The remaining 2 quiescent positive pressure receptors were excited and the remaining 2 tonic positive pressure receptors were unaffected by CO_2. These effects were usually concentration-dependent with 9% CO_2 causing significantly greater responses than 5% for both continuously applied and expiratory CO_2.

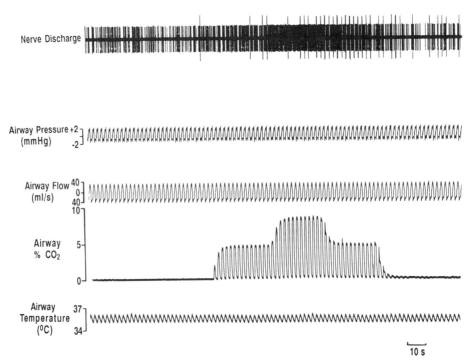

Figure 1. The effect of 5 and 9% CO_2 applied during expiration only on a cold receptor (nerve discharge). The larger spike was not functionally identified.

DISCUSSION

The present data suggest that laryngeal receptors responding to mechanical and thermal stimuli are also sensitive to the level of CO_2 in the airway lumen during expiration. Bartlett and Knuth (1992) have shown that pulses of 3, 5 and 10% CO_2 alter superior laryngeal nerve afferent activity in the cat. However, the receptors involved were not functionally identified and were not tested with CO_2 whilst simultaneously in receipt of the mechanical, thermal and other stimuli associated with a normal respiratory cycle.

Intralaryngeal CO_2 reflexly inhibits breathing (Boushey and Richardson, 1973) and affects UA muscle activity (Nolan et al., 1990; Bartlett et al., 1992). Therefore, the sensitivity of laryngeal receptors to expired CO_2 may contribute to the control of breathing and UA muscle activity, especially in conditions of altered end-tidal CO_2 concentration.

Supported by the Health Research Board (Ireland) and the Wellcome Trust.

REFERENCES

Anderson, J. W., Sant'Ambrogio, F. B., Orani, G. P., Sant'Ambrogio, G., & Mathew, O.P. (1990). Carbon dioxide-responsive laryngeal receptors in the dog. Respir. Physiol. 82, 217-226.

Bartlett, Jr., D. & Knuth, S.L. (1992). Responses of laryngeal receptors to intralaryngeal CO_2 in the cat. J. Physiol. 457, 187-193.

Bartlett Jr., D., Knuth, S.L. & Leiter, J.C. (1992). Alteration of ventilatory activity by intralaryngeal CO_2 in the cat. J. Physiol. 457, 177-185.

Boushey, H.A. & Richardson, P.S. (1973). The reflex effects of intralaryngeal carbon dioxide on the pattern of breathing. J. Physiol. 228, 181-191.

Boushey, H.A., Richardson, P.S., Widdicombe, J. G. & Wise, J.C.M. (1974). The response of laryngeal afferent fibres to mechanical and chemical stimuli. J. Physiol. 240, 153-175.

Bradford, A., Nolan, P., McKeogh, D., Bannon, C. & O'Regan, R.G. (1990a). The responses of superior laryngeal nerve afferent fibres to laryngeal airway CO_2 concentration in the anaesthetized cat. Exp. Physiol. 75, 267-270.

Bradford, A., Bannon, C., Nolan, P & O'Regan, R.G. (1990b). A study of the effects of airway carbon dioxide (P_{aw} CO_2) on superior laryngeal nerve afferents using an isolated, artificially ventilated closed laryngeal preparation in the anaesthetized cat. In "Chemoreceptors and Chemoreflexes." H. Acker et al., ed. Plenum Press, New York.

Nolan, P., Bradford, A., O'Regan, R.G. & McKeogh, D. (1990). The effects of changes in laryngeal airway CO_2 concentration on genioglossus muscle activity in the anaesthetized cat. Exp. Physiol. 75, 271-274.

THE EFFECTS OF AIRWAY CO$_2$ AND COOLING ON VENTILATION AND UPPER AIRWAY RESISTANCE IN ANAESTHETIZED RATS

Aidan K. Curran, Kenneth D. O'Halloran and Aidan Bradford.

Department of Physiology, Royal College of Surgeons in Ireland, St. Stephen's Green, Dublin 2, Ireland

INTRODUCTION

Upper airway (UA) luminal CO$_2$ modulates the activity of superior laryngeal nerve afferents (Boushey et al., 1974; Bradford et al., 1990) and affects breathing and UA muscle activity through a superior laryngeal nerve-mediated reflex (Nolan et al., 1990). Therefore, airway CO$_2$ may influence the patency of the UA, especially in obstructive apnoea and other circumstances of altered UA CO$_2$ concentration. However, the effects of UA luminal CO$_2$ on airway patency have not been studied.

UA cooling also alters the activity of superior laryngeal nerve afferents (Sant'Ambrogio et al., 1986) and inhibits breathing through a laryngeal reflex (Orani et al., 1991) but the effects of cold air on breathing and on UA resistance have not been studied in the rat. The purpose of the present investigation is to compare the effects of cool air and CO$_2$ on ventilation and on UA resistance in anaesthetized rats.

METHODS

Experiments were performed on 18 supine, adult, male, anaesthetized (chloralose, 100 mg/kg; urethane 1000 mg/kg I.P), Wistar rats. Animals breathed spontaneously through a cannula inserted into a low-cervical tracheostomy. Spontaneous tracheal airflow was recorded using a pneumotachograph connected to this cannula. A constant flow of gas (10ml/s/kg) was delivered rostrally to the UA through another cannula inserted into the trachea to lie just rostral to the glottis. A second pneumotachograph was placed in series with this cannula to record UA airflow. The nose was sealed. Spontaneous tracheal airflow and UA airflow, pressure and temperature were continuously recorded. Upper airway resistance was calculated from UA pressure and flow values. Warmed (36°C), humidified air containing 0, 5 and 10% CO$_2$ or cool (26°C), room humidity air were applied to the UA in an expiratory direction. Data were analysed using Student's paired t-tests with p $<$ 0.05 taken as significant.

Arterial Chemoreceptors: Cell to System
Edited by R. O'Regan *et al*, Plenum Press, New York, 1994

RESULTS

Switching from warm air to warm air containing 5 or 10% CO_2 had no significant effects on tracheal airflow or UA resistance. However, cool air caused a substantial fall in UA resistance (-44.0 ± 3.3% SEM of control) and in peak inspiratory flow (-13.0 ± 3.3% SEM of control). Cutting both superior laryngeal nerves abolished the inhibitory effect on breathing and significantly attenuated the effect of cool air on UA resistance (-33.0 ± 3.1% SEM of warm air control).

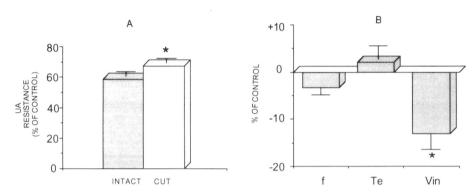

Figure 1. A shows the effect of cool air on upper airway (UA) resistance before (intact, n= 11) and after (cut, n=5) superior laryngeal nerve section. B shows the effect of cool air on UA resistance (expressed as a % of warm air control), respiratory frequency (f, n=13), expiratory time (Te, n=13) and peak inspiratory flow (Vin, n=13) in animals with intact superior laryngeal nerves. n= number of animals. ∗ p < 0.05.

DISCUSSION

These data indicate that UA luminal CO_2 does not reflexly influence UA resistance in the anaesthetized rat. Using a similar technique for applying CO_2 to the UA, it has been shown that CO_2 alters superior laryngeal nerve afferent activity in the anaesthetized dog (Anderson et al., 1990) and in the anaesthetized or decerebrate cat (Bartlett & Knuth, 1992) and modulates UA muscle motor nerve activity (Bartlett et al, 1992a; Bartlett et al, 1992b) in decerebrate, paralyzed, vagotomized cats. However, it cannot be concluded that UA CO_2 does not influence UA patency because excitation of UA dilator muscles may act to stiffen the airway and prevent collapse without actually dilating the airway and reducing resistance.

Cool air substantially reduced UA resistance and slightly inhibited breathing. Superior laryngeal nerve section abolished the effect on breathing and somewhat reduced the effect on UA resistance. This indicates that a part of the effect on UA resistance is due to a laryngeal reflex, either directly affecting UA muscle activity (see Ukabam et al., 1992) or indirectly due to effects secondary to the inhibition of breathing.

We propose that the large residual effect on UA resistance following superior laryngeal section may be mainly due to an effect of cold air on mucosal blood flow (see Wasicko et al., 1991).

Supported by the Health Research Board and The Royal College of Surgeons in Ireland.

REFERENCES

Anderson, J. W., Sant'Ambrogio, F. B., Orani, G.P., Sant'Ambrogio, G & Mathew, O.P. (1990). Carbon dioxide-responsive laryngeal receptors in the dog. Respir. Physiol. 82: 217-226.

Bartlett Jr., D. & Knuth, S.L. (1992). Responses of laryngeal receptors to intralaryngeal CO_2 in the cat. J. Physiol. 457: 187-193.

Bartlett Jr., D., Knuth, S.L. & Gdovin, M.J. (1992a). Influence of laryngeal CO_2 on respiratory activities of motor nerves to accessory muscles. Respir. Physiol. 90: 289-297.

Bartlett Jr., D., Knuth, S. L. & Leiter, J.C. (1992b). Alteration of ventilatory activity by intralaryngeal CO_2 in the cat. J. Physiol. 457: 177-185.

Boushey, H.A., Richardson, P.S., Widdicombe J.G. & Wise, J.C.N. (1974). The response of laryngeal afferent fibres to mechanical and chemical stimuli. J. Physiol. 240:153-175.

Bradford, A., Nolan, P., McKeogh, D., Bannon, C. & O'Regan, R.G. (1990). The responses of superior laryngeal nerve afferent fibres to laryngeal airway CO_2 concentration in the anaesthetized cat. Exp. Physiol. 75: 267-270.

Orani, G.P., Anderson, J.W., Sant'Ambrogio, G. & Sant'Ambrogio, F. B. (1991). Upper airway cooling and l-menthol reduce ventilation in the guinea pig. J. Appl. Physiol. 70 (5):2080-2086.

Nolan, P., Bradford, A., O'Regan, R.G., & McKeogh, D. (1990) The effects of changes in laryngeal airway CO_2 concentration on genioglossus muscle activity in the anaesthetized cat. Exp. Physiol. 75:271-274

Sant'Ambrogio, G., Brambilla-Sant'Ambrogio, F. & Mathew, O.P. (1986). Effect of cold air on laryngeal mechanoreceptors in the dog. Respir. Physiol. 64:45-56.

Ukabam, C.U., Knuth, S.L. & Bartlett Jr., D. (1992). Phrenic and hypoglossal neural responses to cold airflow in the upper airway. Respir. Physiol. 87, 157-164.

Wasicko, M.J., Leiter, J.C., Erlichman, J.S., Strobel, R.J. & Bartlett Jr., D. (1991). Nasal and pharyngeal resistance after topical mucosal vasoconstriction in normal humans. Am. Rev. Respir. Dis. 144: 1048-1052.

THE EFFECTS OF LARYNGEAL CO_2 AND COOLING ON VENTILATION AND LARYNGEAL RESISTANCE IN THE ANAESTHETIZED RAT

Kenneth D. O'Halloran, Aidan K. Curran, and Aidan Bradford

Department of Physiology, Royal College of Surgeons in Ireland, St. Stephen's Green, Dublin 2, Ireland

INTRODUCTION

Superior laryngeal nerve afferent activity is altered by upper airway CO_2 (Bradford et al., 1990) and cold air (Sant'Ambrogio et al., 1986). Ventilation and upper airway muscle activity are also influenced by upper airway CO_2 (Nolan et al., 1990) and cold air (Ukabam et al., 1992) through a superior laryngeal nerve-dependent reflex. These responses may be important in the regulation of upper airway patency. The larynx is a major site of upper airway resistance but the effects of CO_2 on laryngeal resistance have not been studied. The purpose of the present investigation is to compare the effects of laryngeal cooling and CO_2 on ventilation and laryngeal resistance in anaesthetized rats.

METHODS

Experiments were performed on 20 adult male Wistar rats, anaesthetized with chloralose and urethane (100mg/kg and 1000 mg/kg respectively I.P.). Animals were placed supine on a heating pad and rectal temperature monitored and maintained at 37°C. Animals were allowed to breathe room air spontaneously through a cannula inserted into a low cervical tracheostomy and connected to a pneumotachograph. A second cannula was inserted through a high cervical tracheostomy to just below the level of the cricoid cartilage. Warmed (35.9 ± 0.4°C), humidified air 0, 5 and 9% CO_2 and cool (29.5 ± 0.7°C), room humidity air were delivered at constant flow (20 ml/s/kg) in an expiratory direction through the cricoid cannula to exit through a pharyngotomy. Spontaneous tracheal airflow and laryngeal airflow, temperature and sub-glottic pressure were continuously recorded. The superior and recurrent laryngeal nerves were preserved intact. Laryngeal resistance was calculated from measurements of laryngeal airflow and pressure. Data were analysed using Student's t tests with $p < 0.05$ taken as significant.

RESULTS

There were typical increases and decreases of laryngeal resistance in phase with expiration and inspiration respectively. Carbon dioxide (5 and 9%) had no significant effect on breathing or on laryngeal resistance (see Fig. 1B) although laryngeal resistance was slightly but non-significantly increased in 6 out of 8 animals. Cool air reduced respiratory frequency (68.8 ± 4.1 SEM % of warm air control, n=14 animals) and peak inspiratory flow (36.9 ± 2.3 SEM %, n=14) and increased expiratory duration (401.7 ± 113.8 SEM %, n=14). These effects were abolished by superior laryngeal nerve section. Cool air significantly decreased laryngeal resistance and this effect was significantly attenuated by superior laryngeal nerve section (see Fig. 1A).

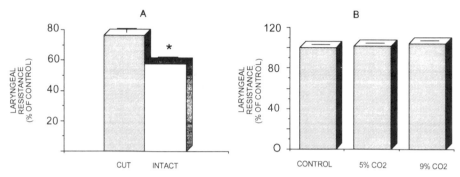

Figure 1. A shows the effect of cool air on laryngeal resistance (expressed as a % of warm air control) before (intact, n=10) and after (cut, n=5) superior laryngeal nerve section. B shows the effect of 5 and 9% CO_2 (n=8) on laryngeal resistance (expressed as a % of warm air control) in animals with intact superior laryngeal nerves. n= number of animals. * $p < 0.05$.

DISCUSSION

In anaesthetized or decerebrate cats, intralaryngeal CO_2 reflexly inhibits breathing (Boushey & Richardson, 1973; Nolan et al., 1990; Bartlett, Knuth & Leiter,1992) and excites the thyroarytenoid muscle, a laryngeal adductor (Bartlett, Knuth, & Gdovin, 1992). The latter response would be expected to increase laryngeal resistance. However, in the present experiments, laryngeal CO_2 had no effect on either breathing or laryngeal resistance although there was a tendency for laryngeal resistance to increase. This unresponsiveness may be due to species and methodological differences and cannot be ascribed to the insensitivity of the preparation since cool air caused marked reductions in ventilation and laryngeal resistance which were totally or partially superior laryngeal nerve-dependent. The inhibitory effect of cold air on breathing has been well described in neonatal animals and has been reported more recently in adult cats (Ukabam et al., 1992) and guinea pigs (Orani et al., 1991). Consistent with these latter studies, the ventilatory inhibition in the rat demonstrated in the present work is a superior laryngeal nerve-dependent reflex.

To our knowledge, the only other study on the effects of cold air on laryngeal resistance was in anaesthetized cats (Jammes et al., 1983) where very cold air (8.8°C) was also shown to decrease resistance. In the present study, cutting the superior laryngeal nerves significantly attenuated the fall in laryngeal resistance caused by cool air, indicating that part of the response is due to a laryngeal reflex, either directly affecting intrinsic laryngeal muscles or indirectly due to effects secondary to the inhibition of breathing.

Upper airway mucosal vascular tone has been shown to have an important influence on upper airway calibre and resistance (Wasicko et al., 1992) The substantial fall in laryngeal resistance caused by cool air in superior laryngeal nerve-sectioned animals may be due to a vasoconstrictor effect of cool air on the vasculature of the laryngeal mucosa leading to a reduction in mucosal thickness and an increase in laryngeal cross-sectional area.

Supported by the Health Research Board (Ireland) and the Royal College of Surgeons in Ireland.

REFERENCES

Bartlett, Jr., D., Knuth, S.L. & Gdovin, M.J. (1992). Influence of laryngeal CO_2 on respiratory activities of motor nerves to accessory muscles. Respir. Physiol. 90, 289-297.

Bartlett Jr., D., Knuth, S.L & Leiter J.C. (1992). Alteration of ventilatory activity by intralaryngeal CO_2 in the cat. J. Physiol. 457, 177-185.

Boushey, H.A., & Richardson, P.S. (1973). The reflex effects of intralaryngeal carbon dioxide on the pattern of breathing. J. Physiol. 228, 181-191.

Bradford, A., Nolan, P., McKeogh, D., Bannon, C. & O'Regan, R.G. (1990). The responses of superior laryngeal nerve afferent fibres to laryngeal airway CO_2 concentration in the anaesthetized cat. Exp. Physiol. 75, 267-270.

Jammes, Y., Barthelemy, P & Delpierre, S. (1983). Respiratory effects of cold air breathing in anaesthetized cats. Respir. Physiol. 54, 41-54.

Orani, G.P., Anderson, J.W., Sant'Ambrogio, G. & Sant'Ambrogio, F.B. (1991). Upper airway cooling and l-menthol reduce ventilation in the guinea pig. J. Appl. Physiol. 70 (5), 2080-2086.

Nolan, P., Bradford, A., O'Regan, R.G., & McKeogh, D. (1990) The effects of changes in laryngeal airway CO_2 concentration on genioglossus muscle activity in the anaesthetized cat. Exp. Physiol. 75:271-274

Sant'Ambrogio, G., Brambilla-Sant'Ambrogio, F & Mathew, O.P. (1986). Effect of cold air on laryngeal mechanoreceptors in the dog. Respir. Physiol. 64, 45-56.

Ukabam, C.U., Knuth, S.L. & Bartlett Jr., D. (1992). Phrenic and hypoglossal neural responses to cold airflow in the upper airway. Respir. Physiol. 87, 157-164.

Wasicko, M.J., Leiter, J.C., Erlichman, J.S., Strobel, R.J. & Bartlett Jr., D. (1991). Nasal and pharyngeal resistance after topical mucosal vasoconstriction in normal humans. Am. Rev. Respir. Dis. 144: 1048-1052.

INDEX